A FIELD MANUAL OF CAMEL DISEASES

A FIELD MANUAL OF CAMEL DISEASES

Traditional and modern health care for the dromedary

Compiled by

Ilse Köhler-Rollefson, Paul Mundy and Evelyn Mathias

Intermediate Technology Publications Ltd
Schumacher Centre for Technology and Development
Bourton Hall, Bourton on Dunsmore, Rugby, Warwickshire CV23 9QZ, UK

Reprinted 2006, 2008
ISBN 978-1-85339-503-1

A catalogue record for this book is available from the British Library.

Intermediate Technology Publications Ltd, is the publishing arm of Intermediate Technology Development Group Ltd. Our mission is to build the skills and capacity of people in developing countries through the dissemination of information in all forms, enabling them to improve the quality of their lives and that of future generations.

The League for Pastoral Peoples is a non-profit organization devoted to advocacy and technical support for pastoralists. Founded in 1992 in Germany, its activities focus on research, training, capacity building and networking in co-operation with partner organizations. LPP seeks to promote the concepts of endogenous livestock development utilizing indigenous animal genetic resources and building on local institutions. For further information, contact: League for Pastoral Peoples, Pragelatostrasse 20, 64372 Ober-Ramstadt, Germany. E-mail: goikr@t-online.de

Typeset by Paul Mundy, Bergisch Gladback, Germany

Disclaimer

This book is intended to assist those working in situations where resources and veterinary services are limited or unavailable. This book only reflects the knowledge and practice of camel herders, veterinary practitioners and the current veterinary literature available. Readers must use their skill and judgement to apply the principles set out in this book to the circumstances in which they find themselves.

The authors, contributors and publisher assume no responsibility for and make no warranty with respect to the results of using the diagnoses and treatments in this book. The authors, contributors and publisher accept no liability for any damage or loss whatsoever resulting from use of or reliance on any information contained in this book.

Since this book will enjoy wide distribution, the veterinary procedures, drugs and doses given here do not and cannot comply with all the veterinary drug laws of each sovereign country. Before performing any procedure, giving veterinary advice or using any animal drugs, readers are responsible for familiarizing themselves with the local laws and regulations that apply to the practice of veterinary medicine and drug use in animals and must practice strict adherence to those laws.

Similarly, this book is not intended to substitute for the complete prescribing information prepared by each manufacturer for each drug. The package insert and directions for use of every drug product should be read, understood and followed before any drug is administered or prescribed.

Contents

Contributors

A brief profile and contact details for each contributor are given under ▷*Contributor's profiles*.

Camel specialists and veterinarians

Hamid Agab, Sudan
Mohamed Fadl Ahmed, Sudan
Darlington Akabwai, Kenya
John Akkara, India
Stephen Ashdown, UK
Muhammad Athar, Pakistan
Set Bornstein, Sweden
Andy Catley, UK
Maurizio Dioli, Italy
Christopher Rashid Field, Kenya
Tarun Kumar Gahlot, India
Andrea Gervelmeyer, Austria
Christian Hülsebusch, Germany
Brigitte Kaufmann, Germany
Ilse Köhler-Rollefson, Germany
B.J. Linquist, Kenya
Evelyn Mathias, Germany
Ghulam Muhammad, Pakistan
Babiker Elhag Musa, Sudan
Augustine Namanda, Kenya
Shravan Singh Rathore, India
Hanwant Singh Rathore, India
Jacob Wanyama, Kenya
Fran White, UK

Artists

Nyotomba Bonaventure, Kenya
Vitthal Kamble, India
Elijah Njoroge, Kenya
Atmaram Pund, India
Richard Wanyiri, Kenya

Organization, editing, desktop publishing

Ilse Köhler-Rollefson, Germany
Paul Mundy, UK
Evelyn Mathias, Germany

Foreword

This field manual on camel diseases is a unique publication, combining traditional and modern treatments for the first time. The authors have listed the most important diseases and conditions in camels, and provide in a simple, concise form a description of the various disease conditions in camels and how to treat them. This approach makes the book very handy for daily use.

This book is an attempt to melt the ice and remove the misunderstanding between local herders and professionals. By providing both traditional and scientific treatments, the authors offer the reader a range of options for treating a sick camel. This type of information has long been lacking in the veterinary profession.

The manual is a serious, practical effort to help camels and their owners. It will be of benefit to veterinarians, professionals, herders and camel owners alike.

Professor Babiker Elhag Musa
Camel Affairs, Diwan of Royal Court
Sultanate of Oman

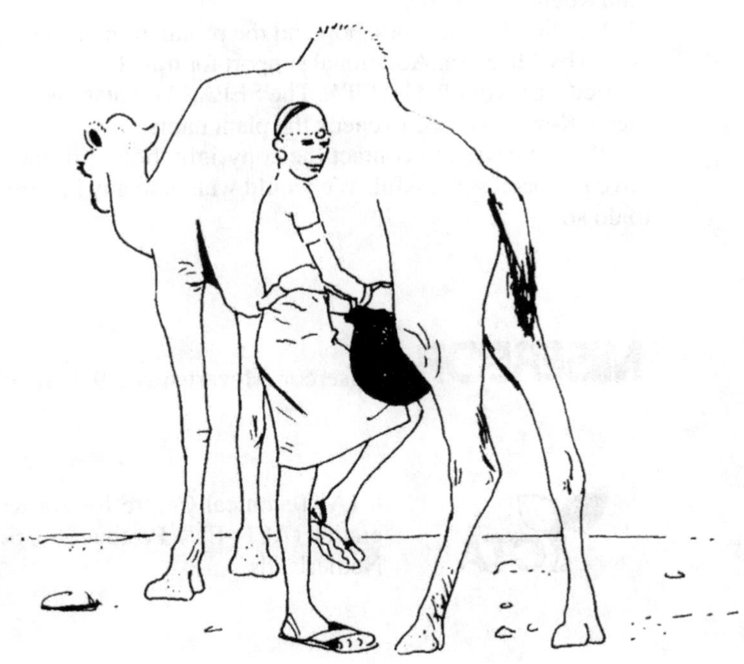

Acknowledgements

The authors would like to thank the many people who contributed directly or indirectly to this book.

In 1997, the BAIF Development Research Foundation hosted an international conference on ethnoveterinary medicine in Pune, India (Mathias et al. 1999), providing an opportunity for most of the contributors to meet and discuss the veterinary medicine of camels in pastoral conditions. Immediately after the conference, the contributors held a 2-day workshop, during which they discussed, wrote and revised many of the manuscripts on which this book is based. Our thanks to BAIF for providing facilities and logistical support for this workshop, and especially to A.L. Joshi and Datta V. Rangnekar for their encouragement, interest and support.

A major part of the contents of this book was compiled during the Pune workshop by a group of camel specialists. These, and additional contributors who were unable to attend the Pune workshop, are listed in the *Contributors* section.

The pictures were drawn by five artists: Vitthal Kamble and Atmaram Pund in India, Nyotomba (Bonnie) Bonaventure, Elijah Njoroge and Richard Wanyiri in Kenya. Jacob Wanyama of ITDG Kenya and Christian Hülsebusch reviewed and commented on most of the pictures.

The following reviewed the book in detail, pointed out errors and suggested corrections, and gave many valuable comments: Hamid Agab, R.S. Broadbent, Maurizio Dioli, David Hadrill, Christiane Herweg, Christian Hülsebusch, Babiker Elhag Musa and Regina Schwabe.

Funding for the workshop and the production of this book was generously provided by Misereor. Additional support for travel expenses for two participants from Africa was provided by CTA. The SEPASAL database of the Royal Botanical Gardens, Kew, was used to check the plant names.

We have tried to contact the copyright holder of the skeleton on page 21 but have not been successful. We would welcome any information that will enable us to do so.

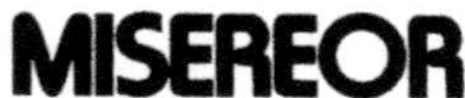

Misereor, Mozartstrasse 9, 52064 Aachen, Germany

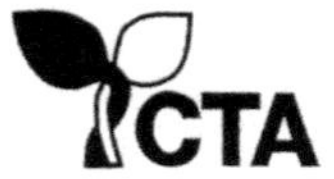

CTA, Technical Centre for Agricultural and Rural Cooperation (ACP–EU), Postbus 380, 6700 AJ Wageningen, The Netherlands

Introduction

The camel has special significance for the frequently drought-stricken arid and semi-arid parts of Africa and Asia. The majority of the world's 19 million camels are kept by pastoral peoples in traditional systems and remote areas. Since these people depend on their animals for food, transport and income, the health and productivity of their camels are vital for their economic survival.

Yet providing these communities with veterinary services according to the western model has proven exceedingly difficult – if not impossible. In part this is due to the lack of infrastructure in the isolated regions where camel pastoralists live. It is also because veterinarians have very limited experience with the particular problems of camels kept under pastoral conditions. Most veterinarians are not well versed in diagnosing and treating even the more common camel diseases. They often find themselves at a loss when they are confronted with sick camels in the field. Relatively little research has been done on camels, and camel medicine is rarely taught at veterinary colleges. Where it is taught, the case material comes from animals used for work in cities. It does not reflect the range of diseases encountered by pastoralists.

Matters are compounded by the lack of suitable information materials on camel diseases. Up to now, the book by Leese, *A treatise on the one-humped camel in health and disease*, published in 1927, remains the most comprehensive source of information on the subject; others are oriented to specific countries or regions. A number of books have emanated from the high-income racing-camel circuit in the Arab and Gulf countries, but they have limited applicability to the pastoral situation. First, racing camels are prone to a different range of diseases to those kept in traditional management systems. Second, these books assume that the veterinarian has high-technology diagnostic and therapeutic facilities – conditions that simply do not exist in pastoral settings with their chronically scarce resources.

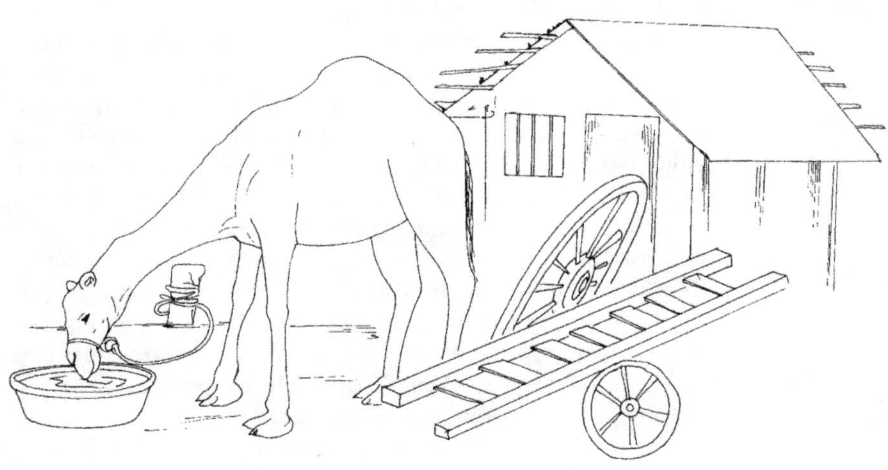

Who is this book for?

This manual aims to fill this gap by providing comprehensive information on camel diseases with special reference to a low-technology environment. It is intended for all those who deal with camels under pastoral or low-income conditions: veterinarians, paraveterinarians, livestock workers, extension workers, NGO staff, teachers and students who work with camel herders and deal with camels. This is a broad group. Accordingly, the text is written in simple language. We have avoided jargon wherever possible: we write 'inject into the muscle' instead of 'intramuscular application', and 'dislocated kneecap' rather than 'luxation of the patella'. It is impossible in a book on animal diseases to avoid using any technical terms. But where a technical term cannot be avoided, we explain it in the text. The glossary provides further explanations of technical terms, or other words that the reader may come across while dealing with camels and their diseases.

The book also contains many line drawings so that it will be useful for those both with and without formal veterinary training.

Some veterinarians may regard the advice on such subjects as surgery, laboratory tests and other procedures as oversimplified, too complex or difficult to do in the field, or not appropriate for people without formal veterinary training. We have included this information for two reasons:

- Readers may be called on to treat a sick camel in a remote location, where they cannot call on the services of a qualified veterinarian. The camel is a valuable one, and it will clearly die if nothing is done. In such a situation, it may be better to attempt a procedure (after consulting with the owner and warning him or her of the dangers), rather than to do nothing. In these instances, the advice in this book may prove useful.
- This book may be used in training courses for veterinarians and paravets. There is, sadly, a major lack of simple, easy-to-understand information on how to perform such procedures as giving an injection or stitching a wound. We hope that the clear, simply written instructions will help students understand these procedures and will lead to fewer mistakes.

Traditional and scientific knowledge

A central purpose of this manual is to draw attention to the extensive body of traditional, or 'ethnoveterinary', knowledge that many camel pastoral societies have accumulated over generations. Pastoralists successfully relied on this knowledge long before the advent of modern veterinary medicine. Herders have a deep knowledge of their animals and their environment, and are able to correctly diagnose and treat many diseases. This traditional knowledge is sufficient to prevent or treat many common afflictions of camels, although it cannot control major epidemics. Unlike modern drugs, ethnoveterinary remedies are locally available, and are usually free. In many instances, they may be the only option available to treat an animal. This manual gives equal status to this knowledge by providing both modern and traditional treatments side by side.

Traditional remedies made from herbal and household ingredients have other advantages over commercially produced medicines. Many chemical preparations used for controlling parasites have dangerous ecological side-effects, as they do not break down, so can accumulate in the environment. In addition, they are toxic when overdosed, and can even cause cancer. Frequent application of antibiotics and trypanocides causes resistance and renders them ineffective. Furthermore, pastoralists have problems with applying purchased medicines

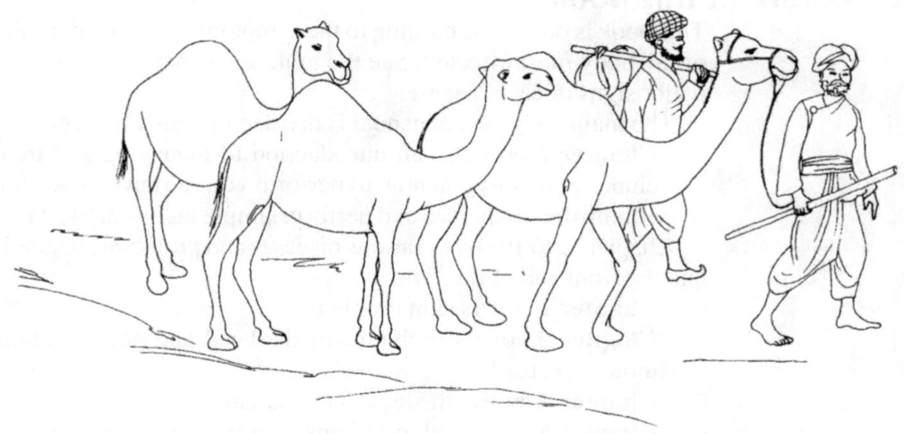

correctly, since they frequently cannot read the instructions and have not developed an awareness about possible side-effects. Hence there is much to be said for keeping traditional knowledge alive.

Relatively little is known about the efficacy of ethnoveterinary treatments. Some are undoubtedly beneficial, and indeed have been tested and have become part of modern scientific practice. Others are more questionable, or indeed may be harmful to the animal or the environment.

Ideally, an academically trained veterinarian should be familiar with the remedies that pastoralists know. Yet this is rarely the case. Unless the veterinarian comes from a pastoralist family, their knowledge and experience do not even overlap; this lies at the root of many misunderstandings. By highlighting ethnoveterinary knowledge, we hope that the manual will improve the often prevailing image of pastoralists as ignorant and uneducated, and that it will contribute to a better understanding, and better communication between pastoralists and academically trained camel specialists.

Local and scientific names

A particular problem relates to the names of diseases and plants in local languages. The scientific classification of diseases relies largely on causal organisms, identified by laboratory tests. Traditional disease names, by contrast, often refer to observable signs of the disease. The two disease classification systems may not always correspond. For example, a skin ailment known as *kharfat* among the Rendille in Kenya may be classified by scientists as lymphadenitis, contagious skin necrosis, or dermatophilosis, depending on the organism causing it. Similarly, herders may recognize two distinct ailments which western medicine classifies as one and the same.

A similar problem occurs with the plants used to treat diseases. Two different plant species may have the same name in the local language, and a single species may have several local names, making it difficult to identify a plant using the scientific species classification.

This difficulty is compounded by the lack of research on camels relative to other livestock. Several diseases widely recognized by herders are not mentioned in the scientific literature, and little research has been done on the effectiveness of the remedies used.

Structure of this book

This book is ordered according to the symptoms or signs of the disease, and the parts of the body most affected. See the table at the beginning of each section for some major signs of each disease.

The main body of the manual is divided into ten chapters:

- **Chapter 1** provides an introduction to managing and treating camels. It includes guidelines on how to perform various basic procedures, such as how to administer medicines and perform simple laboratory tests.

Chapters 2 to 10 cover various diseases and problems, beginning with the outside and the front end of the camel.

- **Chapter 2** covers skin problems.
- **Chapter 3** covers problems of the head and neck (including the eyes, ears, mouth and teeth).
- **Chapter 4** covers the legs, feet and tail.
- **Chapter 5** deals with problems affecting the nose and lungs (respiratory diseases) .
- **Chapter 6** covers diarrhoea and other problems that affect the stomach and intestines (gastro-intestinal diseases).
- **Chapter 7** deals with infectious diseases that affect the body as a whole (those affecting mainly one part of the body are dealt with in the relevant section).
- **Chapter 8** covers a range of other, non-infectious diseases not covered elsewhere, including red urine, poisoning and pica.
- **Chapter 9** deals with reproduction (both females and males).
- **Chapter 10** covers the care of newborn calves and problems relating to them.

Each of the sections in Chapters 2 to 10 has the same structure. Each deals with a single problem or disease, as reflected in the title of the section. This is then followed by the names of the disease in local languages, along with a short description. The text then lists the signs of each disease, its cause, and possibly a list of similar diseases. This is followed by a list of measures that may prevent the disease, and a list of treatments (⊳*How to read a treatment*).

The **appendices** give the ethnic names for the diseases in the book and for medicinal and poisonous plants; a list of common medicines and their dosages; units of measurement; profiles of contributors; a glossary of technical terms; a list of the books used to compile this manual, other useful reading materials and resource organizations; and an index.

Cross-references to other sections of the book are marked with the symbol '⊳'.

Caution

This manual does not cover all aspects of camels, and it is impossible to learn how to treat these complex, valuable animals from a book alone. The book should be seen as an aid to memory and practice, rather than a substitute. The novice can best learn about camels through observation and hands-on experience under the guidance of experienced practitioners and herders.

Veterinarians are rare in camel-herding areas, and veterinarians who specialize in camels are rarer. If you are not a veterinarian yourself, find out if there is one nearby, and ask if you can call on his or her help in difficult cases. Experienced herders and traditional healers also know a lot about camels and may be able to help.

In preparing this book, the authors put a lot of effort into checking the validity and efficacy of the treatments, and rejected many treatments because they felt they would be ineffective or even harmful. But it was not possible to check all the treatments listed. Readers should therefore use them with caution, using their own best judgement. Just because a treatment is included here does not mean that the contributors or authors recommend it; merely that pastoralists or veterinarians use it to treat a certain disease. The authors and publisher cannot be held liable for any problems that may arise from applying the practices in this book.

If you discover an error, or if you have additional information that may be useful for future editions of this book, please contact Ilse Köhler-Rollefson at Pragelatostrasse 20, 64372 Ober-Ramstadt, Germany; tel +49-6154-53642, 52309; fax +49-6154-53642; email gorikr@t-online.de.

How this book was compiled

The material for this book was originally compiled by a group of about 20 camel specialists at an intensive, 2-day workshop in Pune, India, in November 1997. Participants included veterinarians and livestock specialists with experience of camels in India, Kenya, Oman, Saudi Arabia, Somalia and Sudan. Several other contributors, including those from Pakistan, were unable to attend the workshop, but later sent manuscripts.

The participants brought with them rough manuscripts on diseases or problems in their own speciality. Other manuscripts were prepared during the workshop itself. During the workshop, the participants presented their papers to small groups, who then discussed and critiqued them. Modifications included the addition or refinement of treatments, local names, and further information on the disease. The organizers originally intended to cover just 20 or so of the most important diseases affecting camels in pastoral conditions, but at the participants' insistence, the range of topics was expanded to cover many afflictions of secondary importance.

During the workshop, participants commissioned the artists present to draw pictures to illustrate each disease, based on photographs they had brought with them. Further pictures were drawn by artists in Kenya after the workshop.

After the workshop, the authors compiled the large amount of information gathered at the workshop, added information from key references (see below), and put the whole into a consistent and easily understandable format. The complete manuscript was reviewed by several camel specialists, and the changes they suggested were incorporated.

Other sources of information

The structure of this book draws on a manual on ethnoveterinary medicine for all livestock species in Kenya, including camels (ITDG and IIRR 1996), which two of the authors (Mundy and Mathias) helped produce. Some of the treatments are taken directly from this manual.

Important sources of information on camels include:

- Evans et al. (1995)
- Gahlot and Chouhan (1992)
- Higgins (1986)
- Kaufmann (1998)
- Manefield and Tinson (1997)
- Projet Cameline (1999)
- Schwartz and Dioli (1992)
- Wernery and Kaaden (1995)
- Wilson (1998)

Schwartz and Dioli (1992) is particularly useful, as it contains some 250 colour photographs of camel diseases and management techniques.

Three books were published after the bulk of this manual had been prepared. *Where there is no vet* by Forse (1999) is an excellent guide to field-level animal health care; it covers camels as well as other major livestock species. *Traitement des maladies du dromadaire* (Projet Cameline 1999) is a booklet written for livestock field assistants and camel herders; it is available in French, Arabic, Amharic and Tifinar (Tamashek). Both of these books use simple language, and like this manual, contain many line drawings. *Selected topics on camelids* (Gahlot 2000) contains 21 chapters on various aspects of dromedaries, Bactrians and South American camelids.

This manual has relied heavily on all the books listed above, as well as on the knowledge and experience of the various contributors. A list of references after each section lists useful sources of information on that topic.

Other useful sources include FAO (1994), Quesenberry (1990) and IIRR's manuals on ethnoveterinary medicine in Asia (IIRR 1994) and paraveterinary medicine (IIRR 1996). While these do not deal with camels, they are useful guides to field-level treatment of livestock diseases, and use an approach similar to that followed in this book.

A complete bibliography and list of other books likely to be useful to people working with camels is provided at the end of the manual (▷*Bibliography and resources*).

This manual is neither perfect nor complete. It very much reflects the geographical origin of its contributors, who came from or have experience in the Indian subcontinent and the Horn of Africa (Kenya, Sudan), with Arabia also being represented. Thus North and West Africa – the French-speaking regions – have not been done justice. Nor have the Bactrian (two-humped) camels of Central Asia.

How to read a treatment

The manual lists both scientific and traditional treatments (where they are known) for each disease. Where possible, we have classified each of the treatments in this manual according to the following categories:

SCI	Standard scientific veterinary practice. Where relevant, these practices are grouped under the heading '*Modern treatments*'.
TRAD+SCI	Common traditional practice, supported by scientific knowledge.
TRAD	Common traditional practice that indigenous healers agree works, but without scientific support. The name of the healers' ethnic group (such as RENDILLE) is given if possible.

Each separate remedy in the *Treatments* sections begins with the symbol 'O'. Where there are several alternatives, you can choose the one that is most appropriate to your situation.

A few remedies, such as that for ▷*Broken jaw*, are complex and consist of a series of steps. These steps are marked with numbers 1, 2, 3, etc.

Most of the treatments are given in recipe form, as in the example below.

Instructions on preparing and applying the medicine

Botanical name of plant

Name of plant in the local language (in this case, Arabic)

O Grind the seeds of *Citrullus colocynthis* (bitter apple, *handal*) and heat them until they form a liquid tar (called *gutran* in Arabic). Rub the tar into the affected area. Repeat this treatment at 2-day intervals until the animal is cured. LAHAWIYIN, RASHAIDA, SHUKRIYA, TRAD

Communities that use this remedy (see maps on pages 2–3)

Type of remedy (see above)
TRAD = *traditional*
SCI = *scientific*
TRAD+SCI = *both*

O	Alternatives in the *Signs, Prevention* and *Treatment* sections.
1, 2, 3, etc.	Steps in a procedure.
▷	Cross-references to other sections of the book.
?	Species or local name is uncertain.

1 Managing and treating camels

Traditional management systems

Camels are kept and bred for many different purposes, and there is great regional diversity in management and production systems. In the Horn of Africa, herders keep camels mainly for their milk. In northern Africa, camels are bred mainly for meat, but also for milk and transport. In India, camels are used as draught animals; milk is a by-product, and they are not used for meat.

The management system depends largely on why camels are kept. If herders aim to maximize reproduction – if they breed camels for meat or transport – they can do this with minimum inputs. They can allow their herds to range freely, and sell off young animals at regular intervals.

If milk is the main goal, then herds have to be supervised; this means a considerable amount of labour. Herds must be divided into milking and non-milking animals, and the young camels have to be kept separate from their mothers for at least part of the day.

Horn of Africa

Pastoralists in the Horn of Africa emphasize milk production, and camel milk is an important part of their diet. They do not generally use camels for riding, although they do sometimes use them as pack animals and for meat. Some groups, such as the Rendille, Gabbra and Turkana, also bleed their camels and consume the blood. They have many traditional beliefs associated with camels. For example, many camel-related transactions can only take place on certain days of the week. Milking can only be done by men who are not sexually active. Twice a year there are large gatherings where people feast on ritually slaughtered, castrated male camels.

Arabia, North and West Africa

Pastoralists in the Arabian Peninsula and northern Africa traditionally used a wide variety of camel products. They used camels for food, and camels were their main means of transport. In some parts of North Africa, the Bedouin have switched to breeding camels to provide meat, especially for poor people in the cities. Camel milk is regarded highly in Arab culture and is now being developed into a health

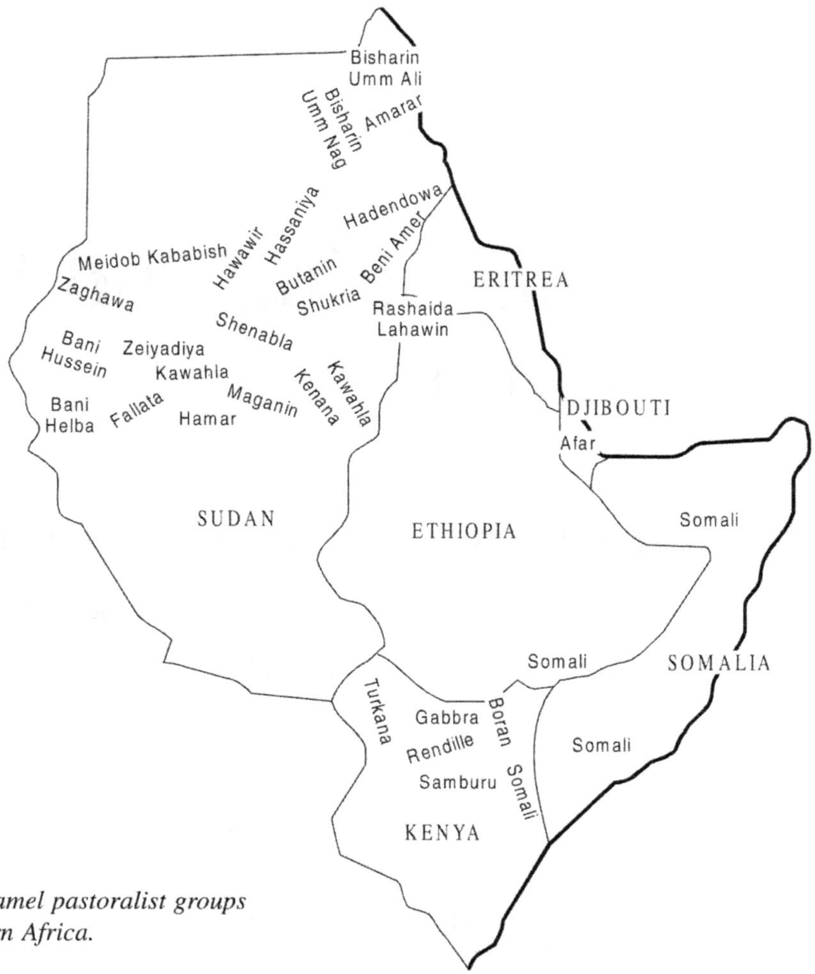

Major camel pastoralist groups in eastern Africa.

food for export into Europe. In the Gulf countries, camel racing has become big business and is a major stimulus for camel breeding. In the Sahel, pastoralists keep camels for their milk and for transport.

South and Central Asia

In South Asia, camels are used mainly for transport, and their food potential is of secondary importance. With the notable exception of the Indian Raika, there are few specialized camel pastoralists, but many sheep- and goat-raisers keep a few camels as pack animals to transport their belongings when they move. In India, the camel is an important draught animal of great value for both rural and urban poor. Use for draught leads to special health problems, such as saddle sores and muscle difficulties.

In the deserts of Central Asia, Bactrian (two-humped) camels range from the Crimea and western Kazakhstan to Mongolia and northern China. They are adapted to the long, cold winters and short summers in these areas. (This book is concerned primarily with dromedaries.)

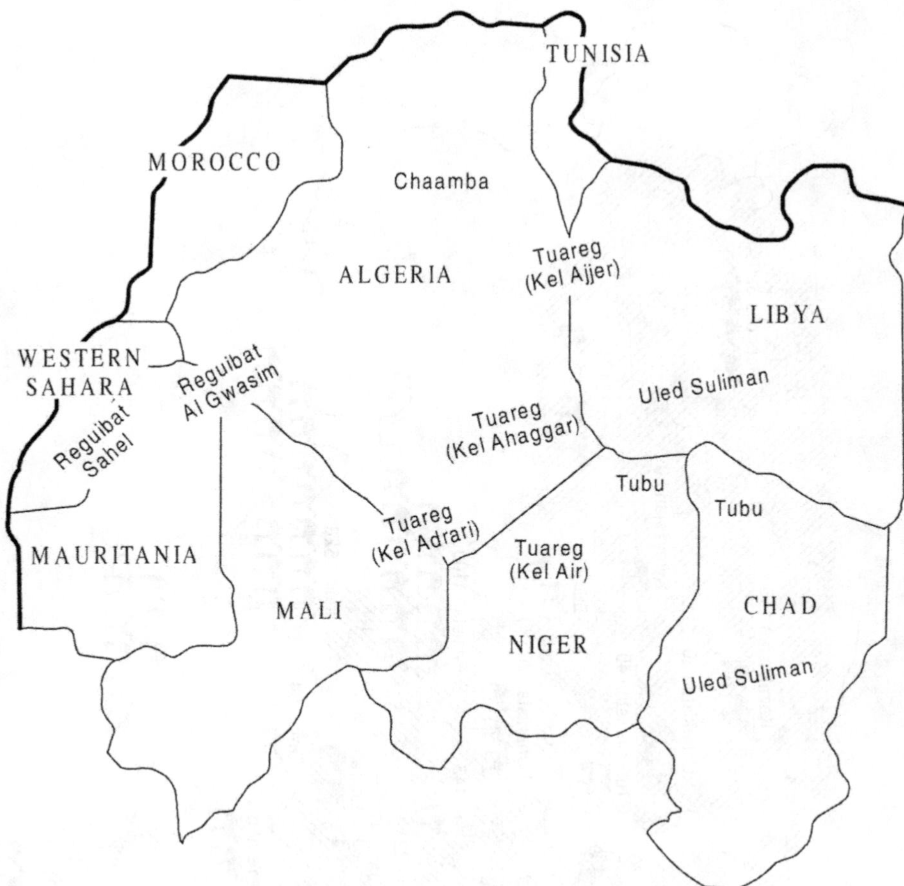

Major camel pastoralist groups in western Africa.

Indigenous knowledge

Over generations, camel pastoralists have accumulated a large body of practical knowledge on all aspects of camel management, breeding and disease control. This knowledge is passed on from generation to generation.

Herding and control

Pastoralists subject camels to varying degrees of control. If milk production is not of concern, then camels are often allowed to range freely. Nevertheless, herders check their movements at regular intervals. They get young animals used to people by waiting for them at wells and feeding them regular titbits.

Herding means letting the camels graze under supervision. The amount of labour needed for this depends on the situation. In an open area where there is no danger from predators, an 8-year-old child can supervise 50–60 animals. However in territory with denser vegetation, several young men will be necessary to control a smaller group of animals. Keeping a herd together requires a good knowledge of camel behaviour.

100,000 camels

20,000-100,000 camels

37 *Number of camels (1996) ('000s)*

Camel distribution

Dromedary

Bactrian

Both

Mongolia 390

China 351

Kazakhstan 156

Kyrgyzstan 50

Tajikistan 50

Uzbekistan 20

Turkmenistan 40

Afghanistan 265

Pakistan 1100

India 1520

Azerbaijan 30

Iran 143

Emirates 160

Oman 94

Qatar 47

Saudi Arabia 422

Yemen 179

Djibouti 62

Ethiopia 1020

Somalia 6100

Eritrea 69

Kenya 810

Egypt 135

Sudan 2950

Tunisia 231

Libya 129

Chad 632

Niger 386

Algeria 115

Mali 327

Morocco 37

W Sahara 99

Mauritania 1087

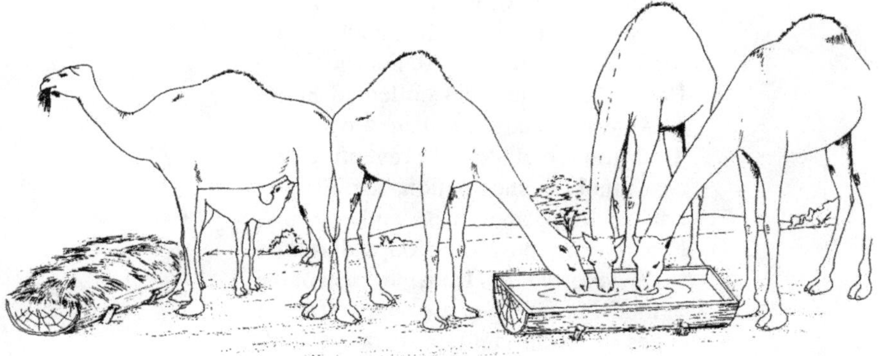

Feeding

Although pastoralists may not know how to calculate a ration, they generally have profound knowledge of the effects certain fodder plants have on the condition and health of their camels. The Kel Adav Tuareg distinguish between 38 grasses and herbs and 24 trees and shrubs; they say that camels eat 47 of these species. They know the effect of these plants on the quantity and taste of the milk, whether they cause bloat, and their salt content. The Rendille have similarly detailed knowledge of 49 plants consumed by camels.

Reproduction

Herders have to choose between optimizing reproduction or production. If milk is the prime objective, then the reproduction rate often suffers. Pastoralists use various methods to maximize their share of the milk: for instance, killing male calves, separating mothers from their calves, preventing suckling by tying up the teats, and controlling breeding to delay the next pregnancy.

Breeds

Animal scientists often state that there has not been much differentiation into camel breeds. But pastoralists have an entirely different view, distinguishing among a large number of camel types. Every ethnic group has a different strain of camel, sometimes several. Although there is little scope for selection among female animals, the male animals are chosen very carefully for certain qualities, such as milk yield of their mother, size, conformation, temperament, etc. Before they use a male animal for further breeding, the Somali critically examine its previous offspring. The ancestry of their camels is a popular topic among pastoralists, and they memorize it in great detail.

Disease control

Western interest in camel diseases dates back only to the colonial period; however, written Arab tradition of camel medicine goes back at least to the twelfth century. Camel pastoralists have independently developed their own concepts, diagnoses and treatments for camel diseases. There have been several studies of the ethnoveterinary knowledge of camel pastoralists, such as the Tuareg, Somali, Pokot (Kenya), Rashaida (Sudan), Ghrib-Bedouin (Tunisia), Reguibat (western Sahara) and Raika (Rajasthan).

The Somali know at least 20 different camel diseases, the Rashaida 22 and the Tuareg more than 30. For the Ghrib Bedouin, researchers collected about 1100 terms relating to camel diseases. Traditional methods of preventing diseases include vaccinations against pox and avoiding areas with endemic diseases. Many pastoral groups diagnose ▻*Trypanosomiasis* from the smell of the animals' urine. They use many different types of traditional treatments, including herbal remedies, bone-setting and branding (▻*Traditional medicines, Branding*).

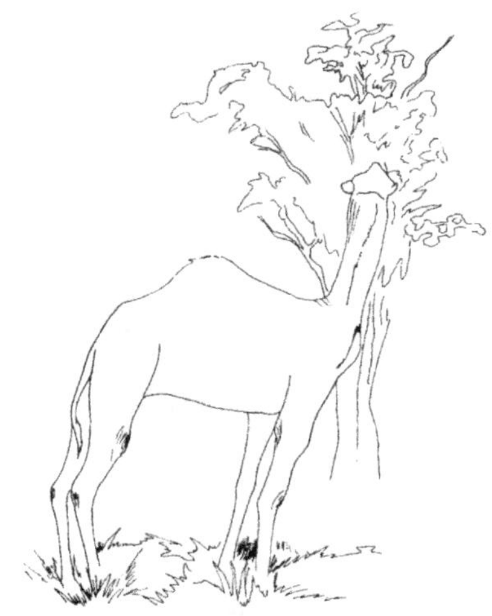

References

Evans et al. (1995) p. 5:1–33; Kaufmann (1998); Klute (1992); Manefield and Tinson (1997) p. 74–5; Rathore (1986) p. 3–61; Sato (1980); Schwartz and Dioli (1992) p. 30–61, 111–41; Wilson (1998) p. 12–31.

How to keep camels healthy

Care of pregnant animals and newborn calves

- Avoid stressing pregnant animals, and do not bleed them to obtain food for people (as is done in some pastoral societies).
- Treat the umbilical cord with iodine or another disinfectant (▻*Navel ill*).
- Make sure the newborn calf drinks the colostrum (the mother's first milk) as soon after birth as possible. Help it if necessary. The colostrum is rich in antibodies and helps build up the calf's resistance to diseases. The colostrum should be undiluted, and no other animal should have suckled the mother for several days before the birth. Many herding societies do not allow the calf to drink the colostrum; this may be one reason that many calves die. Note, however, that drinking too much colostrum may give the calf diarrhoea.
- Make sure the mother accepts the calf and allows it to drink (▻*Poor mothering and fostering, Care of newborn calves*).

Feeding

Camels are adapted to desert plants and shrubs with a high fibre content. As long as they can forage for themselves on range vegetation, they rarely have stomach and gut problems. Problems arise if they are stall-fed with concentrate and lack access to roughage.

Cut, green feed, such as maize, millet, sorghum, legumes, grass and loppings from trees make excellent fodder. These can be supplemented with:

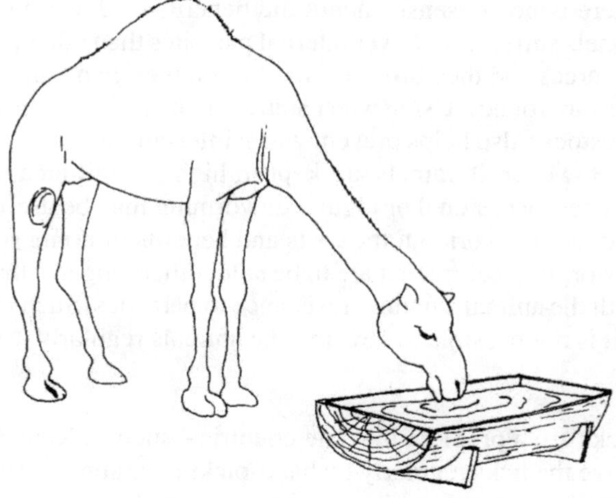

- Ground grain, beans and grams.
- Oilseed and oilseed cake.
- Dates and crushed date stones.
- Jaggery (palm sugar), brown sugar or molasses mixed up with other ingredients as a tonic.

Some pastoralists offer other feeds, such as sardines or meat items, to build up a camel's fat store before heavy work or a long journey.

A typical daily diet for a large (600 kg) Indian working camel is about 2 kg of grain, and 9–18 kg of green feed or 7 kg of hay or straw, and some salt.

Valuable animals, such as pregnant and milking females, calves, breeding males and working animals, need extra feed.

Water

The amount of water a camel needs varies according to the conditions. Camels can go for long periods without water, and they generally need less water than other livestock. During the rainy season, if given green fodder they can get all the water they need from the feed. When thirsty, they can drink 80–100 litres of water at a time.

Different breeds of camels need different amounts of water. Somali camels can rarely go longer than 7–9 days without water, while Rendille camels can go 12–14 days.

Some pastoralists train their camels to go without water during the dry season for at least 7 days. This enables them to forage further away from the watering-place than other livestock.

Salt

Camels require large amounts of salt in their diet. You can provide it by grazing them on vegetation with a high salt content, feeding with additional salt, or by watering the camels at salty springs or wells.

Do not allow confined camels free access to salt blocks, as they may become addicted to licking them. Instead, give loose salt, or mix it with the feed or water. You may also need to give additional minerals to avoid mineral deficiency (▷*Pica*).

Deworming

There is no consensus about the benefits of deworming. It is often believed that camels suffer from fewer internal parasites than other livestock because they live in dry areas and they browse from trees rather than graze on grass (where most parasites are found). Using water sources that are free from faeces (from camels or other livestock) also helps prevent worm infestations.

However, if camels are kept in high-rainfall areas or use contaminated water sources, occasional or regular deworming may be useful. Before deciding whether to deworm, work out the costs and benefits of doing so. Some people recommend deworming calves that are to be sold; others suggest that deworming may interfere with the animal's natural resistance to parasites. Such interference may be a danger if it is not possible to deworm the animals regularly (▷*Internal parasites*).

Tick control

Ticks are a problem in some countries, such as Kenya. Here it is necessary to remove the ticks regularly by hand-picking or applying acaricides. This is especially important for calves. The calf enclosures should be shifted every month, and tick-infested grazing areas must be avoided (▷*Ticks*).

Trypanosomiasis prevention

If at all possible, do not graze camels in areas with many biting flies carrying trypanosomiasis. While avoiding flies completely is not possible, camel pastoralists avoid infested areas during the seasons and times of the day when the flies are most active. Limit the number of fly bites by using fly repellents, especially in the rainy season when there are many biting flies (▷*Bites and stings*).

In infested areas, camel pastoralists are keen to have their camels treated to prevent trypanosomiasis. Quinapyramine chloride prevents camels from catching the disease; it should be given before, or at the beginning of, the rainy season. Some scientists recommend administering it 3–4 weeks after the onset of rains, at the time when danger of infection is highest. However, medication is expensive, so compare the costs and benefits before making a decision (▷*Trypanosomiasis*).

Vaccination

Vaccinations are available in some countries against ▷*Anthrax* and ▷*Blackquarter* ('Blanthrax'), ▷*Haemorrhagic septicaemia* and ▷*Haemorrhagic enteritis*. Some camel pastoralists use a traditional method of vaccinating camels against ▷*Pox*. Consider protecting valuable animals, such as breeding bulls, against ▷*Rabies*.

Care of sick camels

Sick camels need special care if they are to recover quickly and completely.

- Keep the sick animal separate from the herd to avoid the disease from spreading to other animals.
- Provide enough good-quality feed, clean water (especially for animals with diarrhoea or fever), shade and shelter from the wind.
- Cover the animal with blankets during cold nights.
- Move animals that cannot stand up once or twice a day to prevent sores.
- Make sure the sick animal gets enough rest: do not move it with the herd, and do not use it for work until it has recovered completely.
- Check on the sick animal regularly. Clean discharge from the eyes, nose and ears, and clean wounds and renew the dressings each day.

- To reduce the risk of spreading disease, the person who takes care of animals with infectious diseases should not handle healthy animals.
- You can build a separate enclosure, or 'hospital' for sick animals. Make sure that this is free of ticks (▷*Ticks*), and that the ground is dry and free of thorns and sharp stones.
- Take special care of sick calves: keep them with their mother if possible, or feed them with milk from a bottle or teapot (▷*Poor mothering and fostering, Care of newborn calves*).

Disease control under ranch conditions

A ranch in Kenya uses the following management routine:

- Use sheep orf vaccine to inoculate young camels against orf (▷*Orf*).
- Inoculate against blackquarter and anthrax (▷*Blackquarter, Anthrax*).
- Deworm if the camel does not grow well (▷*Internal parasites [worms]*).
- Vaccinate against haemorrhagic septicaemia if necessary (▷*Haemorrhagic septicaemia*).
- Treat against trypanosomiasis if necessary* (▷*Trypanosomiasis*).
- Control nasal bot-flies (▷*Nasal bots*).
- Treat wounds, abscesses and skin diseases* (▷*Wounds and burns, Skin abscesses*).
- Feed with salt and minerals*.
- Clip the ears of young camels to show their month and year of birth (▷*Estimating a camel's weight and age*).
- Brand the camels with their owner's mark and their individual identification number*.
- Keep detailed records of the animals' performance*.

A nearby ranch with Somali-breed camels and employing skilled Somali herders uses only those items in the list above marked *.

References

Evans et al. (1995) p. 5:33; Higgins (1986) p. 16–21; ITDG and IIRR (1996) p. 22–7; Manefield and Tinson (1997) p. 171–6; Rathore (1986) p. 34–49; Schwartz and Dioli (1992) p. 150–1; Wilson (1998) p. 72–6.

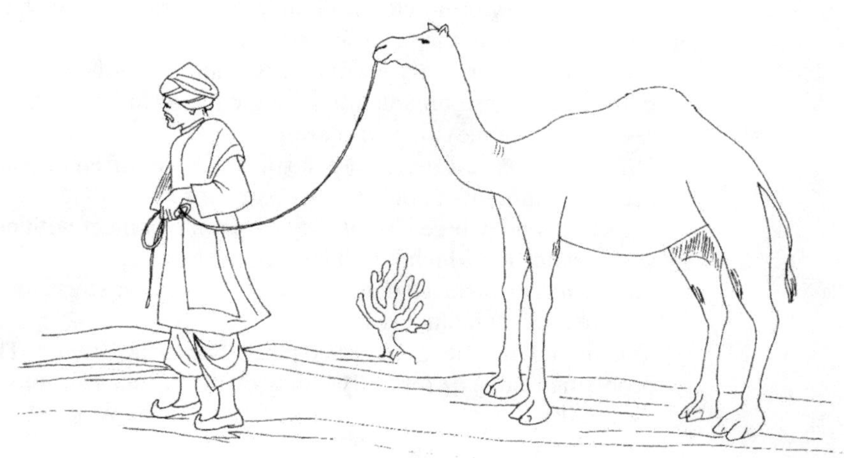

Common diseases

The most common diseases of camels, and the ones you are most likely to encounter in the field, are probably:

- *Trypanosomiasis*
- *Mange*
- *Pox* and *Orf*
- *Wounds and burns*
- *Calf diarrhoea*, *Salmonellosis* and *Colibacillosis*
- *Ticks*
- *Ringworm*
- *Wry neck*
- *Abscesses* (especially on the lymph nodes)
- *Foot problems*

Factors affecting disease occurrence

The occurrence of diseases is influenced by the management pattern, environmental conditions, and possibly genetic resistance (▷*How to keep camels healthy*). Many diseases occur in certain places and at certain times of the year. For example:

- Trypanosomiasis is carried by biting flies, so occurs in areas infested by flies and mainly during the rainy season. It is rarely a problem in desert areas (▷*Trypanosomiasis*).
- Ticks undermine camels' health in East Africa, but are less important in India (▷*Ticks*).
- In milk-oriented systems, a greater percentage of calves might die than in systems that try to maximize reproduction (▷*Care of newborn calves*).
- Mange is important mostly in areas with cold winters and in wetter areas (with over 300 mm of rain a year). It seems to be comparatively rare nearer to the Equator (▷*Mange*).

Camels that are kept under nomadic conditions are generally much healthier than those kept in sedentary systems. Mange, ticks and internal parasites are some of the most likely problems to occur if the camels stay in the same night enclosure or resting-place for a long period.

Disease resistance

Local breeds of camels have been exposed to the same disease-causing organisms (bacteria, viruses, worms, etc.) for hundreds of years, so they have often developed a natural resistance to them. However:

- Some animals are only partially resistant if they have not been exposed to a particular disease organism for long enough for them to become completely resistant (immune) to the disease.
- Different disease-causing organisms occur in different places, and an animal acquires immunity to only those organisms found in its area. When this animal is moved somewhere else, it may come into contact with new diseases or disease strains, for which it will have no resistance.
- An animal's resistance may decrease if it is under stress (due to transportation, bad weather, or malnourishment).
- The animal may never have had resistance to the disease. This is particularly a problem in calves, especially if they do not get enough colostrum (the mother's first milk).

Diseases that people can catch from camels

Zoonotic diseases, zoonoses

Some diseases can spread from animals to people, or from people to animals. These diseases are called 'zoonoses'. Some of them can kill people; others are less serious.

Precautions

- Wash your hands after handling animals and before eating.
- Always cook meat properly.
- Have your animals vaccinated if a particular disease is a problem in your area.
- Use latrines to prevent diseases from spreading via human faeces.
- Be especially careful when handling animals that are ill or have died from one of the diseases listed below. Do not touch the body fluids (blood, pus, saliva, etc.) from these animals, as these may contain the organisms that cause the disease.
- If you must handle infected animals or carcasses, wear plastic bags on your hands like gloves, and wash your hands thoroughly with soap afterwards.
- Dispose of carcasses, and aborted foetuses and their placenta, by burning or burying them. If you bury them, put thorn bushes over the place to prevent dogs or wild animals from digging them up.
- After slaughtering a healthy animal for meat, burn or bury the organs not used for human consumption (such as the lungs) so dogs or wild animals cannot eat them. This helps prevent the spread of diseases such as ▷*Hydatid disease*.

Skin

- **Mange (scabies)**. People can catch mange from camels, but this is not common. In people, camel mange usually heals by itself (▷*Mange*).
- **Ringworm.** A common skin disease in camels, caused by a fungus. People who handle infected animals often become infected (▷*Ringworm*).

Nose and lungs

- **Hydatid disease**. Camels are important carriers of a tapeworm that infests dogs and hyenas. In some areas, nearly all the camels carry the tapeworm cysts. People cannot get the disease directly from camels, but from dogs that eat the uncooked internal organs of an infected camel. People (especially children) can catch the disease easily by eating the tapeworm eggs in the dog faeces, for instance if they do not wash their hands. Hydatid is a serious disease in people, and may cause death (▷*Hydatid disease*).
- **Influenza.** A viral disease of the respiratory system, the 'flu' (▷*Problems of the nose and lungs*). It is possible that camel flu is transmissible to people.

- **Tuberculosis.** While it is not common in camels, tuberculosis can be transmitted from infected camels to people in the animal's saliva, milk, droplets in the breath, or through contaminated water.

Stomach and intestines

- **Salmonellosis** is a common disease carried by apparently healthy camels. People can catch salmonellosis through contaminated surroundings, from flies, and by eating infected meat or drinking infected milk. It is a very serious disease for small children (▻*Salmonellosis*).

Infectious diseases

- **Anthrax** kills infected people unless it is treated promptly. People catch it by breathing in spores containing the anthrax bacteria, through skin contact, or by eating or drinking contaminated food (▻*Anthrax*).
- **Brucellosis** can be transmitted from animals (cattle, sheep, goats) to people via the milk, aborted foetuses and discharge from the vagina. Although camels may get infected with brucellosis, they develop only mild symptoms, if any. Camel pastoralists in India and in Kenya drink raw camel milk without fear of infection, although they boil the milk of other animals.
- **Crimean-Congo haemorrhagic fever.** A viral disease carried by ticks. It is very dangerous to people, but camels do not show any signs of illness. It is thought that people catch it by breathing in the virus.
- **Leptospirosis.** A rare disease in camels, causing blood in the urine and abortions. It usually causes mild, influenza (flu)-like signs in people. It is transmitted via the urine.
- **Orf.** Causes skin disease in people (▻*Orf*).
- **Plague.** A very serious disease in people, causing only mild signs in camels. It is transmitted through infected meat, milk, skins, saliva and body fluids.
- **Q-fever.** Causes severe influenza-like symptoms in people, but no noticeable disease in camels. It is transmitted via tick bites, breathing in dust from the dung, or eating or touching contaminated meat and other animal products.
- **Rabies.** Rabies is a very dangerous disease. If you are bitten by a camel (or another animal) that may have rabies, get treatment immediately. If you wait until the signs of rabies appear, it is too late. Camel bites should be seen as potentially dangerous in areas where rabies is common. This is particularly important if the camel is behaving unusually when it bites you, or if it dies within 7–10 days (▻*Rabies*).
- **Rift Valley fever.** Camels do not show signs of the disease (except for abortions) (▻*Rift Valley fever*).
- **Toxoplasmosis.** May cause abortions, pus in the throat and difficult breathing in camels. People catch the disease by handling or eating raw or undercooked meat. It can cause mild fever in people, and can make pregnant women abort.

References

FAO (1994) p. 229–48; Forse (1999) p. 6–8; IIRR (1996) vol. 3, p. 52–60; ITDG and IIRR (1996) p. 15; Manefield and Tinson (1997) p. 296–9.

How to examine a camel

It can be difficult to determine what disease a sick camel has. You need to examine it carefully, checking for typical signs of disease, as well as other, less usual signs (▷*Diagnosing and treating diseases*).

Patient's history

Take notes on the following information about the sick camel.

About the animal

- The animal's age and sex.
- Its individual habits or characteristics.
- The animal's mother, and whether the animal has been weaned (if it is a calf).
- Where was it acquired? Where did it come from?
- What diseases has it had in the past?
- Has it been vaccinated (against which diseases)?
- When was it last watered and fed? When did it last urinate and defecate?
- Has it been treated with any medicines? If so, what were the results?

About the herd

- How many animals are there in the herd?
- Are other animals infected? Has any animal died from this disease?

About the disease

- How did the disease start? How long has it lasted?
- What are the disease signs (for example, does the animal eat, is it hot, does it have diarrhoea)?
- Which signs appeared first, and which ones later?
- How does the owner or caretaker think the animal got the disease?
- Which disease does the owner or caretaker suspect?

About the surroundings

- Where is the animal kept? Is the enclosure clean? How long has it been in use?
- Where has the animal been grazing?
- Has it been moved recently (or if bought recently, where did it come from)?
- Check also the feeding and water troughs, harnesses and other things that are used by or with the animal.

Physical examination

Examine the camel first from a distance to observe its behaviour and general appearance. Then do a close-up examination from head to toe and check out individual organs. Pay attention to the following (again, write down notes if possible).

Behaviour and appearance

- Unusual behaviour (e.g., lying down at odd hours, lack of appetite, eating strange things, weakness, dullness, tiredness, lameness, scratching).
- Difficulty in breathing.
- Coughing. To get the camel to cough so you can listen to it, offer it some water or feed on the ground so that it lowers its head.

- Difficulty in walking, or unusual posture.
- Swelling of joints.
- The animal's appetite, feeding and ruminating (chewing the cud). Lack of appetite is most apparent while the animal is out at pasture. Sick camels may still eat fodder that is placed in front of them, but lack the energy for grazing.
- The temperature of different body parts (your forehead is more temperature-sensitive than your hands). See below for how to take an animal's temperature.
- The breathing rate. See below for how to measure this.
- The animal's heartbeat. See below for how to take a camel's pulse.
- The hump.

Skin

- Unusual appearance of the skin and hair.
- Presence of parasites on the skin.
- Elasticity of the skin: pull a skin-fold up and check how long it takes until the skin is flat again; the less elastic, the longer it takes.
- Presence of oedema (swelling).
- Swelling or ▻*Abscesses on the lymph nodes.*

Mouth, nose and ears

- Colour of the skin inside the mouth and nose. This should be pink. If the animal has a fever, the colour will be redder and darker. If it is pale or whitish, this is a sign of anaemia.
- Discharge from the nose: one nostril (sinus infection) or both (respiratory infection)? Discharge watery, bloody, or thick and yellowish?
- Discharge from one or both ears.
- Smell from the animal's mouth.

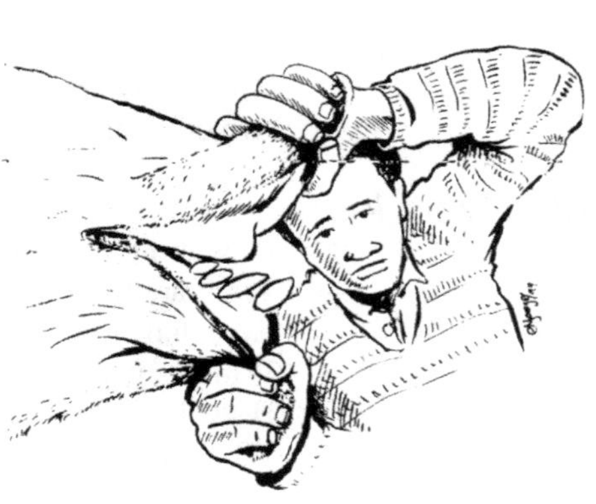

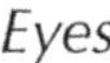

Eyes

- Tears or other discharge in the eyes.
- Colour of the skin under the eyelid: one eye only (local inflammation) or both eyes (more general disorder)?
- Swelling of the eyelids.

Faeces and urine

- Colour and odour of urine (both fresh and dry encrusted on tail hairs).
- Colour, consistency and odour of dung or diarrhoea. Normal dung is hard, round, oval and green. Camels fed with dry feed produce black pellets.
- Appearance of worms in the faeces.
- Colour of the skin inside the anus.
- Discharge from the vagina: blood may be a sign of abortion. After calving, the normal discharge is red or brownish for several days.

Milk

- Colour, odour, and consistency of milk.

Taking the body temperature

1. Tie one end of a string to the thermometer and the other end to a clothes-peg. Shake the thermometer to bring the mercury level below the normal temperature of the animal. If necessary, grease the thermometer with Vaseline or oil to make insertion easier.
2. It is best, although not essential, to take the temperature when the animal is sitting and is restrained securely by its handler. Hold the tail firmly or tie it to the side and insert the bulb of the thermometer 3–5 cm into the rectum. Clip the clothes-peg to the hair at the base of the animal's tail to prevent the thermometer from getting lost.

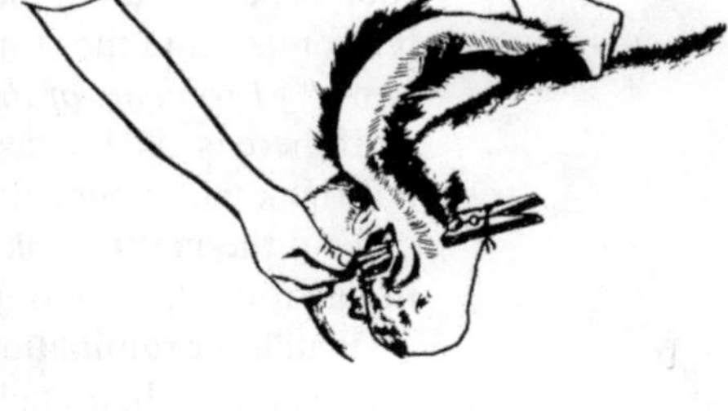

Peg and string tied to thermometer.

3. Leave the thermometer in position for about 3 minutes.

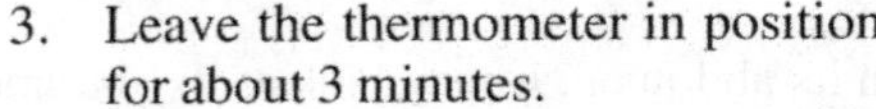

4. Take the thermometer out and read the temperature.
5. Shake the thermometer again to bring the mercury back into the bulb, then clean it and put it back into its case.

The normal temperature is 37.5°C, but a camel's body temperature varies up to 6 degrees (34.2°–40.7°C) during the day. It is low in the morning and higher in the evening. This variation is larger if the animal has not been watered for many days.

The body temperature tends to be higher in young camels and in pregnant and lactating females. (The normal body temperature of humans is about 37°C.)

Signs of fever include dull and half-closed eyes, water running from the eyes, increased pulse and breathing rate, loss of appetite, and reduced urine and milk.

Taking the heart rate (pulse)

You can feel a camel's pulse with your fingers:

- On the underside of the tail, near the root (only in young animals).
- Inside the hind leg, about 18 cm above the point of the hock (although this location may be dirty and crusted with urine).
- Behind the knee on the front leg. (You are least likely to be kicked if you measure the pulse here.)

You can also listen to the heart rate with a stethoscope in the armpit (in the angle behind the front leg).

A healthy camel's heart beats about 30–50 times a minute: slower than humans (60–70 times a minute).

If the camel has a fever, the pulse becomes hard, fast and wiry.

Measuring the breathing rate

You can see a camel breathe by standing behind it and watching its sides move (particularly the right side).

To feel the breathing, put your hand against the side of its body, just behind the ribcage. Measure the breathing rate while the camel is at rest (not right after exercise or work).

Healthy camels breathe silently and barely noticeably, except after physical exertion. A healthy camel at rest breathes 5–12 times a minute in cool temperatures, and 8–24 times a minute on hot days. Young camels under 3 months of age breathe 14–16 times a minute. (An adult human breathes about 10–12 times a minute.)

Checking the rumen and gut

Check the activity of the rumen with a stethoscope placed on the left side of the abdomen, behind the rib cage. Listen for 2–3 minutes. Normally you can hear 3–4 sounds per minute if the camel is ruminating (otherwise you hear only the sound of fermentation in the stomach). If you hear no sound, the animal has digestive problems (▷*Problems of the stomach and intestines*).

If there is excess gas in the camel's gut, you can see it on the **left** flank. Poke the left flank with your fingers to check for gas, fluid or impaction (blockage).

Feel the **right** flank for swellings or pain which could be due to constipation, impaction, a hernia, or pregnancy.

Watch for rumination, especially during the night and in the morning, when the camels are in their enclosure. A camel that ruminates does not have a serious systemic disease or fever.

If the camel has pain in its abdomen, it may kick at its abdomen frequently, sit down and stand up often, shift its position when it is lying down, and bleat.

Taking samples

In order to confirm that a camel has a particular disease, it may be necessary to take samples of the dung, urine, blood or body tissue for further testing in the laboratory (▷*How to collect samples for testing*).

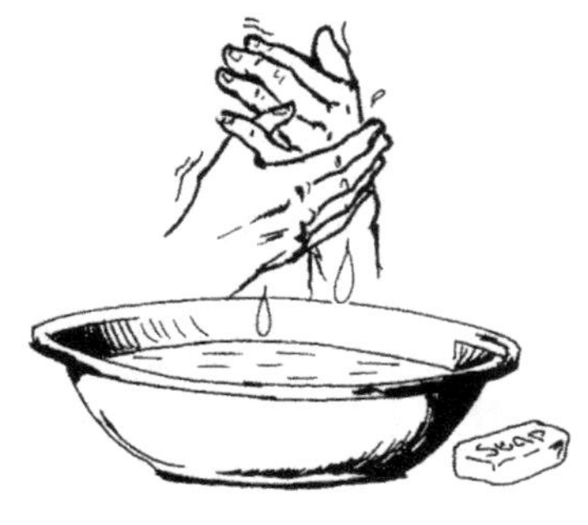

Hygiene

After examining the animal, wash your hands with soap and water, and use disinfectant if you have any scratches on your hands. If you suspect a serious, infectious disease or one that people can catch (such as anthrax), bathe and wash your clothes as soon as possible (▷*Diseases that people can catch from camels*).

Asking a specialist for help

If you need to call in someone else (an expert veterinarian or an experienced healer) to treat a sick animal, insist that he or she comes personally to look at the animal, rather than just relying on a second-hand description. For calves, the specialist should examine the mother too. It is best for the specialist to see the whole herd as well as the sick individual, since he or she may be able to detect disease signs that might otherwise be easily overlooked.

Give the specialist as much detailed information as you can about the animal. This is easy if you have made notes about each of the items above.

References

Evans et al. (1995) p. 4:1–2; FAO (1994) p. 15–21; Higgins (1986) p. 27–9; Köhler-Rollefson (1991) p. 3; Manefield and Tinson (1997) p. 1–6.

Diagnosing and treating diseases

Examine the sick camel and its surroundings carefully, and question the owner (▷*How to examine a camel*).

First look at the general signs (fever, weakness, lack of appetite, diarrhoea, etc.). Then try to narrow down the range of possible diseases by checking for signs that are more specific to particular diseases (e.g., blood in the faeces, pimples on the lips, abortion). Double-check for signs of the disease you suspect. Check also for signs that are *not* present: for example, many diseases cause diarrhoea, but diarrhoea without fever may well be worm infestation (▷*Intestinal parasites [worms]*), while diarrhoea with fever is more likely to be a bacterial disease (▷*Infectious diseases* and *Diarrhoea*).

The tables at the beginning of each chapter in this book list the major disease signs. More specific signs are listed in the sections on each disease. Check also any cross-references in these sections.

Ask the owner or a local healer what the disease is called in the local language. You can look this word up in the section ▷*Disease names in local languages* to help you locate the disease in the book. You should not rely totally on the local name, though, as the owner's diagnosis may not be correct, and the local name may refer to more than one disease.

Difficulties in diagnosing

It can be difficult to decide what disease a sick camel has.

- The animal may show only some of the signs of the disease (in fact, it is rare to see all of the characteristic signs at the same time).
- The same disease may produce different signs in different animals.
- Different diseases may produce the same signs.
- A camel may be suffering from more than one disease, and the signs may mask or reinforce each other.
- Because they are generally placid animals, camels often do not show much distress, even if seriously ill. This complicates diagnosis, especially if the camel suffers from a general, systemic illness that affects its whole body and not one particular organ.
- Some of the less common diseases are not mentioned in this book.

Common disease signs

The following signs can be caused by many different types of disease:

- Weakness.
- Dullness.
- Tiredness.
- Lack of appetite.
- Lying down at unusual times.
- Fever (see below).
- Rapid heartbeat.

If you see these signs, check for other, more specific signs that will help you determine the disease and correct treatment.

Arriving at the correct diagnosis is often a matter of experience. Often a major sign is accompanied by several others; taken together, they give you an idea about which disease you are facing and so how to treat it.

Signs of fever

- High body temperature.
- Fast pulse, sweating.
- Standing with head down and still.
- Dull, half-closed eyes; watery eyes.
- Camel does not ruminate (chew the cud).

Signs of dehydration (lack of water)

- Pinch a fold of skin and let it go: it returns only slowly to its normal position.

Signs of anaemia (loss of blood, or lack of blood)

- Skin inside mouth and nose is pale or whitish.
- The conjunctiva (the membranes around the eye) are pale.

Signs of pain

- Neck erect and stiff, sometimes quickly lowering and raising the neck.
- Watery eyes.
- Sitting uneasily, shifting body around.
- Grunting when breathing or ruminating.

Normal in camels

- Shrunken hump (in females suckling a calf). Can also be a sign of ▷*Trypanosomiasis*, *Mange*, *Internal parasites (worms)*, *Teeth problems*, and chronic stomach and gut diseases (▷*Problems of the stomach and intestines*).
- Grinding of teeth, foam in mouth: normal after eating salt or in male camels during the rut (▷*Rutting*).

Laboratory tests

You may decide to take a sample to test in the laboratory so you can confirm the diagnosis (▷*How to collect samples for testing* and *Checking for diseases in the laboratory*). But even if you are able to do laboratory tests, these may not always identify the disease. For example, the mites that cause ▷*Mange* are very hard to find under a microscope, so a laboratory test may be negative even though the camel actually may have this disease. In many cases you may not have access to a laboratory, or you cannot wait for the test results as the camel needs treatment urgently.

Tentative diagnosis

Often you will not be sure exactly what the disease is. In such cases, you should decide what the disease *probably* is, and treat that. This is called 'tentative diagnosis'.

If the treatment works, continue using it (if necessary). If it does not work, try another remedy. In practice, this method is often the only one possible, especially for hard-to-diagnose problems such as ▷*Skin problems*, *Infectious diseases*, *Diarrhoea* and *Coughs, colds and pneumonia*.

Acute versus chronic diseases

It is important to distinguish between 'acute' and 'chronic' forms of a disease. The animal may have an acute form of the disease to begin with. It should be treated immediately. After an acute disease, the animal (if it has not died) either recovers or develops a chronic (long-lasting) form of the disease. You have more time to reach the correct diagnosis and treat the animal accordingly.

	Signs	Treatment
Acute disease	o Disease lasts 1–10 days o High fever o Severe signs	o Requires immediate action. Try a tentative treatment without delay
Chronic disease	o Less severe signs o Disease lasts a long time o Weakness, loss of condition and weight o Lower production (less work, less milk) o Possibly no fever, or only at some times	o Examine more carefully (e.g., time-consuming lab tests) to determine correct treatment

Choosing a treatment

When you have decided what disease the camel (probably) has, you can choose a treatment. Discuss with the owner what treatments might be used, how effective they are, whether they are available, and how much they cost. The most appropriate treatment depends on the particular situation. Is modern medicine available, at an affordable price? Is the animal seriously ill, or is there time to try a traditional alternative before having to resort to expensive drugs? How confident are you and the owner that the traditional method will work? How much is the animal worth, in relation to the cost of the treatment and its probable success? See ▷*Using the right amount of medicine* for how to calculate dosages.

Broad-spectrum medicines

Some medicines (such as ivermectin and broad-spectrum antibiotics) are effective against several diseases, so have been used extensively. However, they may be expensive, and over-use may lead to the disease organism becoming resistant to the medicine – making the disease harder to treat in the future. Use them sparingly. ▷*Common medicines* gives further guidance.

Medicines to avoid

Certain cattle medicines are (or may be) poisonous for camels, or are dangerous for pregnant females. ▷*Common medicines* contains a list of these.

Follow the law

Laws in many countries prohibit people without a qualification in veterinary medicine from using certain types of medicines, such as antibiotics. These laws are designed to protect human and animal health, and to prevent organisms from becoming resistant to medicines that are misused.

References

Forse (1999) p. 109–39; Manefield and Tinson (1997) p. 1–15.

Parts of a camel

The diagrams below show the main parts of a camel's anatomy and skeleton. For the teeth, see ▷*Estimating a camel's weight and age*. For the eyes, see ▷*Eye problems*. For the location of the main lymph nodes, see ▷*Abscesses on the lymph nodes*.

Anatomy

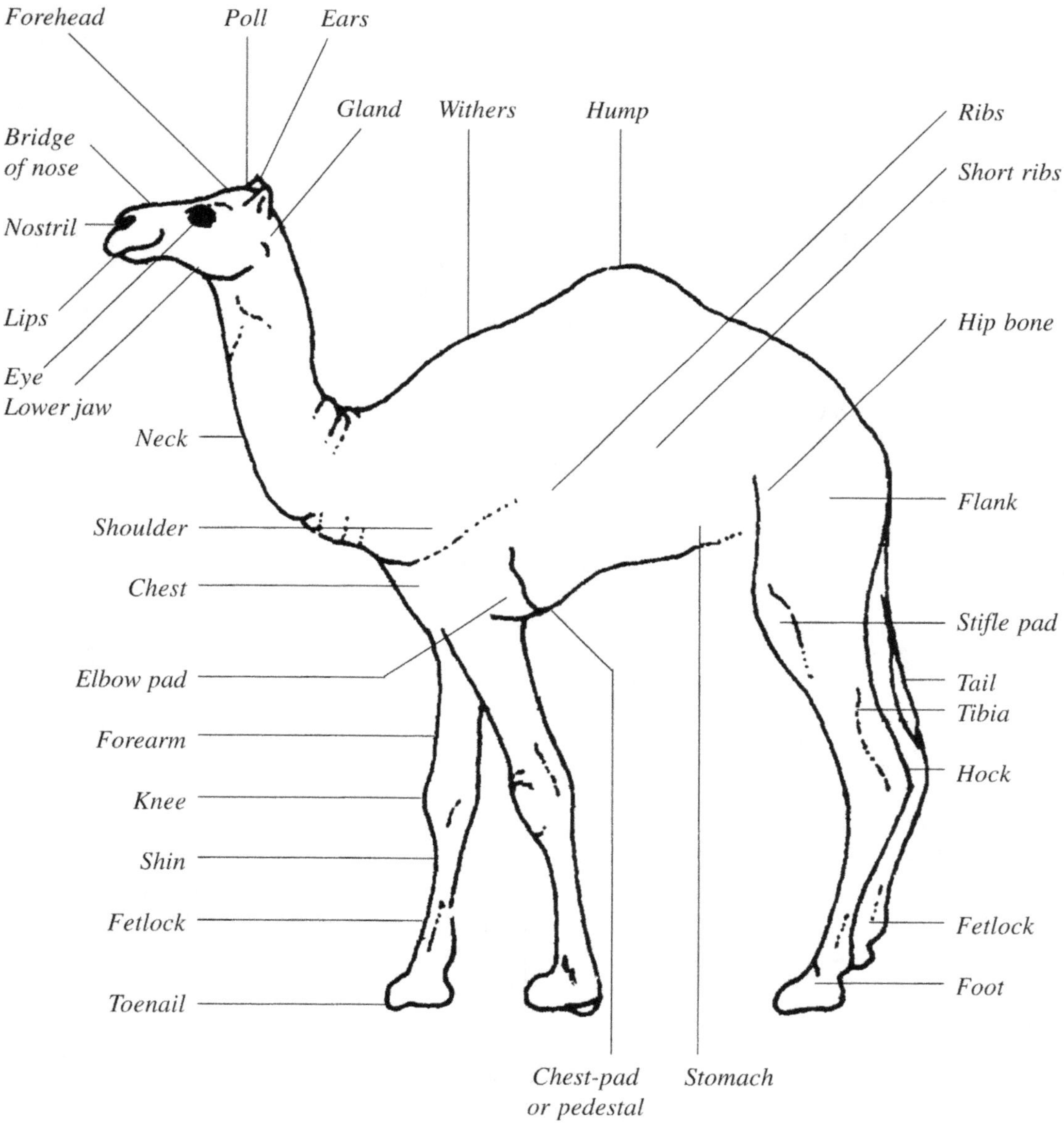

Forehead
Poll
Ears
Gland
Withers
Hump
Ribs
Short ribs
Bridge of nose
Nostril
Lips
Eye
Lower jaw
Hip bone
Neck
Shoulder
Flank
Chest
Stifle pad
Elbow pad
Tail
Tibia
Forearm
Hock
Knee
Shin
Fetlock
Fetlock
Toenail
Foot
Chest-pad or pedestal
Stomach

***Source**: Acland (1932) in Evans et al. (1995).*

Skeleton

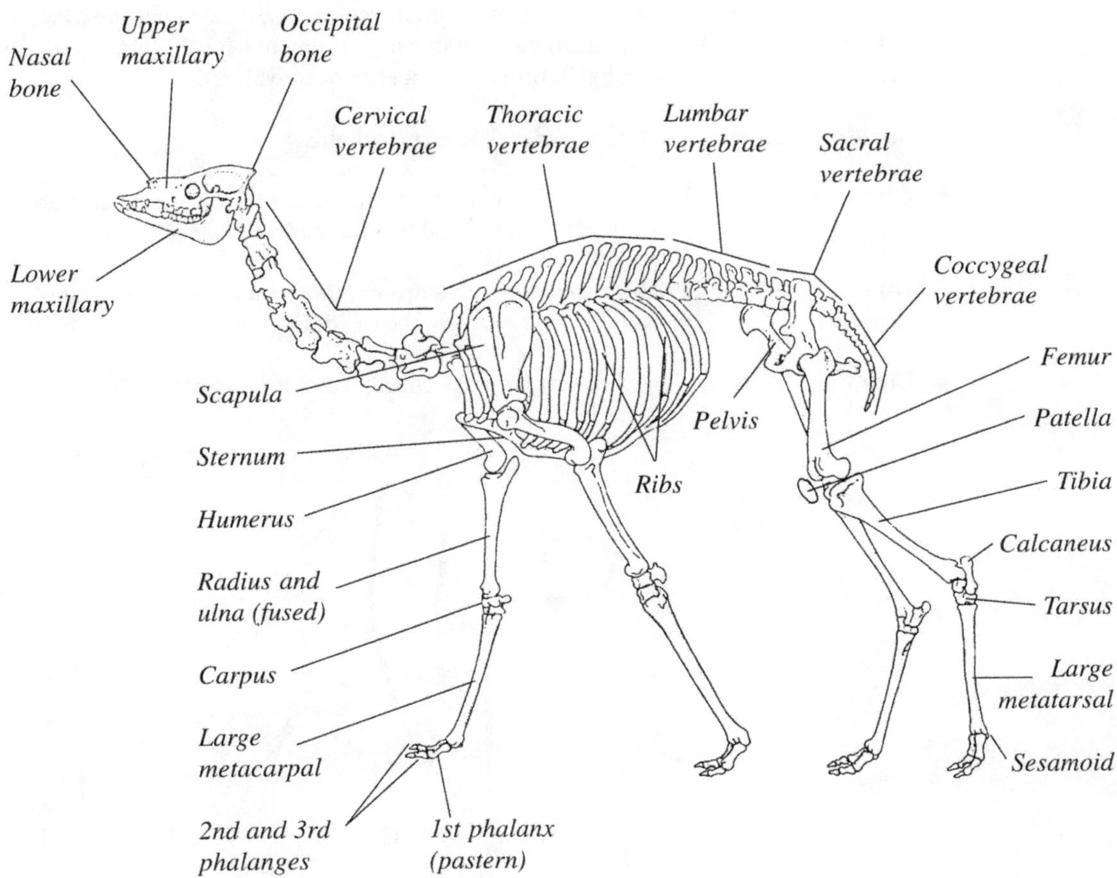

Source: *Kingdon, J. (1979). East African Mammals, vol. 3 part B: Large Mammals. Academic Press, London, in Evans et al. (1995).*

References

Evans et al. (1995) p. 6:2–5.

Estimating a camel's weight and age

Weight

Newborn calves weigh 26–51 kg (an average of 30–40 kg). A mature camel weighs 400–800 kg. Camels reach their mature weights at between 4 and 9 years of age, depending on their feeding and management: usually earlier under more intensive management, and later under extensive pastoral conditions. Males reach their mature weight at about 8 years of age.

The amount of medicine to use often depends on how much the camel weighs. You may also want to know an animal's weight if it is to be bought or sold.

If you do not have scales to weigh the animal, you can use a tape measure to work out roughly the body weight from three simple measurements. It is best to take these measurements in the morning, before the camel has been watered.

Shoulder height Height of the shoulder (in metres).

Chest girth Distance (in metres) around the camel's chest, measured in front of the hump and behind the front legs and chest-pad.

Hump girth Distance (in metres) around the camel's body, measured at its widest point, from the top of the hump around the belly.

Live weight (in kg) = Shoulder height × chest girth × hump girth × 50.

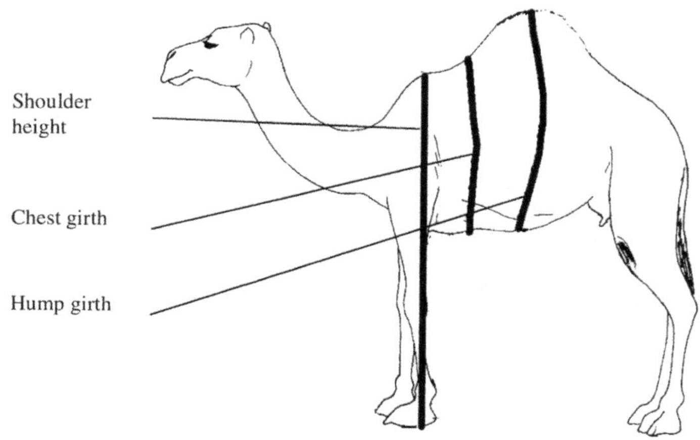

Example

Shoulder height	= 1.95 m
Chest girth	= 2.00 m
Hump girth	= 2.20 m
Live weight	= 1.95 × 2.00 × 2.20 × 50 kg = 429 kg

▷*Using the right amount of medicine* for how to calculate the amount of medicine based on the body weight.

Age

Camels can live to about 40 years of age, but by the time they reach 30, their teeth are often so worn that they can no longer feed. Their useful working lives are from 6 to 15–20 years (for breeding bulls, 7 to 13–15 years).

Camel herders usually know how old each of their animals is. However, it may be necessary to check the age if the animal is being bought or sold, when treating it, or when deciding whether to use it for breeding.

You can tell how old a camel is by looking at its teeth, especially during their first 9 years of life. Hold the upper and lower lips and pull them apart (or ask the owner to do this for you). Look at the teeth from the front and side.

Check for the number of teeth of each type, whether they are milk teeth (smaller) or permanent teeth (larger), and how worn they are:

- **Incisors**: the flat teeth in the lower jaw at the front of the mouth.
- **Canines**: the pointed teeth or 'tushes', which can grow very large in males. Bulls use them as weapons in fights with other males.
- A pointed **'wolf's tooth'** (first premolar) on each side of the upper and lower jaw.
- **Premolars and molars** (cheek teeth): flatter teeth for chewing.

Young camels have 22 'deciduous' or **milk teeth**:
- 1 incisor, 1 canine and 3 premolars on each side of the upper jaw,
- 3 incisors, 1 canine and 2 premolars on each side in the lower jaw.

Older camels have 34 **permanent teeth**:
- 1 incisor, 1 canine, 3 premolars and 3 molars on each side of the upper jaw,
- 3 incisors, 1 canine, 2 premolars and 3 molars on each side in the lower jaw.

Normally it is only necessary to look at the incisors and canines in order to estimate a camel's age. It is difficult to see the premolars and molars because they are set far back in the mouth.

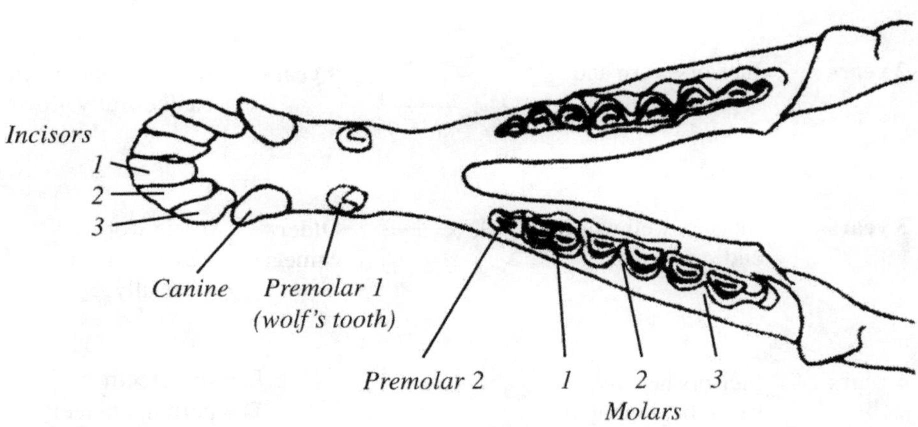

Position of teeth in the lower jaw of an adult camel.

Checking the teeth to determine age is accurate until the camel is about 9 years old. The teeth of older camels wear differently because they eat different things, so looking at their teeth is not as reliable. You should also take into account other factors, such as the animal's appearance, its sexual maturity, the number of calvings (for females), grey hairs and skin texture.

A frequent mistake is to confuse a 3-year-old camel with one that is 7 years old, since both have a full set of front teeth. A 4-year-old may also be confused with an older camel, since both have heavily worn teeth. But 3- and 4-year-olds still have their milk teeth, which are smaller than the permanent teeth, and are thinner at the base. Also look at the animal's appearance to confirm its age.

Camels that browse on trees and shrubs all the time wear their teeth down quickly. In some areas, 6–7-year-old camels have only stump incisors.

Development of front teeth in the lower jaw

Birth	No teeth	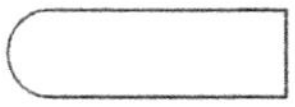	**5 years**	First permanent teeth (incisors 1) emerged	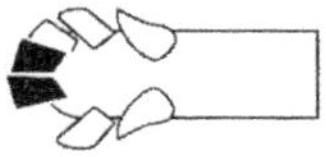
1 month	2 pairs of incisors, 3rd pair emerging	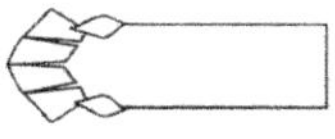	**6 years**	Permanent incisors 2 emerged and grown	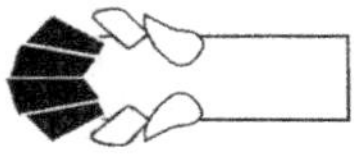
3 months	Canines emerging	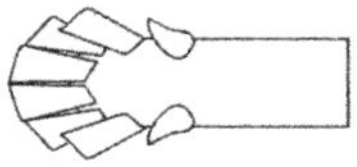	**7 years**	Permanent incisors 3 emerged and grown; permanent canines emerging	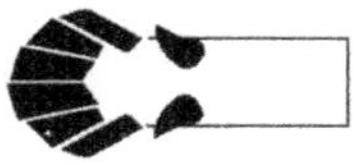
1 year	Canines and all 3 pairs of incisors grown	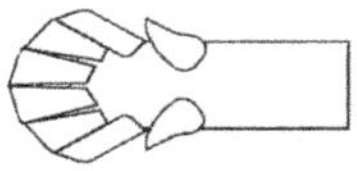	**8 years**	Incisors worn, canines half grown	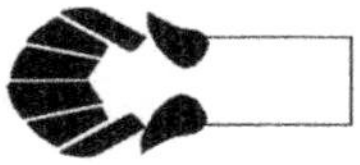
2 years	Incisors worn and separated	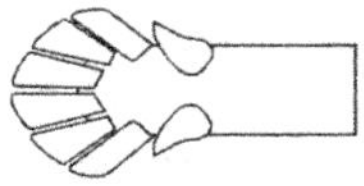	**9 years**	Incisors more worn, canines fully grown	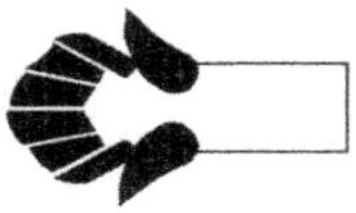
3 years	Incisors well worn and separated	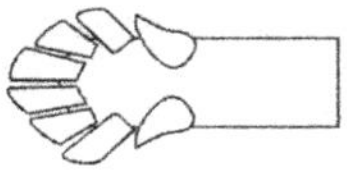	**Older camels**	Teeth worn, incisors stand vertically	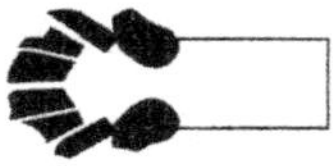
4 years	Incisors heavily worn, beginning to fall out	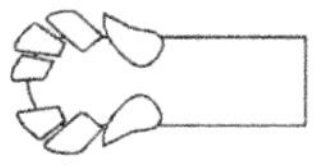		□ = milk teeth ■ = permanent teeth	

Age at which milk teeth and permanent teeth appear

Tooth	Lower jaw		Upper jaw	
	Milk teeth	**Permanent teeth**	**Milk teeth**	**Permanent teeth**
Incisor 1	2 weeks	4.5–5 years	None	None
Incisor 2	2 weeks	5.5–6 years	None (stays in gums)	None
Incisor 3	1–3 months	6.5–7 years	2–4 months; not always present	5.5–7 years
Canine	2–4 months	6–7 years	2–4 months	6–7 years
Premolar 1	1 month	6.5–7.5 years	ca 1 month	6.5–7.5 years
Premolar 2	1 month	5–5.5 years	ca 1 month	5–5.5 years
Premolar 3	None	None	ca 1 month	5–5.5 years
Molar 1	None	12–15 months	None	12–15 months
Molar 2	None	2.5–3 years	None	2.5–3 years
Molar 3	None	5–5.5 years	None	5–5.5 years

Adapted from Schwartz and Dioli (1992)

References

Evans et al. (1995) p. 6:8–12, 8:2; FAO (1994) p. 170–4 (has ageing method using cheek teeth); Forse (1999) p. 315; Higgins (1986) p. 34–7; Köhler-Rollefson (1991) p. 3; Leese (1927) p. 29, 134; Manefield and Tinson (1997) p. 22; Projet Cameline (1999) p. 60; Rathore (1986) p. 89–91; Schwartz and Dioli (1992) p. 74, 95–8, 107–10 (contains colour photographs of camels' teeth at various ages); Wilson (1998) p. 80–3, 115.

Equipment and medicines

Keep a kit of equipment and medicines ready so you can leave immediately if some kind of emergency arises. A sturdy cloth or leather bag is the handiest container; some people use containers made from sheet metal. After returning from the field, make sure that you refill all the medicines and other supplies that you have used.

Here is a list of the main types of equipment, supplies and medicine you will need in the field. For certain problems (especially for complicated surgery), you will need more specialized equipment and specific types of medicine.

Commonly used equipment

- Veterinary syringes (5, 10 and 20 ml).
- Syringe needles (disposable or non-disposable): 25 and 37 mm, 16 and 18 gauge (▷*Administering medicines*).
- Clinical thermometer.
- Forceps: for holding tissues during surgery.
- Scissors: for surgery and taking samples.
- Needles: for stitching.
- Scalpel handle and blades (or razor blade or sharp knife).
- Plastic or glass containers with lids (e.g., jam jars or film canisters): for collecting samples.
- Measuring container: for measuring medicines.
- Measuring spoons.
- Strong knife: for trimming nails, etc.
- Drenching bottle.
- Indelible marker pen.
- Notebook and pen: for recording cases treated.
- Strong bag: for carrying equipment.
- Pair of plastic or rubber gloves.
- Pocket flashlight: to check inside mouth.

Other equipment

- Balling gun: to put pills into the animal's throat (▷*Administering medicines*).
- Rubber pipe: 3 m long, to put medicine into the animal's stomach (▷*Administering medicines*).
- Reinforced plastic tube: to put into mouth to stop animal from biting on stomach tube (▷*Administering medicines*).
- Funnel.
- Trocar and cannula: to pierce rumen to release gas in case of bloat (▷*Bloat*).
- Instrument tray and cover: for keeping instruments clean.
- Branding irons.
- Stethoscope.
- Drip equipment.

Equipment usually available in the field

- Ropes for restraining animals.
- Buckets.
- Bottles.
- Blankets.

Supplies

- Thread (silk or nylon): for stitching the skin.
- Catgut: for stitching internal tissues.
- Cotton wool.
- Distilled water.
- 70% alcohol.
- Soap.
- Bandages.

Medicines

See ▷*Common medicines* for a more complete list and names of commercial medicines. Note that in many countries, only veterinarians are allowed to use certain medicines (especially antibiotics and vaccines).

- Antiseptic (e.g., tincture of iodine, Savlon, Dettol, hydrogen peroxide, potassium permanganate): for cleaning and disinfecting wounds.
- Turpentine or Maggacite: to kill maggots.
- Wound ointment (e.g., Ectosep, Himax, Lorexane).
- Liquid paraffin, castor oil, or magnesium sulphate: for constipation.
- Trypanocide.
- Dewormer (e.g., Panacur).
- Antihistamine (e.g., Avil).
- Mange treatment (e.g., Butox, Ivomec).
- Cough ointment or powder (e.g., Caflon, Catcough).
- Preparation against diarrhoea (e.g., Neblon).
- Eye drops (e.g., Ciplox).
- Pain-killing medicine (e.g., Diclovet).
- Antibiotics (e.g., injectable penicillin and tetracycline).
- Vaccines.
- EDTA or sodium citrate: to stop blood from coagulating.

Only for the vet

- Sedative (e.g., xylazine).
- Drip fluid (Ringer's lactate, glucose, sodium chloride).
- Corticosteroid.
- Anaesthetic (e.g., lignocaine hydrochloride).

Portable laboratory

- Microscope, lens, objectives.
- Microscope slides and cover slips.
- Battery centrifuge and centrifuge tubes: to test for skin parasites, etc.
- Mini-haematocrit centrifuge and capillaries: to test blood samples.
- Test tubes.
- Spatula and plate (or pestle and mortar): for grinding medicines.
- Strainer: for faecal samples.
- Cups or glasses: for sedimenting faecal samples.
- Pressure cooker: for sterilizing equipment.

References

FAO (1994) p. 260–2; Forse (1999) p. 9–13; IIRR (1996) vol. 1, p. 11; Quesenberry (1990) p. 226–7.

Traditional medicines

Many camel herders have a detailed knowledge of medicinal plants and how to use them to treat particular diseases. Many of these herbal medicines are effective at treating particular diseases, or at least help relieve the symptoms. However, they are often less effective than modern medicines, and some may be ineffective or even harmful.

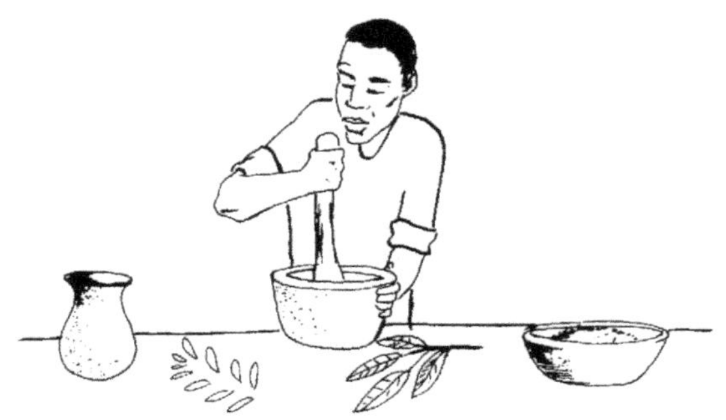

Relatively little scientific research has been done on camel diseases. Much remains to be learned about the types of herbal medicines used and their effectiveness.

Certain people in a society know a lot about traditional medicines: they are able to identify which plants are useful against particular diseases, and use them to prepare and administer medicines. These people are often elderly, having learned their skills over many years of apprenticeship, observation and experiment. The owners of sick animals often go to them first, before (or as well as) seeking outside help. These indigenous specialists can be very valuable allies for the veterinarian or paraveterinarian in treating animals, or in alerting the authorities about a disease outbreak.

The application of traditional medicines may be accompanied by special rituals or magic. Some practices may be secret. (This is true also of 'modern' societies: for example, people pray for recovery from illness, and veterinarians and other scientists are often reluctant to share their knowledge with lay people for fear of it being misused.)

Guidelines for traditional medicines

- **Learn the local names of diseases.** The local disease names may not match one-on-one with the scientific names: several diseases may be grouped together under the same name, or the same disease may have several different names. Learn these names, and learn which traditional remedies are used to treat which diseases. This will help you communicate better with the local people.
- **Show respect for traditional knowledge,** and work with the indigenous healers, not against them. Often, a traditional treatment using herbal medicine may be enough to treat a disease. Or it may be possible to combine traditional medicines with modern treatments.
- **Be cautious about trying to stop people from using traditional practices:** they may be an important feature of the society's culture, and may be very difficult to change. In general, do not try to stop a practice

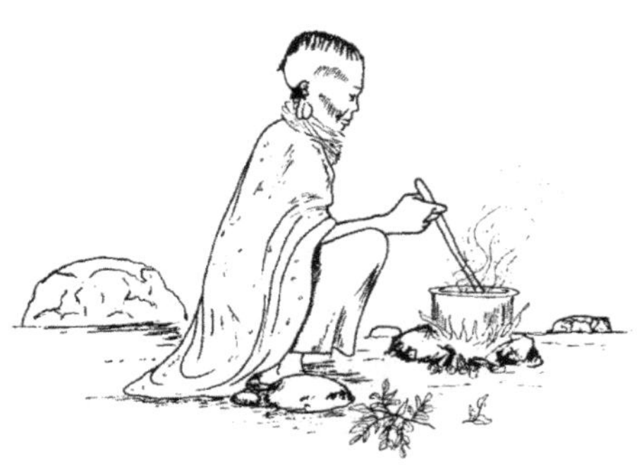

	Traditional medicines	Modern medicines
Advantages	○ Cheap (or free) and locally available ○ People are familiar with them and know how to use them ○ Useful for many minor ailments	○ (Often) treat underlying cause as well as symptoms ○ Quick-acting and effective ○ May be simple to apply ○ People often prefer them to traditional remedies
Disadvantages	○ May treat symptoms rather than the underlying cause of a disease ○ May be slow-acting and less effective than modern medicines ○ May be ineffective or harmful ○ May be complex to prepare and apply ○ The plant part needed may be unavailable in some places or at certain times of the year ○ The effectiveness of a plant may differ from place to place or in different seasons	○ May be expensive or unavailable ○ Require specialist knowledge (veterinary training) ○ May require special equipment ○ May have legal restrictions on who can use them (e.g., only qualified veterinarians) ○ Many fake or adulterated medicines on the market

unless it actually causes serious harm or prevents the owner from seeking a more appropriate treatment for the sick animal.

Traditional or modern medicines?

The choice between traditional and modern medicines will depend on many things, including the disease and its severity, the value of the animal, the availability and price of medicines, the amount of money available, and your (and the owner's) confidence that the medicine will be effective. Keep a ready supply of modern medicines, but also know which traditional medicines are useful, and be prepared to use them if appropriate.

Identifying plants

- Make sure that you know exactly which plants to use to treat a problem. Different plant species look similar and may have the same name; and the same plant may be called by different names. (In this book, where the name is not certain, it is marked with a '?')
- Ask indigenous specialists to show you the plants they use to treat particular diseases. Ask them what the plants are called in the local languages.
- If possible, find out the scientific name of the plant. Institutions such as the National Museums of Kenya and the National Herbarium in Addis Ababa can help identify unknown plants. Universities, research centres and national park authorities are other good sources of such information.

Effectiveness

The effectiveness of a plant medicine depends on many different factors:

- **The plant part used:** roots, stem, branches, flowers, leaves, fruits, seeds. Certain parts of a plant may contain lots of active ingredient, while others may have little or none at all.

- **When the plant is collected.** Both the season and the time of day affect the amount of certain ingredients in the plant. In general, collect plant parts in the morning or on a sunny day. Some plants or plant parts (e.g., flowers, seeds) are available only at certain times of the year.
- **The place it is collected.** Soil and climate can have a major influence on the effectiveness of plant medicines.
- **Disease.** Do not use any plant parts that are mouldy or discoloured.
- **Handling and storage.** If you need to store the plant parts for future use, dry them in the shade, if possible – not in the direct sun or over a fire. Protect the dried ingredients from mould or pests by putting them in a closed jar or tin. Write the plant name and the date of collection on the container, and keep it away from the sun.

Plant parts

For the most effective herbal medicine, you should generally collect:

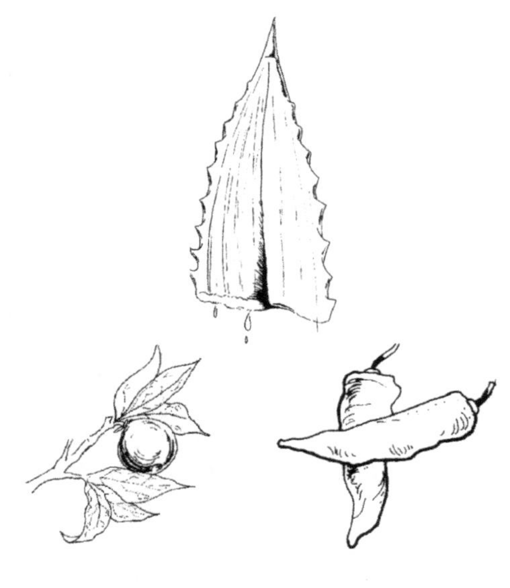

- **Leaves and stems:** During the daytime and when the plant is about to bloom.
- **Seeds:** From completely ripe fruits (if the fruits dry out and split open to scatter their seeds when they are ripe, collect the fruits as soon as they start ripening).
- **Fruit:** Before the fruit matures completely.
- **Flowers that smell:** When the flower buds are just about to open and in the morning when the sun is low.
- **Other flowers:** When they are in full bloom.
- **Bark:** When the plants are in bloom or are growing vigorously. Strip off bark from one side of a tree—not from all the way around the trunk, as this may kill the tree.
- **Roots:** Before the plant starts flowering.

Preparing herbal medicines

Herbal medicines can be made in many different ways. Here are the most common:

Boiling

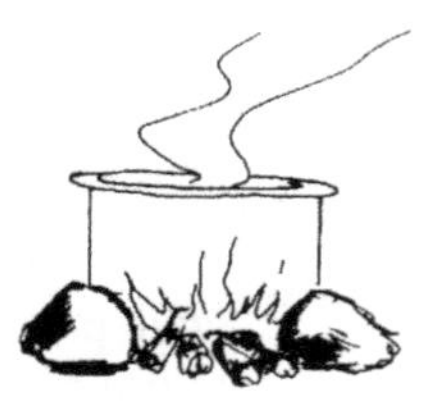

Chop up the plant parts (if necessary) and boil them for 15–20 minutes in a pot of water. Some healers recommend boiling until only half of the water is left.

Allow the liquid to cool and strain it through a clean cloth before using it.

Some plant materials, especially those that are hard and dry, must be soaked in water before boiling. A medicine that is prepared by boiling is called a 'decoction'.

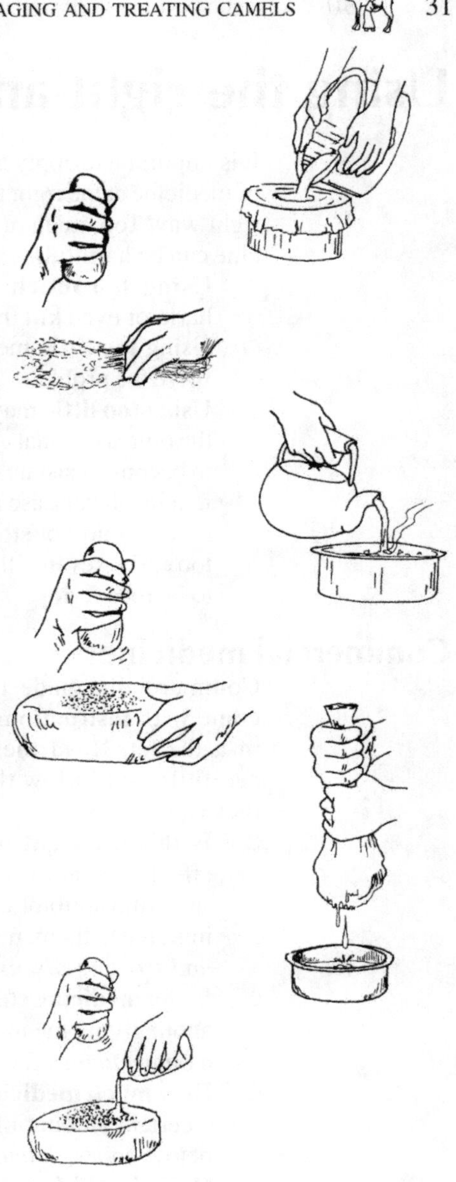

Soaking

Soaking is another method of extracting the medicinal ingredients from the plant. Put the plant part in a pot and pour hot or cold water over it, then allow it to stand. Put a lid on the pot to stop the ingredients from escaping into the air. After several hours, strain the liquid through a clean cloth.

A medicine prepared by soaking plant materials is called an 'infusion'.

Powder

Pound and grind dried plant materials into a coarse or fine powder. You can sift the powder through a tea-strainer to get the required particle size.

Juice

Pound fresh plant materials and strain through a cloth or tea-strainer to get the juice. Or you can just squeeze the plant parts to get the juice.

Paste

Make a paste by grinding the plant materials (either fresh or dry), together with a little oil or water if necessary.

Bolus

A bolus is a solid ball of medicine that is easy to pop into an animal's mouth. Pound fresh or dried plant materials with just enough liquid (such as honey, or flour and water) to bind it together. Roll it into shape with your hands.

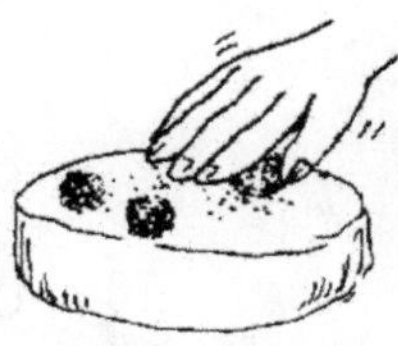

References

Domingo (1998); IIRR (1994) vol. 1, p. 12–19; ITDG and IIRR (1996) p. 2–7; McCorkle et al. (1996) p. 1–23; Wanyama (1997) vol. 2.

Using the right amount of medicine

It is important to apply the right amount of medicine at the right times, and in the right way. Too much or too little medicine can be harmful:

- Using **too much** medicine may harm or even kill the animal.
- Using **too little** medicine may not solve the problem.
- Using **too little** may allow some of the organisms that cause the disease to become resistant to the medicine, making the disease more difficult to treat. So do not stop the treatment too early – even if the animal seems to be recovering.

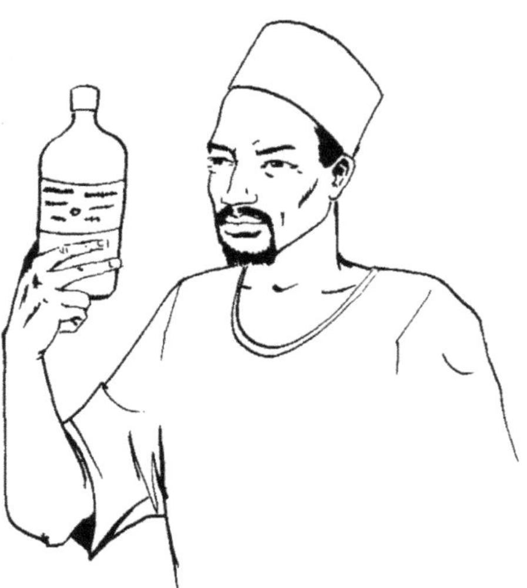

Commercial medicines

Commercially made medicines may come with instructions on the box or in a leaflet. Read these instructions carefully and follow them fully. Use only the recommended dosages. Answer these questions:

- **Is this the right medicine for the disease?** Note that many medicines are effective against a large range of diseases. However, do not overuse broad-spectrum antibiotics or other medicines, as the disease organisms may become immune to them, making the disease harder to treat in the future (▷*Diagnosing and treating diseases*).
- **Is the medicine suitable for the sick animal?** Check especially for warnings about giving the medicine to calves, pregnant or milking animals. See ▷*Common medicines* for a list of medicines that should not be used on camels.
- **How much medicine should I use?** The medicine label might tell you to apply a certain amount of medicine per kilogram of the animal's body weight. See below under *Calculating dosages.*
- **How should I give the medicine?** In the mouth, mixed with the feed, rubbed into the skin, or injected (under the skin, into the muscle, or into a vein)? You may have to mix some medicines yourself from powder or concentrated solution before giving them (▷*Administering medicines*).
- **When should I give the medicine?** Once only, once a day, twice a day, more often? In the morning, before or after feeding or milking, or at night?
- **When should I stop giving the medicine?** With some medicines, you should stop treatment when the animal recovers. With others (especially antibiotics), you should continue the treatment for a certain period, even if the animal seems to have got better. This is to make sure that all of the organisms causing the disease have been killed. For advice on how long to give antibiotics, see ▷*Common medicines.*

If you are not sure about the answers to these questions, ask someone with more experience. Experienced livestock raisers, veterinarians, doctors, nurses and shopkeepers who sell medicines can often give useful advice.

Indigenous medicines

Dosages for indigenous medicines are often imprecise and vary widely from healer to healer and from place to place. For many, it is not important to get the precise dosage, but be careful: some plants are poisonous, so the exact dosage is important. Ask an indigenous healer for help in preparing and using these medicines (▷*Traditional medicines*).

Calculating dosages

The amount of medicine to use may depend on several factors:

- **The type and stage of the disease.** More severe cases may need more medicine, but this is not always the case.
- **The weight of the animal.** You may have to calculate the amount of medicine from the animal's body weight. Larger, heavier animals usually need more medicine than small or young ones (▷*Estimating a camel's weight and age*).
- **The type, composition and concentration of the medicine.** Medicines come in different formulations (liquid, tablets, capsules, powders). Different companies may make the same medicine with different strengths.

The strength of a medicine depends on how much **active ingredient** (**a.i.**) it contains. The active ingredient is the substance that cures or prevents the disease. The medicine may also contain water, substances to make the tablet stick together, and other ingredients. For example, some tablets contain 5 mg of the active ingredient; others might contain 10 mg or more. Check the label carefully to make sure you know how much medicine to give. See ▷*Units of measurement* for some common measures you can use for medicines.

Unless otherwise stated, the amounts in this book are for single applications.

Many medicines are designed for use with cattle, but can also be used to treat the same diseases in camels. They often do not have any instructions for how to use them with camels. In general, use the same amounts as for cattle.

Caution: Some cattle medicines (including Berenil, Levamisole and griseofulvin) are ineffective or harmful to camels. Do not use them (▷*Common medicines*).

Calculating dosage based on body weight

Some medicine labels tell you very clearly how much medicine to apply for a certain type of animal, such as newborn calves. Such cases are easy: just follow the instructions on the label.

Sometimes you have to do some simple arithmetic. You might have to estimate the animal's weight and then calculate the amount of medicine needed (▷*Estimating a camel's weight and age*).

It's best to write down the animal's weight, the dosage, and any other information you need on a notepad, as in the examples below. That way you can recheck your calculation (or ask someone else to check you haven't made a mistake). If necessary, use a pocket calculator.

It is better to be safe than to give the wrong dosage. See ▷*Units of measurement* for more help on measuring medicines.

Examples of calculating dosages

Example 1

The medicine label says to use a dosage of 5 ml/10 kg body weight. The animal weighs 429 kg.

Animal's weight	= 429 kg
Dosage	= 5 ml/10 kg body weight
Amount of medicine to apply	= 429 × 5 ÷ 10
	= 214.5 ml
	= about 210 ml.

Example 2

Some medicines come in solutions of (for example) 2%. It can be a bit more complicated to calculate dosages for these.

The medicine you want to use comes in a 2% solution. The label says to use a dosage of 0.25 mg active ingredient per kg body weight. The animal weighs 429 kg (▷*Estimating a camel's weight and age*).

Remember

- 1 litre of water weighs 1 kg.
- 1 millilitre (1 ml) of water weighs 1 g.
- 1/1000 ml of water weighs 1 mg.

A concentration of 2% means there are 2 mg of the active ingredient in every 100 mg (0.1 ml) of the medicine, or 0.02 mg of active ingredient in every 1 mg of medicine.

Animal's weight	= 429 kg
Dosage	= 0.25 mg a.i./kg body weight
Medicine concentration	= 2%
	= 0.02 mg in 1 mg
Amount of medicine to apply	= 429 × 0.25 ÷ 0.02
	= 5362.5 mg
	= about 5.4 g
	= 5.4 ml of medicine.

References

Forse (1999) p. 311–14; IIRR (1996) vol. 1, p. 12–19; Quesenberry (1990) p. 237–9.

Administering medicines

How to give a medicine depends on the nature of the illness and the type of medicine. The main methods are injection, in the mouth and on the skin. Other methods include in the nose, eyes, ears, vagina, anus, or udder.

Injection

Injecting is a quick and convenient way of giving medicines. It is used for antibiotics and vaccines, as well as for other types of medicines (such as ivermectin against mange). It is sometimes called 'parenteral administration'.

Ways of injecting

Medicines can be injected into the muscle, under the skin, or into the vein (using a syringe or a drip). Check the medicine label to find out which way you should inject the medicine.

Where injected	Also called	Features
Into the muscle	Intramuscular i.m., i/m	Easy to do Most drugs are injected this way Medicine is taken up by the body quickly
Under the skin	Subcutaneous s.c., s/c	Less painful; easy to do Used only for certain medicines Medicine is taken up by the body slowly
Into the vein	Intravenous i.v., i/v	To give large amounts of medicine Medicine gets into the bloodstream immediately Requires extra care
Into the vein through a drip	Drip, intravenous i.v., i/v	To give large amounts of fluid to a dehydrated animal

Syringes

You can use reusable or disposable syringes and needles. Each has advantages and disadvantages (see the table on the next page).

Syringes come in several sizes. For most purposes, you can use a 20 ml syringe. Smaller syringes (5 and 10 ml) may be useful to inject small amounts of medicine.

Needles come in different lengths and widths ('gauges', measured as 'G' numbers). A needle with a low G number is broad, while a high G number is narrow. For most camel work, 16G and 18G needles should be adequate. Use a needle 2.5 cm long for injecting into the muscle, and 3.7 cm long for injecting into the vein. The needle should be sharp and not bent. Make sure that it fits the type of syringe you have.

	Reusable syringe and needles	Disposable syringe and needles
Advantages	○ Cheap (after initial expense)	○ Convenient ○ Reduces risk of contamination
Disadvantages	○ Must be sterilized after each use ○ Needles may become blunt	○ Relatively expensive because new syringe and needle are needed for each injection ○ Used needles and syringes must be disposed of safely

Make sure that the syringe and needle are always sterile to avoid spreading disease from one animal to another. Hold the needle by its base, and don't touch the point or the shaft of the needle with your hand or anything else. See below on how to disinfect a syringe. Before using a reusable syringe and needle, rinse them in boiled, cooled water to wash off any disinfectant.

Filling the syringe with ready-prepared medicine

Some medicines come ready to inject. Others must be mixed before they are injected. Follow these instructions for medicines that come **ready to inject**.

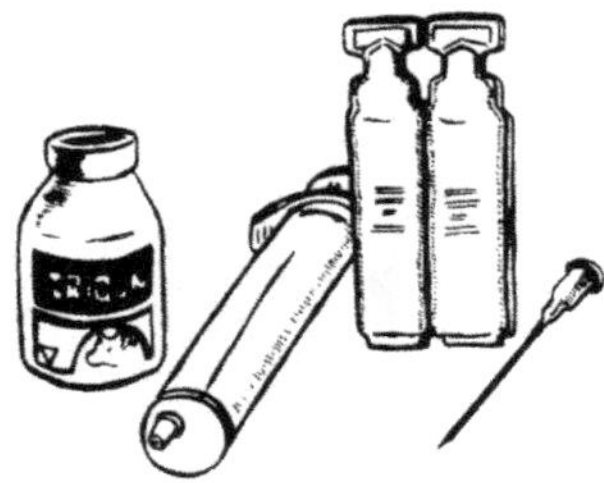

1. Put the needle on the syringe and draw back the plunger to fill the syringe barrel with air.
2. Push the needle through the rubber stopper of the bottle containing the medicine.
3. Hold the bottle upside-down.
4. Press the plunger to push some air from the syringe into the stoppered bottle.
5. Pull the plunger to suck in some liquid.
6. Continue pumping like this until you have enough medicine in the syringe.
7. Pull the needle out of the stopper and hold the syringe upside-down. Push the plunger to remove the air (until liquid comes out of the needle). You are now ready to inject the medicine.

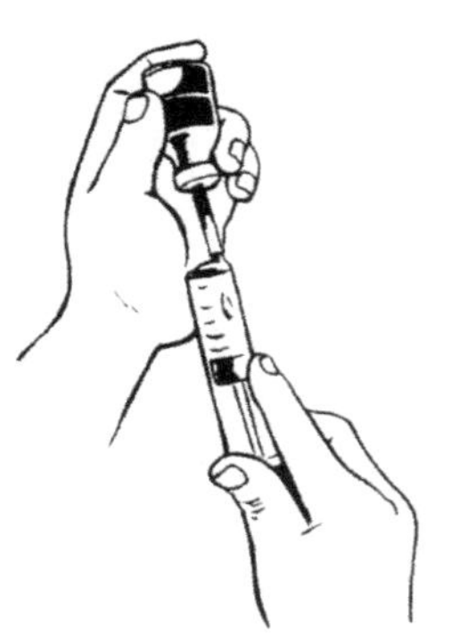

Filling the syringe with medicine that must be mixed

Some medicines **must be mixed** with distilled water or special solvent before they are injected. These medicines come in two separate bottles: one containing the solvent or water, and another with the medicine itself (usually a powder).

1. Attach the needle to the syringe.
2. Push the needle through the rubber stopper into the bottle containing the solvent.
3. Hold the bottle upside-down and fill the syringe with the right amount of solvent.
4. Shake the bottle containing the medicine powder.
5. Inject the solvent into the medicine bottle.
6. Shake the medicine bottle to dissolve all the powder.
7. Fill the syringe with the dissolved medicine (see above).
8. Pull the needle out of the stopper and hold the syringe upside-down. Push the plunger to remove all the air (until liquid comes out of the needle). You are now ready to inject the medicine.

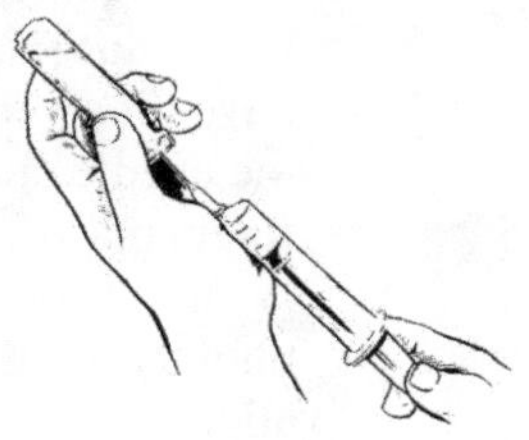

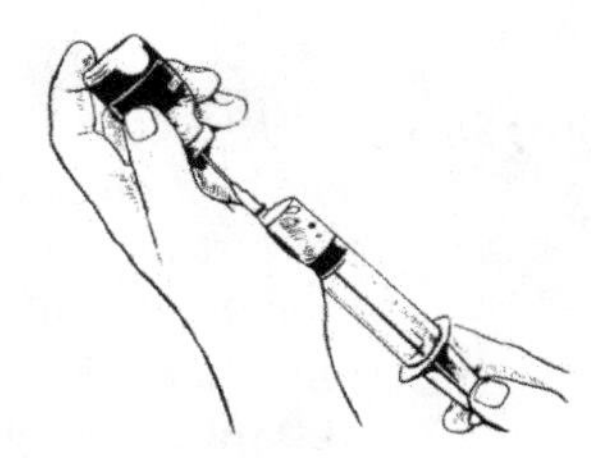

Preparing the injection site

Before injecting, make sure that the injection site is clean. You may need to clip the hair and use a piece of cotton wool dipped in alcohol or another antiseptic to clean the site.

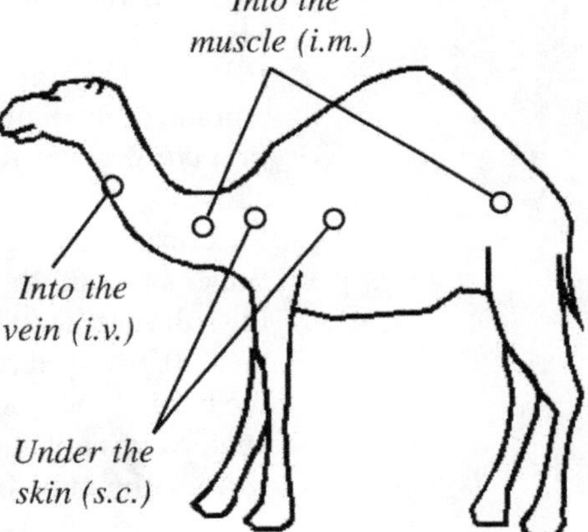

Where to inject a camel.

Injecting into the muscle

This is the commonest and easiest method of injecting. You should not inject more than 15–20 ml in one place; if you have more medicine than this, inject it in two separate places. The most usual injection sites are in the muscles of the neck and at the top of the back legs.

1. Restrain the animal (▷*Restraining*).
2. Fill the syringe with the right amount of medicine (see above).
3. Prepare the site for injection (see above).
4. Take the needle off the syringe, and hold it between your first finger and your thumb, with your hand clenched.
5. Hit the injection site two or three times with the side of your fist.
6. On the next strike, turn your fist to plunge the point of the needle through the skin and firmly and deeply into the muscle (be careful not to hit a bone).

7. Attach the syringe to the needle.
8. Draw back the plunger a little. If blood appears in the syringe, you have hit a vein. In such cases, take the needle out and put it in at a different place.
9. If no blood appears, press the plunger gently but firmly to inject all the medicine into the muscle.
10. Take the syringe and needle out and rub the skin to minimize the swelling.

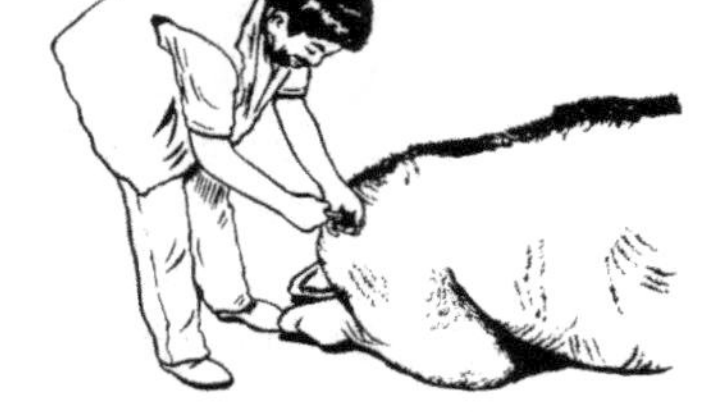

Injecting under the skin

The best places to inject under the skin are just in front of the shoulder, or behind the shoulder, as the camel's skin is loose here. Do not inject more than 50–100 ml in one place; if you have more medicine than this, inject it in two separate places.

1. Restrain the animal (▷*Restraining*).
2. Fill the syringe with the right amount of medicine (see above).
3. Prepare the site for injection (see above).
4. Pick up a fold of skin between your finger and thumb.
5. Push the needle (with no syringe attached) firmly through the skin at the base of the fold. Make sure the needle does not come out the other side of the skin fold. The needle should move fairly easily from side to side under the skin.
6. Attach the syringe to the needle.
7. Inject the medicine.
8. Take the needle out and rub the skin to prevent leakage and to help the medicine be absorbed.

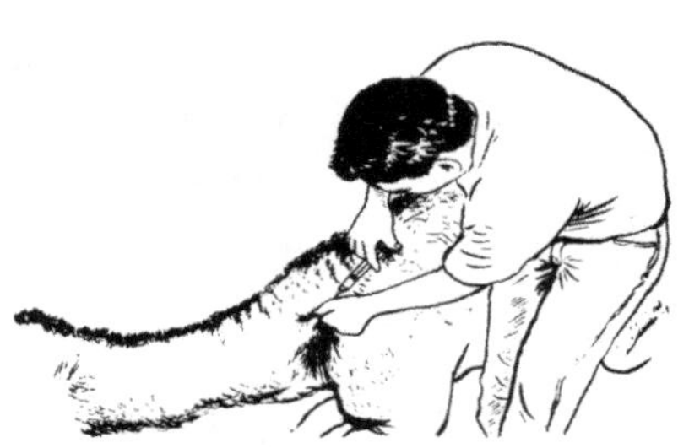

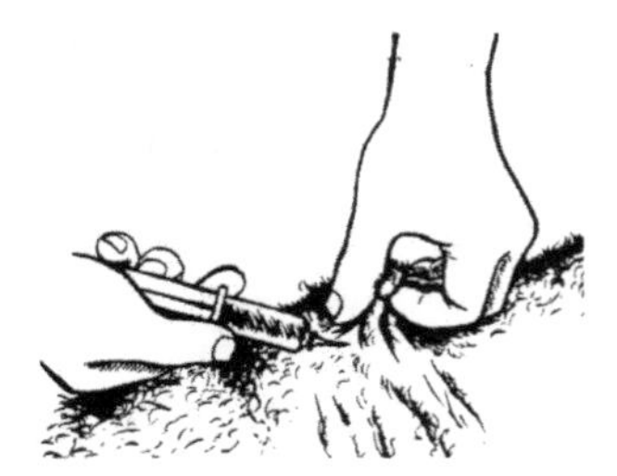

Injecting into the vein

Intravenous injections are given only for certain types of medicines and if a quick reaction is needed (for example, in an emergency). Give the injection into the jugular vein (the large vein in the neck).

Some intravenous drugs can be very irritating, and can damage the tissue, if they are wrongly injected outside the vein. It is important to make sure that most of the needle, and not just its tip, is inside the vein.

1. Restrain the animal (▷*Restraining*).

2. Fill the syringe with the right amount of medicine (see above).
3. Prepare the site for injection (see above).
4. Apply pressure on the vein to make it swell so you can find it easily. You can do this by pressing your hand on the vein below where you will inject, or by tying a rope fairly tightly around the base of the neck.
5. Push the needle (with no syringe attached) slant-wise into the vein, with the point of the needle towards the animal's head (not its body). If you have hit the vein, some blood will come out of the needle. If there is no blood, pull the needle out and try again.
6. Attach the syringe to the needle.
7. Take the pressure off the vein (by removing your hand or untying the rope) to allow the blood to flow.
8. Slowly inject the medicine.
9. Take the needle out and press on the skin with your finger until any bleeding stops.

Giving a drip

A 'drip' is a large amount of liquid, injected slowly into the vein. Drips are used to treat animals that have been severely dehydrated by diarrhoea or other causes.

You will need a bottle (or several bottles) of the intravenous liquid, a special flexible plastic tube with a drip and hollow needle at one end and a clamp in the middle, and two sterile syringe needles (one of which must fit on the end of the tube).

Give a drip into the jugular vein (the large vein on the neck).

1. Restrain the animal and tie its head to make sure it cannot move and dislodge the needle or tube (▷*Restraining*).
2. Push the tube needle through the bottle stopper, hold the bottle upside-down so the liquid drips into the drip container and runs through the tube. When the tube is full of liquid (with no air bubbles), adjust the clamp to stop the flow. Ask someone to hold the bottle and tube until you need it.
3. Prepare the site for injection (see above). Apply pressure on the vein to make it swell so you can find it easily. You can do this by pressing your hand on the vein, or by tying a rope fairly tightly around the base of the neck.

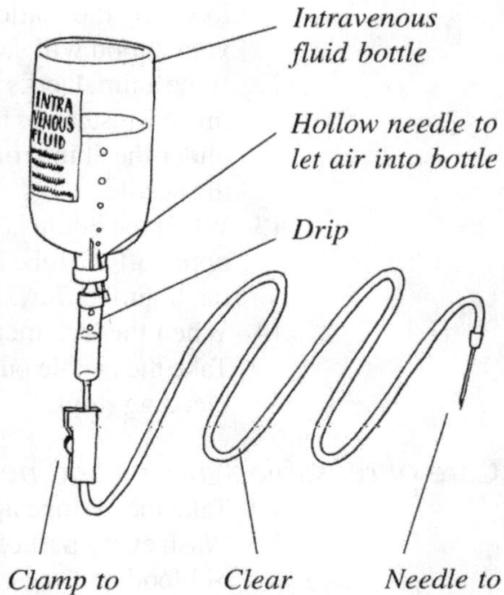

Equipment needed to give a drip.

4. Push one of the syringe needles slantwise into the jugular vein, in the direction of the camel's head. If you have hit the vein, some blood will come out of the needle. If there is no blood, pull the needle out and try again.
5. Attach the end of the tube to the needle, and hold the needle in place using a piece of sticky tape.
6. Ask someone to hold the bottle up (or hang it from a tree) so it is well above the level of the camel's head. The bottle must be kept up all the time while the drip is being given.
7. Release the clamp so the liquid can start flowing into the vein.
8. Take the pressure off the vein (by removing your hand or untying the rope) to allow the blood to flow.
9. If the intravenous liquid comes in a bottle made of stiff plastic or glass, push the second syringe needle through the bottle stopper to allow air to bubble into the bottle (see picture on the previous page). This is not necessary if the bottle is a plastic one that collapses as it empties. For stiff bottles, the liquid will stop flowing if air cannot get into the bottle.
10. Frequently check that the liquid is flowing at the right speed (you can count the number of drops in a minute). You can control how fast the liquid drips into the tube by adjusting the clamp.
11. Also check regularly that the needle is in place in the vein. You can do this by lowering the bottle to below the height of the needle. If the needle is still in the vein, blood will start to flow up the tube.
12. If the animal jerks its head, the needle can become dislodged. If it goes into the muscle instead of the vein, the drip will slow down, and there will be a swelling under the skin around the needle. If this happens, stop the drip and reposition the needle.
13. When the bottle is nearly empty, stop the flow by adjusting the clamp, take the bottle off the tube and attach a full one, and then open the clamp again to allow the liquid to flow.
14. When the treatment is finished, tighten the clamp to stop the liquid flowing. Take the needle out of the vein, and press on the skin with your finger until any bleeding stops.

Care of reusable syringes and needles

1. Take the syringe apart.
2. Wash every part of the syringe and needles in clean water to remove any trace of blood or dirt.
3. Put in a pot of water and boil for 20 minutes, or soak in 1 part chlorine (Clorox) mixed with 7 parts of water.
4. Pour the water off and dry the syringe and needle in a sterilized pan. Touch the syringe only on the plunger, and the needle only at its base.

5. Put the syringe back together again and keep it in a dry, clean place (you can wrap it in a clean cloth).
6. Keep the needles in a sterile bottle, if possible with a little 70% alcohol in it.
7. When it is time to use the syringe and needle again, rinse them with boiled, cooled water to wash off all traces of the disinfectant. You can apply a very small amount of mineral oil (glycerine or Vaseline) around the plunger to make it move smoothly and to prevent medicine from leaking out when you press the plunger hard.

Do not boil plastic syringes. Instead, put them in a disinfectant such as Savlon water (▷*Common medicines*), then rinse with boiled, cooled water. Allow them to dry and store in a clean place.

In the mouth

Some medicines are meant for the sick animal to swallow. They are sometimes called 'oral medication'. 'In the mouth' is sometimes written as 'per os' or 'p.o.' You can make the animal swallow the medicine by:

- Forcing the animal to drink (this is called 'drenching').
- Force-feeding.
- Mixing the medicine with the feed or water.
- Through a stomach tube.

Forcing the animal to drink ('drenching')

To drench a camel, you need a long-necked bottle (preferably made of plastic, in case the camel bites it and breaks it), a drenching gun, a cup or a jar. If you use a glass bottle, you can attach a piece of plastic or rubber tube to the neck so only the tube enters the camel's mouth.

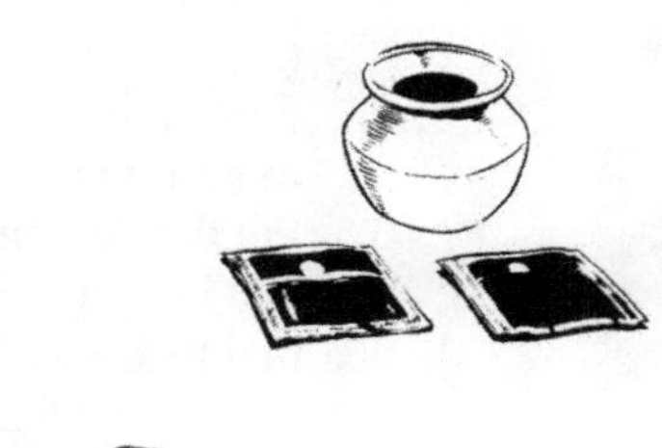

1. If the medicine is a powder, mix it with a little water.
2. Put the medicine in the bottle.
3. Tie the animal's forelegs firmly together and make the animal sit down (▷*Restraining*).
4. Ask the handler to grasp the upper lip with one hand and the lower lip with the other, and force the animal's head back so the mouth is pointed upwards.

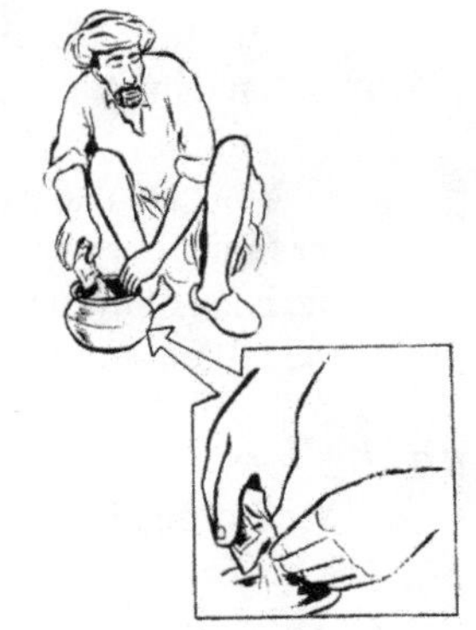

5. Push the bottle neck into the side of the camel's mouth where there are no teeth, and pour some medicine onto the back of the tongue. Allow the animal to swallow the medicine before pouring more in.
6. If the camel does not swallow, have the handler shake its head from side to side, or gently massage its throat.

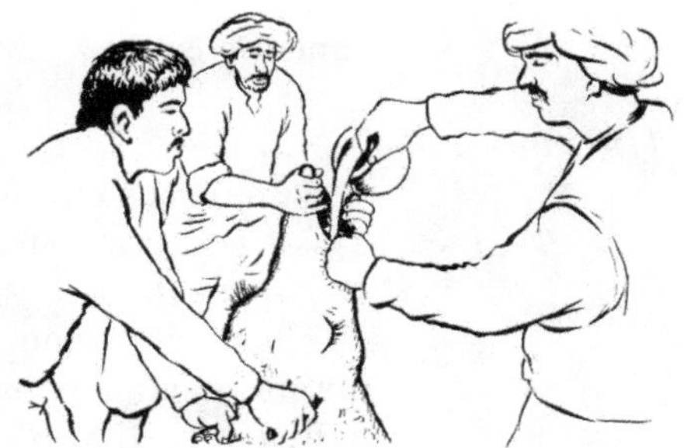

Force-feeding

You force-feed medicines that come as pills, pastes, capsules or boluses. You do it in a similar way to drenching (see above). Dipping the medicine in oil or water makes it easier to swallow.

1. Tie the animal's forelegs firmly together and make the animal sit down (▷*Restraining*).
2. Force the animal's head back so the mouth is pointed upwards.
3. Put the medicine on the back of the tongue, as far back as possible.
4. The animal should swallow the medicine immediately. You can drench with 300–500 ml of water to help it swallow (see above). If it starts to cough, lower its head to prevent it from choking.

For pills, capsules and boluses, you can make a simple 'balling gun' out of a plastic tube and a stick that slides through it. Smooth the end of the tube with a file or sandpaper to remove any sharp edges. To prevent the stick from coming out of the tube and stabbing the animal at the back of the throat, tie something around it at the right place to stop it from sliding too far through the tube.

1. Tie the animal's forelegs firmly together and make the animal sit down (▷*Restraining*).
2. Force the animal's head back so the mouth is pointed upwards.
3. Put the tube in the animal's mouth, and hold it tight to prevent the animal from swallowing it.
4. Put the medicine in the free end of the tube, and push it through the tube and into the animal's mouth with the stick.

You can also use the tube to administer tablets or capsules. Put the tube into the back of the animal's mouth, and drop the tablet or capsule into the open end.

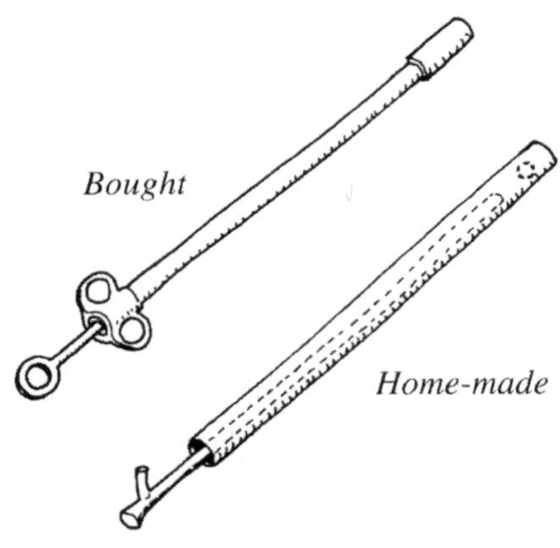

Balling guns

Mixed with the feed

Medicines for camels are not usually mixed with the feed, as camels normally look for their own food. An exception is anti-worm medicine ('anthelmintic'), which is often mixed with mineral mixtures. You can also put medicines into a ball of dates, or mix it with molasses, date juice or honey, to encourage the camel to eat it.

Through a stomach tube

Use a stomach tube to put liquids or medicines directly into the camel's stomach. This is necessary only if the camel cannot swallow by itself, as in ▷*Bloat* or *Haemorrhagic enteritis*.

For an adult camel, you will need a heavy-walled, flexible plastic or rubber tubing, about 3 m long. To prevent the camel from biting the stomach tube, you will also need a shorter piece of reinforced plastic tubing, about 45 cm long, wide enough so that the stomach tube can pass through it easily. Smooth the ends of both tubes with sandpaper or a file to make sure they do not cut the camel's throat. You will also need a funnel to pour liquids into the free end of the tube.

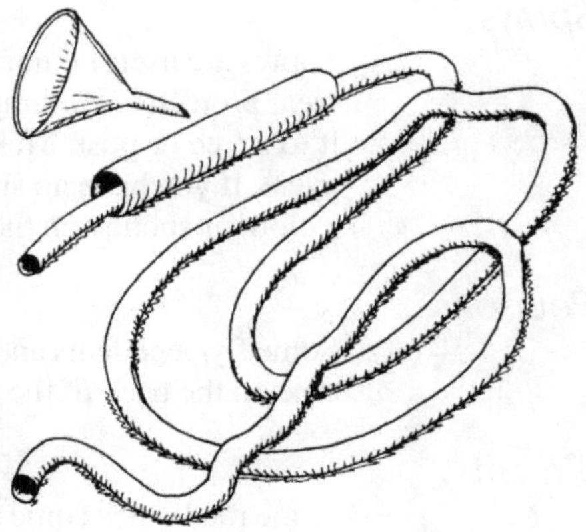
Stomach tube

1. Tie the animal's forelegs firmly together and make the animal sit down (▷*Restraining*).
2. Have someone hold the upper lip or nose with one hand, and the lower lip with the other. Keep the mouth level.
3. Push the short tube into the side of the camel's mouth, above the tongue.
4. Oil the stomach tube with KY jelly or paraffin jelly.
5. Thread the end of the stomach tube through the short tube and into the animal's throat. The camel should begin to swallow, making it easier to push the tube in.
6. Continue pushing the tube down the throat. Make sure it is in the gullet, not the windpipe. You should be able to see a bulge in the left side of the neck as the tube moves down the gullet, and once the tube reaches the rumen, you should be able to smell the gases in the rumen.
7. Pour the medicine into the free end of the tube using the funnel.

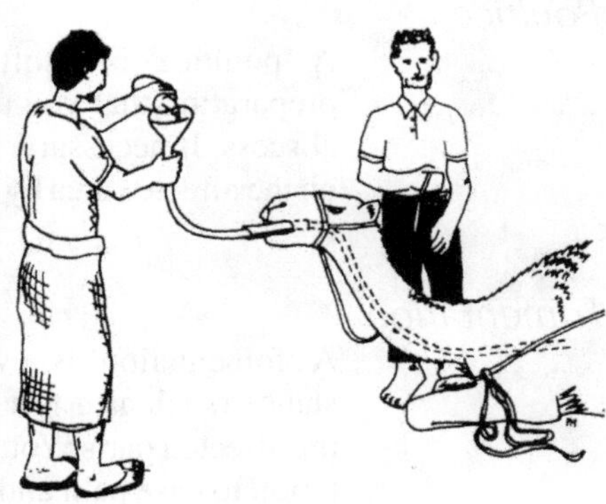

Instead of the shorter tube, you can use a gag (a piece of wood with a hole in it) to keep the camel's mouth open and prevent it from chewing on the tube. Put the gag in the camel's mouth and push the tube through the hole.

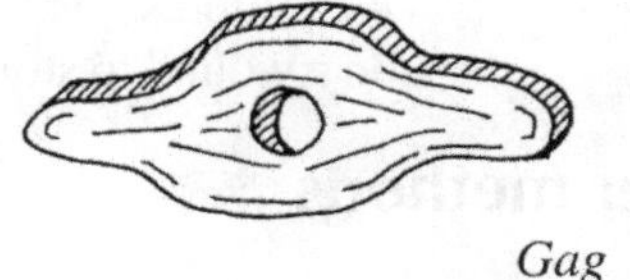
Gag

On the skin

Medicines to be applied on the skin include dips, sprays, dusting powder, pour-ons, creams, poultices, fomentations and compresses.

- **Sprays, dusting powder and pour-ons** are used mainly against ticks and other skin parasites. Before using them, give the camels enough to drink so they do not try to lick or drink the water mixed with the poison. Protect yourself against coming into contact with the poison (▷*Handling medicines and pesticides*).
- **Creams, poultices, fomentations, compresses and direct application** are often used to treat wounds and abscesses, and in traditional treatments.

Sprays

Sprays are useful if not too many animals are to be treated. Everyone nearby should wear protective clothing and a mask during spraying. Make the animal stand and tie it to a tree or post. Make sure that you spray all parts of the animal (but avoid the eyes). If you have no spray pump, you can apply the pesticide with a brush, or with a cloth or sponge on the end of a stick.

Pour-ons

Some fly-repellents and tick treatments come as 'pour-ons'. You just pour the medicine on the back of the animal.

Cream

Some medicines come as a ready-made cream. Traditional healers often make their own creams by pounding medicinal herbs and mixing them with a little cooking oil or ghee.

Poultice

A 'poultice' is a soft, usually heated, preparation that you apply to a sore or abscess. If necessary, keep the poultice on the affected area by tying a cloth over it.

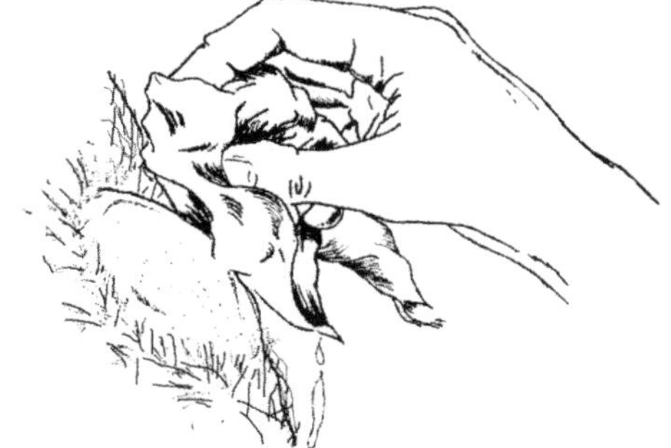

Fomentation

A 'fomentation' is a warm, moist substance (such as a wet cloth) applied to the affected parts. You can use a fomentation to ease pain and swellings.

Compress

A 'compress' is like a fomentation but is dry. An example is a warm stone pressed on a wound to stop bleeding.

Other methods

In the ears

Clean out the ear with a swab, and drop the medicine into the ear canal.

In the eyes

Apply the medicine directly onto the eyeball under the eyelid. For liquids, use a straw or dropper to drop the medicine between the eyeball and the lower eyelid.

To apply eye ointment, hold down the lower eyelid and squeeze some medicine between the eyelid and the eyeball. Make sure that the tip of the tube does not touch the eye.

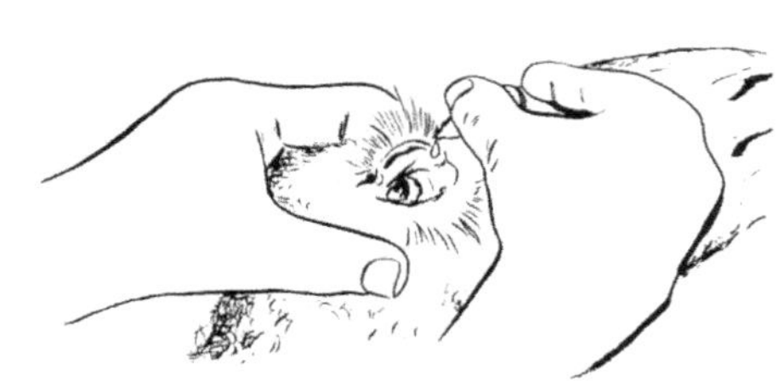

In the vagina or uterus

Applying medicine in the vagina (birth canal) or uterus (womb) is used for female animals that have an infection in the birth canal, for example after a retained placenta or other birthing difficulties. Do not touch the cervix (the narrow opening leading into the uterus) or put medicine in the uterus if the animal is pregnant, or you may introduce an infection that is dangerous for the mother and calf.

1. Clean the animal's vulva with soap and warm water.
2. Put a glove or a clean plastic bag on your hand (this is necessary to protect yourself from diseases like brucellosis).
3. Take the medicine and cup your hand into a cone shape.
4. Push your hand into the animal's vagina, and if necessary, through the cervix.
5. Leave the medicine inside and slowly pull your hand out.

Enema

An enema is a liquid medicine that is put in the animal's anus. It is most often used for ▻*Constipation*. Enemas usually come in a tube with a plunger, like a syringe.

1. Make the animal sit down and restrain it (▻*Restraining*).
2. Ask someone to hold the tail.
3. Insert the nozzle of the enema package carefully into the rectum, and press the plunger to squeeze the medicine into the anus.

You can also use a syringe (without a needle) to squirt liquid into the anus.

In the udder

Medicines are applied into the udder to treat ▻*Mastitis*. The medicine comes in a tube with a nozzle and a plunger, like a syringe without a needle. It is difficult to apply this medicine as the camel's teat has two small holes, not one as in cattle. The holes are small, so it may be difficult and painful for the animal to insert the nozzle. Select a tube with a fine nozzle, and treat both holes in the teat.

1. Milk the udder out if possible.
2. Sedate and restrain the animal (▻*Sedation and anaesthesia*, *Restraining*).
3. Clean and disinfect the teat and the nozzle of the teat tube with Savlon or another antiseptic.
4. Insert the nozzle of the tube into the holes in the teat.
5. Push the plunger to squeeze the ointment into the udder.
6. Close the teat with your hand, and massage the udder.

If it is too difficult to apply the medicine in this way, you can inject antibiotics instead (▻*Common medicines*).

References

FAO (1994) p. 263–9, 272–3; Forse (1999) p. 315–24; Higgins (1986) p. 36–9; IIRR (1994) vol. 1, p. 20–7; IIRR (1996) vol. 1 p. 25–35; ITDG and IIRR (1996) p. 8–11; Manefield and Tinson (1997) p. 77–8, 135–6, 153, 249; Projet Cameline (1999) p. 10–11; Quesenberry (1990) p. 231–6; Rathore (1986) p. 199; Schwartz and Dioli (1992) p. 137–8, 148.

Branding

Firing, using the hot iron, cauterizing
***Dam dena* (Hindi), *kay* (Arabic, Tunisia)**

Applying a hot iron is probably the most widely used traditional treatment method by camel pastoralists. It is practised among the Raika in India, the Bedouin in North Africa, the Tuareg in West Africa, the Somali and others in East Africa.

Conventional veterinarians in Europe used to use branding regularly, for example to treat joint and leg problems in horses. They usually now regard branding as cruel, inefficient and harmful. But for some diseases at least, it has some underlying rationale, supported by science. Applying a red-hot iron turns a chronic condition into an acute one, thus activating the body's defence mechanism. It results in increased blood circulation that can lead to a healing process.

Caution: the use of branding is controversial. It should be used only as a last resort when no other treatment options are available.

Branding can be either organ-specific or systemic. Herders and healers use it mostly to treat joint and muscle afflictions (such as wry neck), as well as skin diseases (such as contagious skin necrosis), abscesses and swollen lymph nodes. But they also use it for internal conditions including diarrhoea, kidney problems, cough and infections of the udder and womb. In some of these cases branding would seem harmful. Yet it seems to help in some cases of vomiting in calves and intestinal obstruction, as well as in joint and muscle problems.

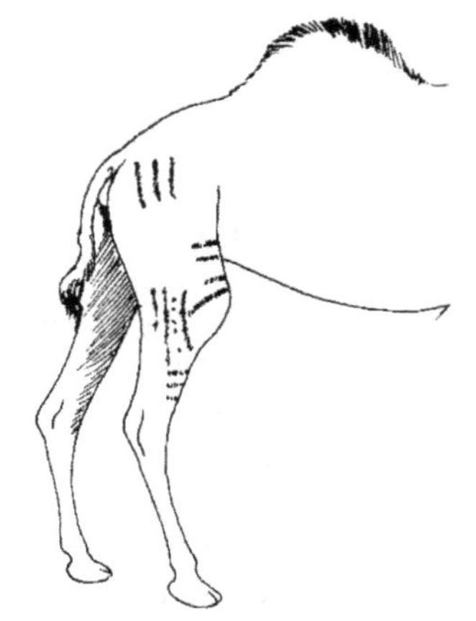

Various tools are used for branding. Strip-firing done with bars that are about 1–3 cm wide is most common, but point-, cross- and ring-firing are also practised. The iron is put into a very hot fire usually made from dung cakes. When the iron is glowing hot, it is pressed onto the skin for 20–60 seconds until the skin turns white. If the procedure is properly done, the burn-marks heal within 2–3 days, leaving smooth, black scars. If the heat or duration of the cauterization are not sufficient, the wounds become red, inflamed and infected, not healing well. ▻*Contagious skin necrosis, Coughs, colds and pneumonia, Skin abscesses* and *Wry neck.*

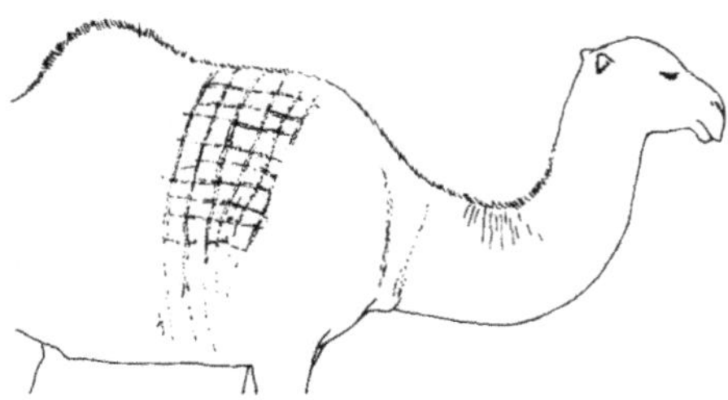

References

Abbas (1996) p. 28–34; Agab (1998); Leese (1927) p. 160; Manefield and Tinson (1997) p. 43; Schwartz and Dioli (1992) p. 130–2, 141.

Restraining

Before you examine or treat a camel, make sure it is restrained properly. This is necessary to avoid injuring the camel, yourself, or the people helping you, and to ensure easy and proper treatment.

There are many different ways to restrain a camel. Which one to use depends on the treatment, the camel's training and its particular nature, and its relationship with its handler. Here are some common methods:

- A well-trained camel needs to be restrained only by holding its head-rope or nose-peg. It will lie down if its handler orders it to.
- Pull on the camel's tail and grab one of its thighs.
- Restrain a small camel by holding its top and bottom lips with both hands and turning its head to one side. If the handler is experienced and the camel well-trained, this is enough when giving an injection. If necessary, you can have a second person hold the camel by its ears. The same method can be used with a large camel if it is in a sitting position.

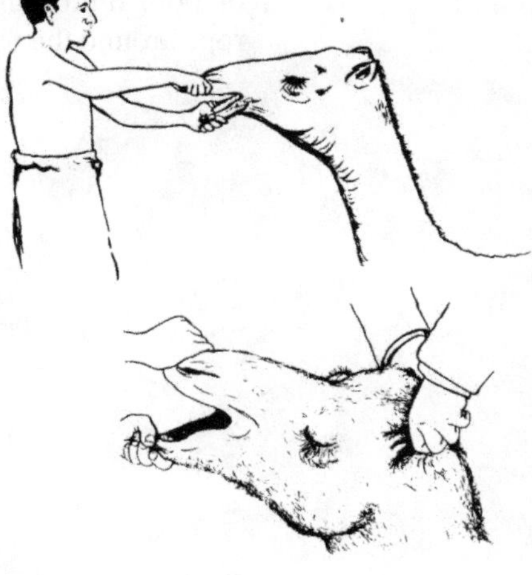

- Hold the camel's lower jaw with a rope running behind the front teeth. Hold the rope in your hands: do not tie it to a tree or post, as a sudden movement can break the camel's jaw (⊳*Broken jaw*).

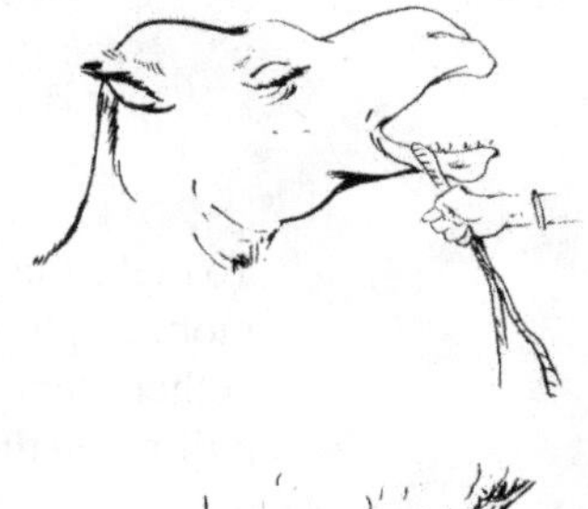

- Make the camel stand on three legs by tying one of its fetlocks to its fore-leg with a rope.

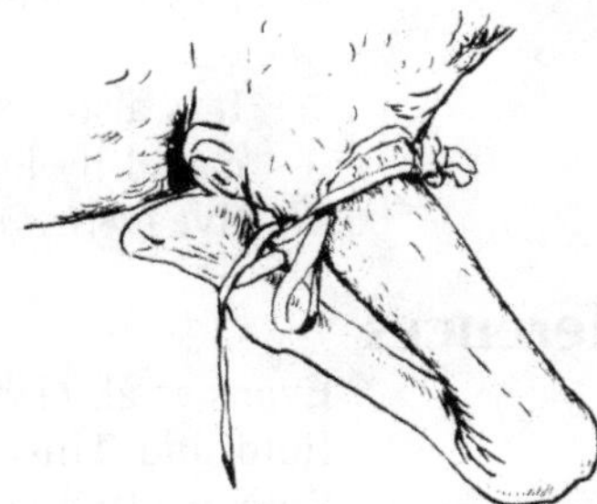

- To restrain a violent animal, tie a rope around its neck and have two people hold the ends, one on each side of the animal. Make sure the camel does not suffocate.

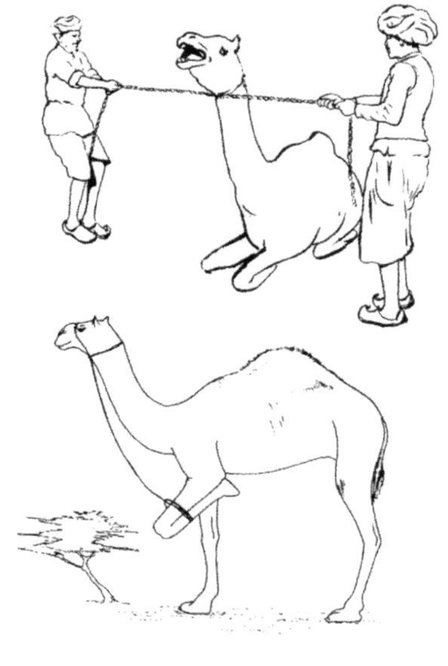

- If the treatment is painful, make the camel lie down by tying one of its fetlocks to its foreleg (as above). Then pull either the other front leg or both hind legs forward with a rope around the fetlocks.

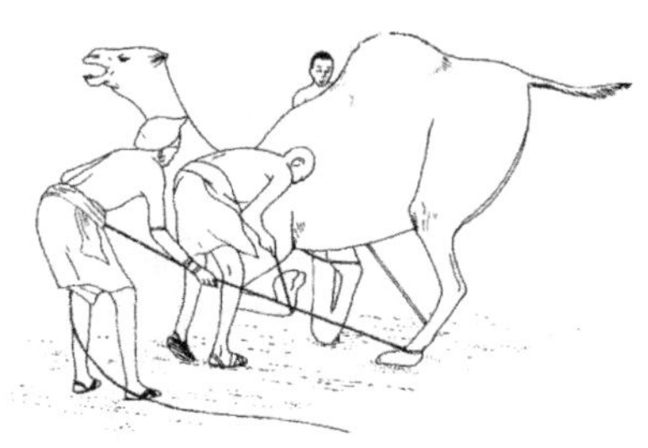

- Tie both front legs together with a rope passing over its neck.

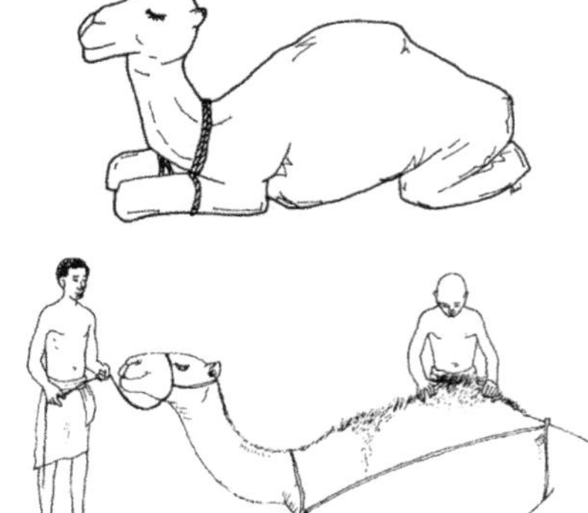

- To make the animal completely immobile, also tie the hind legs together. Bend the neck to the side by pulling on the head-rope.
- It is also possible to immobilize a camel by injecting it with a sedative (▷*Sedation and anaesthesia*).

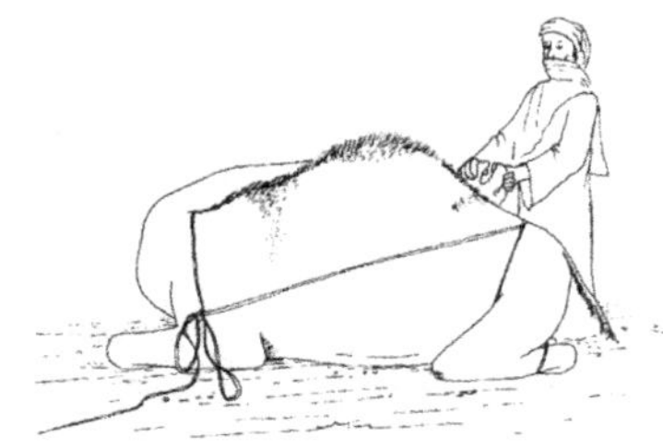

References

Evans et al. (1995) p. 4.3–4.5; Manefield and Tinson (1997) p. 214–18; Rathore (1986) p. 197–9; Schwartz and Dioli (1992) p. 123–8, 139–40.

Sedation and anaesthesia

Sometimes it is advisable to sedate camels for minor and major surgery or to do more painful examinations.

'**Sedatives**' are drugs that reduce anxiety and make the animal easier to handle. Some of them also reduce pain or relax the muscles.

Sedatives that do not make the animal drowsy are called '**tranquillizers**'.

An '**anaesthetic**' is a medicine that stops all feeling. It makes the animal (or the part of the body it is applied to) numb. *Example*: a dentist may use a local anaesthetic (see below) to kill the pain while taking out your tooth.

An '**analgesic**' is a medicine that reduces pain but does not cause numbness. *Example*: people take an aspirin if they have a headache.

Types of anaesthesia

- **General anaesthesia** makes the animal lose consciousness and stops it from feeling pain anywhere in the body. It is rarely necessary to put camels into general anaesthesia, especially in the field.
- **Regional anaesthesia** stops pain in part of the body while the animal stays conscious and remains standing. Use it for surgical procedures in the genital area, such as replacing a ▷*Prolapse of the vagina or womb*. Do it by injecting a local anaesthetic into the 'spinal canal' (see *Epidural anaesthesia* below).
- **Local anaesthesia** stops pain only in the area where it is injected. It is used for sewing ('suturing') wounds and for other minor operations.

Before and after sedation

To make sure the camel does not bring up the contents of the rumen and choke on them, do not allow it to eat for 24–36 hours before the operation, and prevent it from drinking for 12 hours beforehand.

Before injecting the sedative, make the camel sit down in the shade and tie it so it cannot get up. Have somebody hold its head so that it cannot move it violently.

After giving the injection, do not disturb the animal until the sedative has taken effect.

If you have completely sedated the camel, bring it back into a sitting position before it wakes up. Tie its head down until it can hold it up by itself. Do not loosen the ropes until the camel is ready to get up by itself. Once it has stood up, it may sway and reel, so you may have to support it by holding the halter and tail.

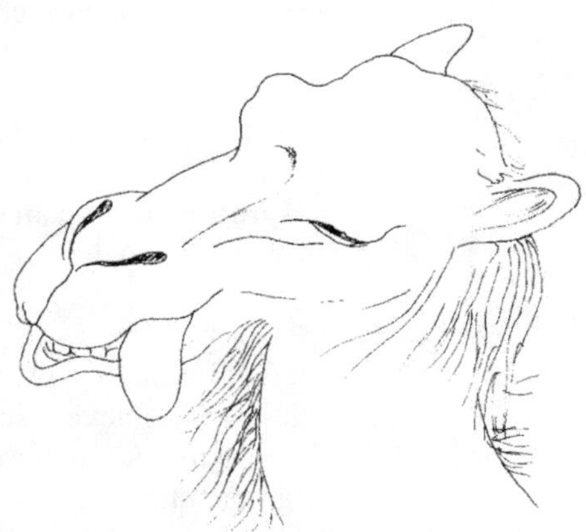

Sedated camel

Medicines for sedation

Xylazine

Xylazine (Rompun) is the main drug used for sedation. It comes as a 2% or 10% solution. Apart from sedating, it also reduces pain and relaxes the muscles. Xylazine is usually injected into the muscle, but can also be given into the vein. How much to use depends on the degree of sedation you want, and on the time required for surgery.

Dosage of xylazine	Length of effect	Purpose
0.25–0.5 mg/kg into the muscle	30–60 minutes	Minor procedures
1–2 mg/kg into the muscle	90 minutes	Immobilization, castration

The sedative usually starts taking effect about 9–15 minutes after it is injected. Make sure the camel is not disturbed during this period. When xylazine starts having its effect, the camel drops its lower lip and closes its eyes. It starts drooling, and its heart slows down.

You can reverse the effect of xylazine by injecting yohimbine HCl (Antagonil) at a dose of 0.25 mg/kg body weight into the vein.

Propionylpromazine

Propionylpromazine (Combelen), at a dosage of 0.2–0.5 mg/kg into the muscle, can also be used to sedate camels. It has a slightly relaxing effect on the muscles, but does not reduce pain, so cannot be used for surgical procedures. Its effects start after about 20 minutes, and last for 2–4 hours. One of the side-effects is an increased heart rate. It can also cause seizures.

Diazepam

Diazepam (Valium), at a dosage of 200–300 mg injected into the vein, tranquillizes the camel for 30–45 minutes. It does not relax the muscles.

Caution: diazepam should not be given to pregnant animals! Use half this dose for young animals.

For painful surgery

For painful surgical procedures, xylazine can be combined with ketamine (Ketanest, Vetalar) to achieve a stronger effect against pain. In this case, xylazine should be given 15 minutes before ketamine. The dosage is 0.4 mg/kg xylazine and 5.0 mg/kg ketamine into the muscle, or 0.25 mg/kg xylazine and 3–5 mg/kg ketamine into the vein. The camel may stay drowsy for up to 2 hours.

Epidural anaesthesia

This is used for surgery in the genital area, for example for ▷*Prolapse of the vagina or womb*.

Move the camel's tail up and down and feel for where the rigid backbone ends and the tail (which can be moved) begins. The gap between these bones is where to give the injection. Clip the hair, and clean and disinfect the skin.

Insert a 20 gauge, 4 cm needle into the gap, at right-angles to the tail. The needle must go between the bones into the 'spinal canal' (the hole that runs along inside the backbone and contains nerves and liquid). Slowly inject 2–5 ml of lignocaine hydrochloride 2% (Lidocaine). This will stop the pain in the genital area for 2 hours. The camel can stay standing.

Caution: epidural anaesthesia should be given only by a veterinarian or experienced person.

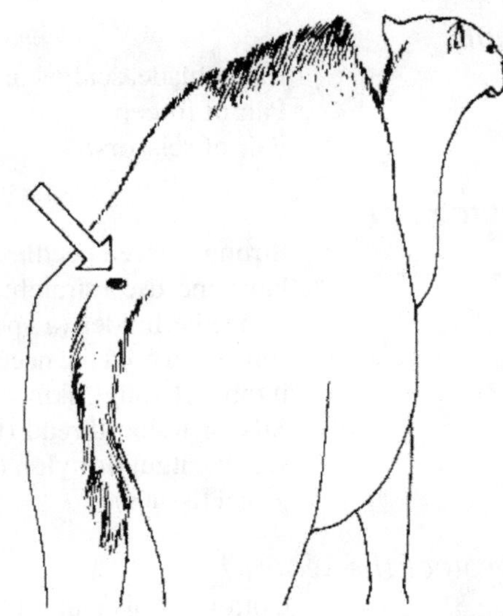

Where to give an epidural anaesthetic

Local anaesthesia

Use lignocaine hydrochloride (Lidocaine) (▷*Surgery*).

References

Allen et al. (1992) p. 341–6; Evans et al. (1995) p. 7:20–1; Gahlot and Chouhan (1992) p. 12–27; Higgins (1986) p. 136–48; Manefield and Tinson (1997) p. 232–4; Rathore (1986) p. 200–3; Schwartz and Dioli (1992) p. 148–50; Wilson (1998) p. 81.

Surgery

Sometimes you have to cut the animal's tissues or stitch its skin in order to:

- Treat a disease (for example, ▷*Skin abscesses*, *Bloat* and *Snake bite*).
- Control breeding, as in castration or during birth (▷*Castration*, *Difficult birth*).
- Treat a wound (▷*Wounds and burns*).
- Prevent injury: trimming the nails and teeth (▷*Teeth problems*).

See the individual sections in this book for details of how to perform surgery for each problem. Learn from a skilled practitioner before trying to do it yourself.

Equipment

The type of equipment you need depends on the type of operation. Below is a list of basic equipment. You may need additional equipment for certain operations. See the relevant section for details.

To keep the animal still and to stop pain

- Syringe, needle, sedative, anaesthetic.
- Ropes.

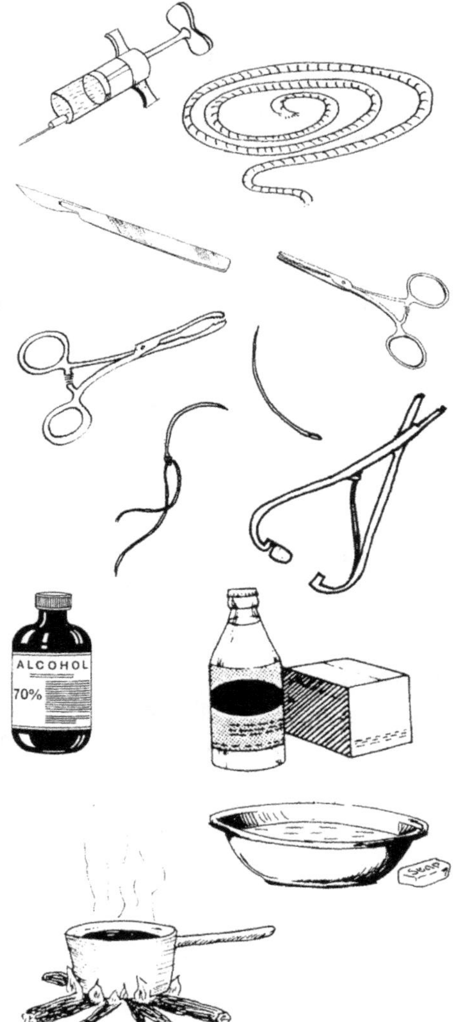

To cut

- Razor blade, scalpel or sharp knife.
- Pair of forceps.
- Pair of scissors.

To stitch

- Strong, curved needle. If you don't have one, use a straight one instead.
- A needle holder (a special pair of forceps to hold the needle and force it through tough skin).
- Silk or nylon thread (to stitch the skin); catgut or nylon (to stitch internal tissues).

To protect the wound

- Cotton wool, clean cloths, bandages.
- Antibiotic (powder, injection).
- Fly repellent (▷*Bites and stings*).

To keep things clean

- Antiseptic liquid (e.g., Dettol, iodine, 0.2–0.5% potassium permanganate solution).
- Metal pans and 70% alcohol to keep tools in.
- Pan with water to boil equipment.
- Clean, boiled water, soap.
- Fire, to boil water or heat the knife to make it sterile.

How to do surgery

Preparation

1. Sedate and restrain the animal so it cannot move and cannot feel pain (▷*Restraining* and *Sedation and anaesthesia*). Tie it so it cannot interfere with the operation, hurt itself, or hurt you while you are operating on it.
2. Clean the skin with soap and a disinfectant.
3. Clip or shave the hair from the injection site (or from the edges of the wound, and clean it properly).
4. Boil the knife in water, or hold it over a flame until it is red-hot, to make sure it is sterile. Allow it to cool before using it.
5. Boil the stitching needle and thread in water, or put them in disinfectant for 20 minutes. Catgut normally comes in a container filled with disinfectant.

Giving a local anaesthetic

1. Fill the syringe with an anaesthetic such as lignocaine hydrochloride (▷*Sedation and anaesthesia* and *Administering medicines*).

2. Insert the syringe needle slant-wise through the skin so it goes under the skin but not into the muscle underneath. Then attach the syringe to the needle.
3. Begin injecting anaesthetic; as you do so, slowly withdraw the needle, so the anaesthetic is distributed along the line where the point of the needle has been, rather than in just one place.
4. Repeat the injection as many times as necessary either side of the line where you plan to make the cut, or around the wound you want to sew closed.

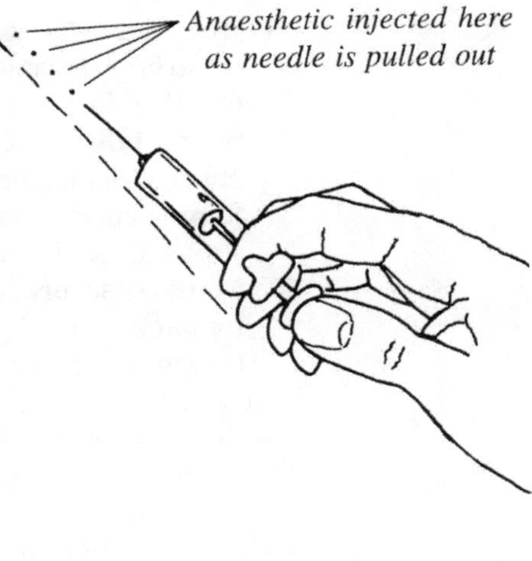

5. Wait for several minutes, then prick the skin with a sharp needle. If the animal does not flinch, you can start the surgery.

Cutting

Cutting the skin or tissue is called 'incision'.

- Use a sterile scalpel, razor or sharp knife.
- During the operation, do not put the knife on the ground. Put it on a clean piece of cloth or a metal tray.

Stopping bleeding

If the wound is bleeding heavily, try to stop the bleeding. You can:

- Press a clean cloth on the wound.
- Tie a bandage around the wound.
- Tie a cloth tightly around the limb above the wound until the bleeding stops. This type of bandage is called a 'tourniquet'. Loosen the bandage for at least 1 minute every 10–15 minutes.
- Heat an iron rod in the fire until it is red-hot. Use it to burn the wound to stop the bleeding.

▷*Wounds and burns* for other ways to stop bleeding.

Stitching

After you have finished cutting, you may have to stitch the tissues together so they heal quickly. This is also called 'suturing'.

Important: you should stitch *only* fresh cuts made during surgery or fresh wounds caused by an accident. *Do not* stitch old wounds, as they will be infected. Do not stitch very deep wounds caused by accidents (e.g., caused by bites or spears), as they may be infected deep inside. It is not necessary to stitch small wounds.

In surgery, you should stitch together each layer of tissue you have cut through.

It is easier to use a curved needle for stitching, but you can also use a straight one.

- Use thread (nylon or silk) for stitching the skin. You will have to take these stitches out when the wound has healed (see below).
- Use catgut for stitching internal tissues. You do not have to take these stitches out, as the body will gradually absorb them.
- Use a needle holder: camel skin is tough!

Use one of the three suture patterns pictured here. Pull each stitch tight enough to bring the edges of the wound together (but do not pull too tight).

- **Simple interrupted suture:** strong, but takes a long time.
- **Simple continuous suture:** not as strong, but quicker to do.
- **Mattress suture:** strong, and good for thick skin.

Tie each suture with a surgical or reef knot so it does not slip. Tie each knot at least three times to make sure it holds.

To practise stitching and tying knots, you can sew together two pieces of leather or a slit cut in a piece of foam rubber.

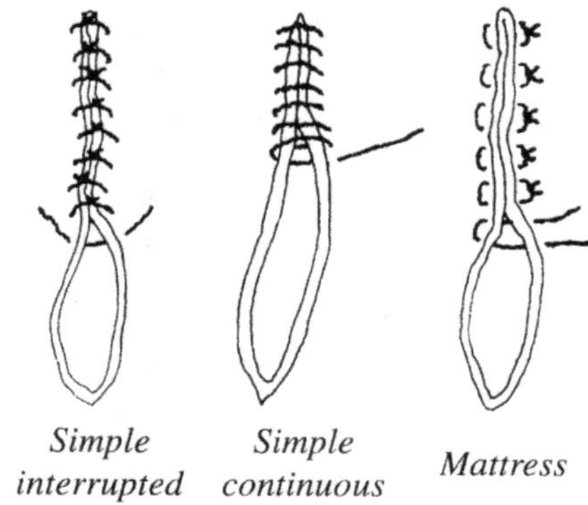

Types of sutures

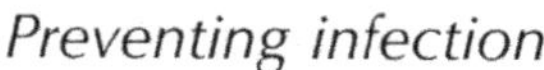

Preventing infection

Treat the wound so it heals quickly and to keep dirt and flies away.

1. Clean the blood from around the wound and allow it to dry.
2. Use an antibiotic such as tetracycline spray or sulphanilamide powder, and a fly repellent to prevent the wound from becoming infected.
3. Put a dressing (such as a clean bandage) on the wound.

▷*Wounds and burns* for further treatment methods.

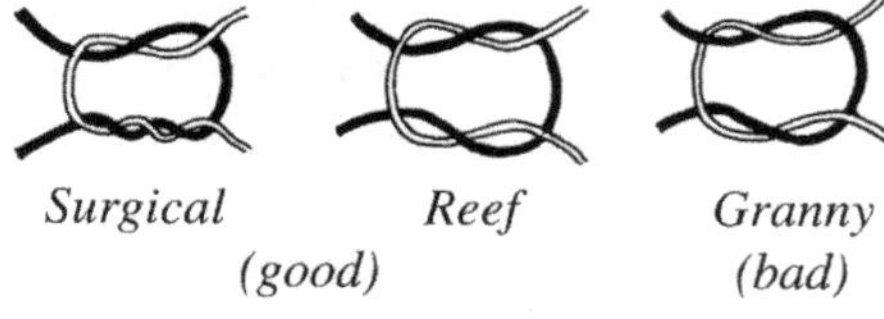

Types of knots

After surgery

Check the stitches and the wound each day. Clean the wound and apply a fresh dressing if necessary.

After 7–10 days

- If the wound has healed, cut the thread and remove the stitches.
- If the wound has not yet healed, clean it carefully. If the wound is infected, remove one or two stitches at the lowest end of the wound to allow any pus to drain out, and inject antibiotics to combat the infection.
- If the wound is completely infected, remove all the stitches, wash it with disinfectant, and allow it to heal as an open wound. Inject antibiotics, and clean the wound each day. Put on a bandage if necessary.

References

Forse (1999) p. 70–2; Gahlot and Chouhan (1992); ITDG and IIRR (1996) p. 60–2; Manefield and Tinson (1997) p. 251; Quesenberry (1990) p. 203–6.

How to collect samples for testing

If you are not sure what disease is making an animal sick, and if a laboratory is nearby, take a sample and send it to a laboratory for testing. The causes of diseases such as ▷*Rabies*, *Anthrax* and *Trypanosomiasis* can be identified for certain only by laboratory tests. If you have the equipment and training, you can perform certain tests yourself (▷*Checking for diseases in the laboratory*).

Depending on the problem, you can collect samples of the camel's:

- Blood (dried, unclotted or serum).
- Faeces.
- Urine.
- Skin and hair.
- Foetus and placenta.
- Body tissue.

Blood and organ-tissue samples can be taken from a newly dead animal to find out why it died. This may be important to prevent other animals from getting the disease. Samples should be taken as quickly as possible. If the sample is taken more than 12 hours after the animal has died, there is less chance that tests will give a useful result.

If the sample may be used to test for bacterial diseases, the equipment and containers you use must be sterile. For other diseases, it is enough to make sure that the equipment and containers you use are clean; they do not have to be completely sterile.

Dangerous diseases

Caution: certain diseases are dangerous for people (▷*Diseases that people can catch from camels*). Do not allow these tissues or the blood to touch your skin. Wear gloves (or plastic bags on your hands), and wash your hands and clothes immediately afterwards. Dispose of the infected tissue by burning or burying it.

If there are any bloody discharges from the nose, mouth or anus, *do not* take samples or cut the carcass open to examine it. The animal may have died of anthrax, and opening it may allow the spores that cause it to escape and contaminate the surroundings, and may expose you to infection by this deadly disease. See ▷*Anthrax* for how to dispose of the carcass safely.

Labelling samples

When you have collected the sample (see below), write a simple code (*A*, *B*, *C*, etc.) on the bottle or bag. Write the following information (on a separate piece of paper so it is easy to refer to in the laboratory):

- The code for the sample (e.g., *A*, *B*, *C*).
- The type of sample (e.g., serum, urine, part of the body the tissues came from).
- The date the sample was taken.
- Name or ear-tag of the animal.
- Name and address of the owner.
- The disease you suspect is causing the illness and the type of test you suggest should be done.
- The history of the disease: signs of the disease, how many animals are affected, how long the disease has lasted, any recent changes (such as changes in grazing or newly introduced animals).
- Your own name and contact details.

Storing and transporting samples

Some types of samples must be kept cold or they will decompose and be useless for testing. Put these in a jar with a screw-top lid (such as a jam jar) and keep them with ice or in a refrigerator. If you need to transport the sample, pack the containers in ice (for example, in a flask or an insulated picnic-box), and make sure the ice is renewed if necessary on the way to the laboratory. During transport, pack the sample tightly and with plenty of absorbent padding so the containers cannot move around or break, and so liquids cannot leak out.

Dried blood film

Used if you need just a few drops of blood, for example to check for **trypanosomiasis** (▷*Trypanosomiasis*).

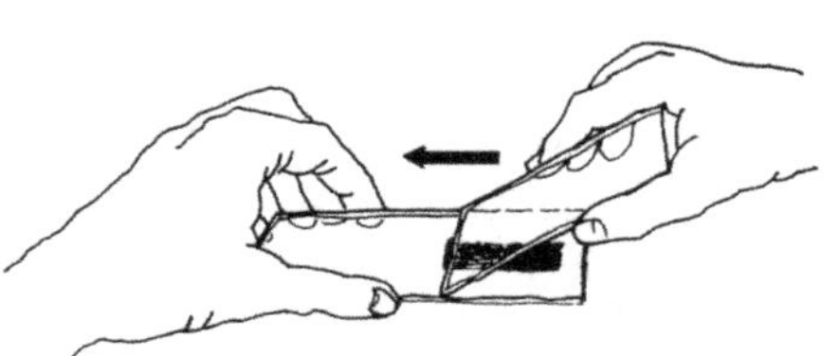

1. Nick the edge of the camel's ear with a pair of sharp scissors or a sharp knife and squeeze the blood out. You can squeeze the drops directly onto a clean microscope slide.
2. Place the straight edge of another clean slide at an angle of 30–40° on the lower slide, just in front of the drop. The drop will spread along the bottom edge of the upper slide.
3. Glide the upper slide evenly forward to form a thin, uniform film on the surface of the lower slide. Prepare two slides from each blood sample in this way.
4. Allow the blood to dry in a shady, dust-free place.
5. Make at least two slides for each animal. You can send these slides to the laboratory. Label the slides and pack them carefully, face-to-face, with matchsticks between them to prevent the dried blood surfaces from touching.

Whole, unclotted blood

Used to test for **trypanosomiasis** and whether the animal has an **infectious disease** (▷*Trypanosomiasis*, *Infectious diseases*).

If you need more than a few drops of blood, use a syringe needle to take a sample. Normally, blood clots quickly when the air touches it. To stop it from clotting, you must use an anticoagulant such as EDTA or heparin. Prepare the blood container by putting a little anticoagulant into it before collecting the blood.

For trypanosomiasis tests, the container must be clean but does not have to be sterile. For other types of tests, make sure it is sterile.

1. Restrain the camel to prevent it from moving.
2. Tie a rope tightly around the camel's neck. Raise the head with the neck straight in front of the body (not bent to one side).
3. Feel for the jugular vein at the side of the throat. You should be able to feel the elastic bulge of this vein about one hand's width from the head.
4. Insert a sterile syringe needle into the vein. Hold a small, clean jar or tube containing some anticoagulant under the needle to catch the blood that comes out. Hold the jar as close as possible to the needle and let the blood run along the inside of the glass without splashing. Catch about 10 ml of blood.
5. Stopper the jar and turn it upside-down several times to mix the blood and anticoagulant. (Don't shake it too much: it may damage the sample and make it useless.)
6. Loosen the rope, and carefully pull the needle out. To stop any bleeding, press

your thumb for several minutes on the skin where you had put in the needle.
7. Keep the blood in a refrigerator (4°C, not frozen) until it can be tested.

If you need a **sterile blood sample**, attach a sterile syringe to the needle before putting the needle into the vein. Collect the blood in the syringe, then inject it slowly through the rubber stopper into a sterile tube containing anticoagulant.

You can also use a special tube called a 'Vacutainer' to collect blood. A Vacutainer is a sealed, sterile tube with a vacuum inside. When the Vacutainer needle is pushed into the vein, the vacuum inside draws in the blood. Vacutainers come with anticoagulant already inside to prevent the blood from clotting. Using Vacutainers is simple and easy, and avoids the risk of contamination.

Blood serum

Used to test for **mineral deficiency** and **infectious diseases** such as brucellosis and ▷*Rift Valley fever*.

Blood serum (the clear liquid that separates from the blood when it clots) is needed to test for antibodies (if bacterial or viral infections are suspected) or to analyse the blood chemistry.

1. Collect the blood from the jugular vein as described under *Whole, unclotted blood* above, but without using any anticoagulant. Instead, put the blood into a sterile, stoppered tube or jar.
2. Put the container in the shade or in the refrigerator and leave the blood to clot for 2–3 hours.
3. Loosen the clot from the wall of the container using a sterile needle.
4. Carefully pour the serum (the clear, yellowish liquid that forms) into another sterile container, leaving the clot behind. Or you can use a sterile syringe and needle, or a pipette, to collect the serum and transfer it to the second container.
5. Store the serum in a refrigerator (4°C) or freezer (–20°C) until it can be tested.

Faeces

Used to test for **intestinal worms** and **liver flukes** (▷*Internal parasites [worms]*).

1. Turn a clean plastic bag inside-out and put it on your hand like a glove.
2. Put the bag-covered hand gently into the animal's anus.
3. Grab some droppings from inside the anus and bring your hand out. Only about 10 g of faeces (less than a cupful) is needed for most tests.
4. Turn the bag the right way round so the droppings are inside it.
5. Tie the neck of the bag closed to keep the faeces in, or put them in a clean, airtight container.
6. Label the bag or container and send it to the laboratory. Keep it cool so the parasite eggs do not decompose or develop into larvae (which are difficult to identify).

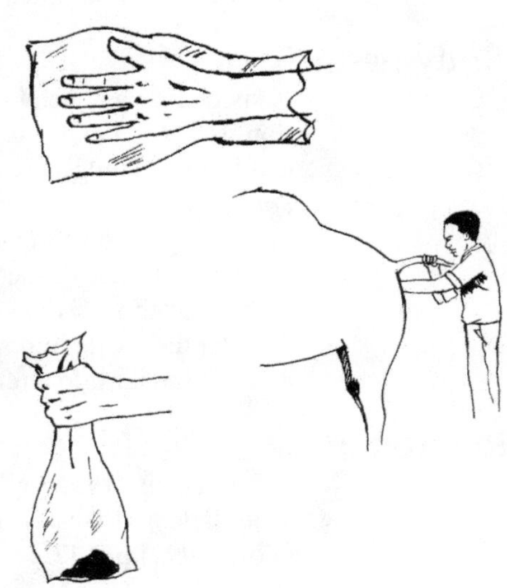

Urine

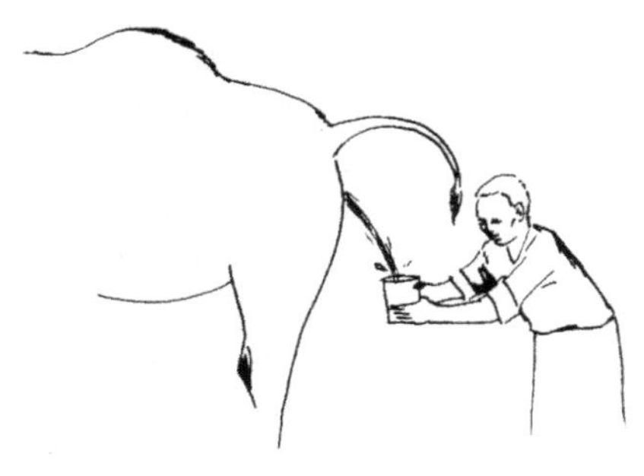

Used to test for **kidney diseases** and the cause of **red urine** (▻*Red urine*).

1. When the camel passes urine, let the first part of the urine pass.
2. Catch the middle part of the urine stream in a clean, wide-mouthed screw-capped jar (such as a jam jar).
3. Screw on the lid.
5. If it will take more than 4 hours before the sample can be tested, freeze it as soon as possible.

Skin and hair

Used to test for **mange** and **ringworm** (▻*Mange, Ringworm*).

1. Scrape the affected skin carefully with a new scalpel. Scrape from the edge of a sore or from a fresh sore (not an old one).
2. Scrape until some blood oozes out of the skin. Let the skin and hair drop into an envelope, jar or small, clean plastic bag.
3. Collect scrapings from three different places.

Foetus and placenta

Used to test for **brucellosis**, one of the causes of abortion (▻*Abortion*). Use the precautions described under *Dangerous diseases* above.

1. Dissect the freshly aborted foetus.
2. Collect the fluid inside the foetus's stomach with a sterile syringe. Put it into a sterile, stoppered jar or tube.
3. Seal the jar with paraffin wax to prevent bacteria from getting in.
4. Collect fluid from the placenta (afterbirth) in the same way. Put it into a separate jar and seal it with paraffin wax.
5. Put the placenta in a plastic bag and tie it securely. Wrap it well to make sure no liquid can leak out.
6. Put all the samples in a refrigerator until they can be tested.

Body tissue

A specialist may need to check certain body parts under the microscope for infection. He or she may ask you to provide a sample of that body part (e.g., a piece of a dead camel's lung). If a dangerous disease is suspected (▻*Diseases that people can catch from camels*), use the precautions described under *Dangerous diseases* above.

1. Cut open the carcass to reveal the organ or body part you need.
2. Cut into the tissue as cleanly as possible using a sharp knife. Cut blocks of tissue about 5 cm across.
3. Put the tissue into a clean, dry jar with a screw lid.
4. Put the jar into a refrigerator until its contents can be tested.

References

Evans et al. (1995) p. 7:38; FAO (1994) p. 270–2; Higgins (1986) p. 29–31; Manefield and Tinson (1997) p. 5–6; Quesenberry (1990) p. 216–25; Schwartz and Dioli (1992) p. 147.

Checking for diseases in the laboratory

With certain types of equipment, it is possible to do some simple tests in the field or in a modest laboratory (▷*Equipment and medicines* and *How to collect samples for testing*).

Disease	Sample type	Type of test	What to look for
Mange	Skin	Microscope	Mites, eggs
Ringworm	Hair, skin	Microscope	Fungal spores
Gut parasites	Faeces	Microscope	Worm eggs
Trypanosomiasis	Blood	Microscope (dry blood film)	Trypanosome parasites
Trypanosomiasis, dipetalonemiasis	Blood	Microscope (wet blood film)	Trypanosome parasites, dipetalonemiasis larvae
Trypanosomiasis	Blood	Micro-centrifuge (packed cell volume, PCV)	Low amount of red blood cells
Trypanosomiasis	Blood	Micro-centrifuge (buffy coat)	Trypanosome parasites
Trypanosomiasis	Blood	Test tube (mercuric chloride)	Protein in blood

Mange

Use this test to check for ▷*Mange*.

Equipment

- Skin scrapings from several parts of the animal (▷*How to collect samples for testing*).
- Test tube, 10% potassium hydroxide solution, microscope slides, cover slips, microscope, centrifuge, centrifuge tubes.

Method

1. Mix the skin scraping with a small amount of 10% potassium hydroxide solution and heat until it is just boiling (or leave to stand for 0.5–1 hour until the skin particles have partly disintegrated).
2. Carefully pour away the liquid (or use a centrifuge to sediment the sample), and spread the sediment on a microscope slide.
3. Cover the slide with a cover slip and examine the sediment under a microscope (40 ×) for the mites and their eggs (see the picture in ▷*Mange*.)

If you cannot see any mites under the microscope:

1. Put some scrapings into a centrifuge tube and add a few ml of 10% potassium hydroxide. Leave at room temperature for 3–6 hours until the dried skin particles have disintegrated.
2. Centrifuge at 3000 revolutions per minute, discard the upper layer, and put one or two drops of sediment on a microscope slide.

3. Use a microscope to check for mites.

If you are unable to check immediately, you can store the centrifuged sample in a refrigerator for up to a few weeks before examining it under a microscope.

Ringworm

Use this test to check for ▷*Ringworm.*

Equipment

- Hair pluckings and skin scrapings from the edge of the suspected ringworm sites.
- Test tube, 10% potassium hydroxide solution, microscope slides, cover slips, microscope.

Method

1. Put the hairs and skin scrapings on a microscope slide and add a few drops of potassium hydroxide.
2. Cover with a cover slip and gently warm for about 10 minutes (or hold it over a flame for a few seconds). If you do not heat it, let the sample stand for 20–30 minutes before you examine it.
3. Examine under a microscope for chains of spherical fungus spores (4–6 μm in diameter) around the hairs. First use the low magnification (10 ×) and then examine suspicious hairs at higher magnification (45 ×).

Gut parasites

Use this test to check for worms in the stomach and intestines (▷*Internal parasites*).

Equipment

- 5 g of faeces (about a teaspoonful).
- Saturated sodium chloride solution: mix 360 g of NaCl (common salt) in 1 litre of warm water, pour into a bottle and store it for use. Alternatively, you can use a saturated sugar solution.
- Sieve with holes measuring 0.5–0.8 mm, such as a tea strainer.
- Pestle and mortar, test tube or small jar, microscope slides, cover slips, microscope.

Method

1. Mix 3–5 g of faeces with 10–15 times as much saturated sodium chloride solution in a mortar, and mix well.
2. Pour the mixture through the sieve into a smaller jar or test tube until the liquid reaches the rim.
3. Put a cover slip onto the mixture (the slip should touch the liquid) and allow to stand for 20–30 minutes.
4. Transfer the cover slip onto a microscope slide and examine under a microscope (ocular 10 ×, objective 4 ×, 10 ×) for eggs.

Instead of using a cover slip, you can make a small loop in the end of a piece of wire (such as a small paperclip) and rest this on the surface of the liquid. The surface tension in the liquid will draw any eggs towards the loop. Take the wire and carefully put the film of liquid that attaches to it onto a microscope slide. Cover with a cover slip. You can then examine the slide under a microscope in the same way as above.

Dry blood film

This is a direct test for ▷*Trypanosomiasis*, since it checks for the trypanosome parasites themselves in the blood. If you see the parasites, you can be sure that the animal has trypanosomiasis. However, the trypanosomes can be hard to see, so if you do not see them, you cannot be certain that the animal does *not* have the disease.

Equipment

- Fresh or unclotted blood sample.
- Microscope slides, methyl alcohol (methanol).
- Microscope, if possible with an immersion objective (a special microscope lens for viewing a slide using immersion oil).
- Immersion oil (a special oil used with a microscope and immersion objective).
- Giemsa solution (a dye to stain the trypanosomes and make them easier to see).

Method

1. Prepare two microscope slides with a dry blood film (▷*How to collect samples for testing*).
2. Cover each entire slide with methyl alcohol for 5 minutes. Shake off the excess alcohol and allow the slides to dry.
3. Put some Giemsa solution on the blood smear so that the whole of the blood film is covered. After 30 minutes, shake off the excess Giemsa solution, or wash the stain away gently with tap water. Allow the slides to dry again.
4. Place each slide on a microscope and examine with immersion oil at 100 × magnification for the trypanosomes. They are longish, thin, whip-like 'flagellates', appearing dark purple among the pale purple blood cells.

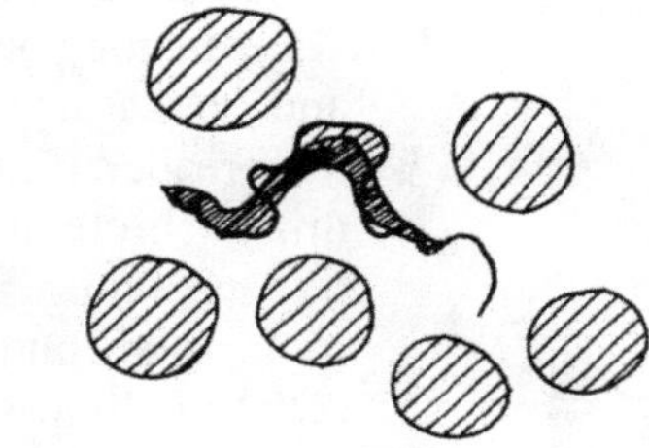

Trypanosome flagellate among circular red blood cells (enlarged)

Wet blood film

Use this test to check for ▷*Trypanosomiasis* and *Dipetalonemiasis*. This is another direct test for trypanosomiasis, although it suffers from the same disadvantage as the dry blood film (see above): the trypanosomes can be hard to see.

Equipment

- Fresh or unclotted blood sample.
- Microscope slide, cover slip, microscope (10 × eyepiece, 25 × objective).

Method

1. Put a small drop of fresh blood onto a glass slide.
2. Apply a cover slip and examine under a microscope. The trypanosomes (or the worm larvae that cause dipetalonemiasis) can be seen wriggling among the blood cells.

Packed cell volume (haematocrit)

Use this test to check for ▷*Trypanosomiasis*. This detects 'anaemia' – a reduction in the number of red blood cells. Anaemia can be caused by trypanosomiasis, but also by several other problems, such as ▷*Ticks* and loss of blood after an accident.

Equipment

- Fresh or unclotted blood sample.
- Mini-haematocrit centrifuge (a piece of equipment that spins tubes containing blood very fast, so separating out the different parts of the blood).
- Capillary tubes (disposable tubes with a very small inside diameter, treated with anticoagulant to stop the blood from clotting).
- Sealant (special material to plug the end of the capillary tubes).
- Haematocrit tube-reader (a scale for reading the centrifuged tubes, which comes with the centrifuge).

Method

1. Draw the blood into a capillary tube and fill to about 1 cm from the end. Wipe the blood from the outside of the tube while it is still wet. Seal the empty end of the tube to stop the blood from coming out.
2. Put the tube in a centrifuge with the sealed end outside and centrifuge for 5 minutes at 10 000–13 000 revolutions per minute, or for 2 minutes at 16 000 revolutions per minute.
3. Take the tube out of the centrifuge and hold it against a haematocrit tube-reader. If the animal has anaemia (which may be caused by trypanosomiasis), the dark portion of the tube contents (the red blood cells) will be less than 0.20 (the normal value for camels is 0.25–0.35, with an average of 0.30).

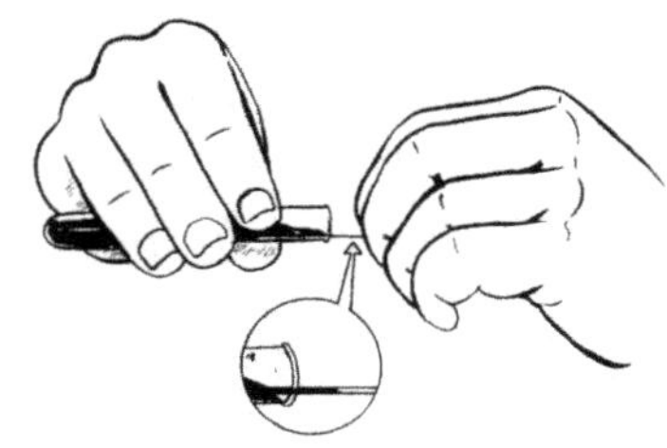

Drawing blood into a capillary tube.

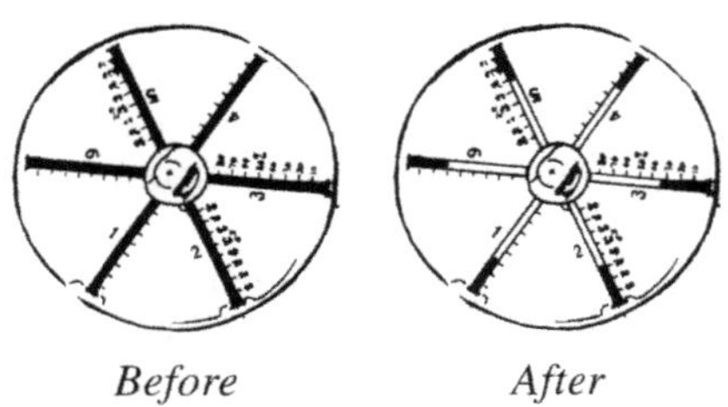

Before *After*

Capillary tubes in mini-centrifuge, before and after centrifuging.

Buffy coat

Use this test to check for ⊳*Trypanosomiasis*. Centrifuging a blood sample makes the trypanosomes collect in the 'buffy coat' – the area between the dark portion in the centrifuge tube (the red blood cells) and the clear part (the blood serum). This makes them easier to see than in a sample that has not been centrifuged.

Equipment

- Fresh or unclotted blood sample.
- Mini-haematocrit centrifuge, capillary tubes, sealant (see *Packed cell volume [haematocrit]* above).
- For the first procedure below: microscope slides, microscope with immersion objective (10 × eyepiece, 20 × objective), immersion oil (see *Dry blood film* above).
- For the alternative procedure below: microscope slides, microscope (10 × eyepiece, 25 × objective), glass-cutter.

Method

1. Prepare the sample and centrifuge (see *Packed cell volume* steps 1–3 above).
2. Place the capillary tube onto a slide, and add a drop of immersion oil.

3. Examine the buffy coat part of the tube under a microscope for trypanosomes.

If you do not have an immersion objective and oil, you can use a standard 10 × objective instead.

Alternative method

1. Prepare the sample and centrifuge as described above.
2. Cut the capillary tube 1 mm below the buffy-coat zone (to include the upper layer of red blood cells).
3. Press out the contents of the cut piece onto a clean slide. Mix and cover with a cover slip (ideally, not too many red blood cells should be included as they may make the trypanosomes harder to see).
4. Examine the slide under a microscope for trypanosomes.

Mercuric chloride test

Use this test to check for ▷*Trypanosomiasis*.

An indirect test for trypanosomiasis: it detects a high level of protein in the blood (one of the effects of trypanosomiasis), rather than the parasites themselves. It is a simple but not very reliable test.

Equipment

- Blood serum (▷*How to collect samples for testing*).
- Freshly prepared solution of 1:25 000 pure mercuric chloride.

Method

1. Collect some blood and allow it to stand for some time until it clots.
2. Take one drop of the clear fluid that forms (the 'serum') and add to 1 ml of mercuric chloride solution. In serum from infected animals, a white precipitate appears almost immediately. In healthy animals, the solution remains clear.

Normal blood values

A laboratory technician can use standard techniques to test the blood of camels. Below are the normal blood values for camels (adapted from Higgins, 1983).

Value	Concentration or range	Average
Red blood cell count (RBC)	3.8–12.6 × 10^{12}/litre	
Haematocrit packed cell volume (PCV)*	0.2–0.35	0.3
White blood cell count (WBC)	12.9–27.2 × 10^{9}/litre	
Neutrophils	21.1–56.3%	38.7%
Lymphocytes	26.5–65.4%	46.0%
Monocytes	0–12.3%	5.7%
Eosinophils	0–18.9%	9.5%

*The packed cell volume depends on when the camel last drank. It is higher if the camel is thirsty.

References

Benjamin (1978) p. 5–14, 25–107; Carter (1986) p. 103–6, 228-31; Evans et al. (1995) p. 7:3, 7:8, 7:10, 7:17; Higgins (1983); Higgins (1986) p. 31–4; Köhler-Rollefson (1991) p. 3; Manefield and Tinson (1997) p. 121–3, 275; Sewell and Brocklesby (1990) p. 210–13; Sloss and Kemp (1978); Soulsby (1982) p. 763–78.

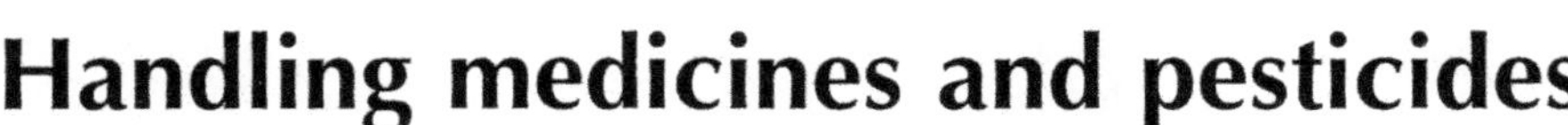

Handling medicines and pesticides

Medicines and pesticides (such as treatments against ticks) can be dangerous. If not used properly, they can harm the sick camel, healthy camels and other animals, people and the environment. Take special care to store them properly, and use them with care.

Storage

- Store medicines and pesticides in a cool, dark, dry place, out of reach of children and animals, and away from human and animal feed. A lockable metal cupboard or box is a good place.
- Make sure the containers are clearly labelled as to what they contain. Keep the instructions with the medicine.
- Some types of medicines, including many vaccines and antibiotics, must be kept cold all the time. Keep them in a refrigerator, or with ice in a thermos flask or an insulated box.
- Many medicines must be used by a certain date (marked on the bottle or box). Regularly check the expiration date of the medicines and throw them away if they have passed this date. If possible, return expired medicines to the pharmacy or veterinarian. If this is not possible, pour the medicines into a hole in the ground (well away from wells or springs), and bury the containers.
- Some medicines come as powder that you must mix with a liquid (such as water). You can keep the powder for a long time, but once it is mixed with the liquid, you have to use it up quickly (usually within a few days), and you may have to store it in a refrigerator. Check the medicine label for information on this.
- Never use cooking pots to store or mix chemicals. Instead, keep a separate container for mixing.
- Keep an emergency supply of important medicines on hand at all times.

Records

- Keep a record of any medicines used, how they were used, where and when.
- Order replacement stock well before you run out of the medicine.

Before use

- Work out how much medicine or pesticide you will need (▷*Using the right amount of medicine*), and prepare only this amount.
- Double-check to make sure you are using the right medicine or pesticide, and that you are using it in the right way. Mistakes can be very costly, as well as harmful for the animal.
- Disinfect syringes and other equipment by boiling them in water for 10 minutes. If you keep the syringe and needles in disinfectant, rinse them with cooled, boiled water to wash off all traces of the disinfectant. ▷*Administering medicines* for how to keep syringes and other equipment sterile.
- Before mixing a pesticide, put gloves (or plastic bags) on your hands and wear protective clothing to prevent any pesticide from splashing onto your skin. If you do get some on your skin, wash it off immediately with soap and water.

Using medicines

- Follow the instructions on the medicine label carefully.
- Always use the recommended dose. Using too much medicine or pesticide may harm or even kill the animal, and may make you ill, too. Using too little may allow the organism that causes the disease become resistant – making the disease harder to treat. ⊳*Using the right amount of medicine* for how to calculate dosages.
- Animals seem to recover from some diseases quite quickly, and you may be tempted to stop the treatment to save money. But the disease may come back, and the bacteria or other organisms that cause it may become resistant to the medicine, making it harder to treat next time. Keep giving the medicine for the recommended length of time – even if the animal seems to have recovered already. This is especially important when using antibiotics.

Using pesticides

- Be careful not to allow any pesticide to touch your skin, or get into your nose, mouth or eyes. Wear protective clothing and gloves, and goggles and face mask if possible, to protect your skin, eyes and mouth, and to prevent you from breathing any in.
- Make other people handling the animals also put on protective clothing.
- Do not eat, smoke or drink while handling pesticides.
- Always use the recommended pesticide dose. Too much pesticide may kill the animal or make it ill. Too little may be ineffective and is a waste of money.
- Try to avoid using pesticides on animals that are under a month old, or if it is ill with another disease (unless treating it against ticks will help it combat the other disease). Use other remedies (such as hand-picking the ticks) instead.

After using pesticides

- Wash yourselves and your clothes well with soap and water after you have used a pesticide.
- Clean all containers and sprayers immediately after use.
- Take care not to damage the environment. Do not pour any unused chemical into rivers or ponds, since it might kill fish or harm people or animals.
- Do not use old pesticide containers for other purposes. Burn empty containers and cardboard boxes in the open, away from animals and people. Or dig a hole far away from any water source and bury the containers in it.
- Do not allow animals near places where you have used chemicals, or allow them to lick or drink from old chemical containers.
- Do not treat an animal just before slaughtering it. The pesticide may stay in the animal's body and contaminate the meat, making it dangerous to eat.
- Do not drink milk from camels for 3 days after treatment with acaricides and certain types of medicine (see the medicine label to check whether it is safe).

References

Forse (1999) p. 339–45; IIRR (1996) vol. 2 p. 59; Projet Cameline (1999) p. 9; Quesenberry (1990) p. 239–40.

Selecting camels

Because camels are such slow breeders, virtually all female camels are used for breeding. This means it is difficult to select females to improve the herd. It is possible to select males, however. Every group of camel-keepers has its own ideas on what constitutes an ideal camel type, so it is impossible to give detailed guidelines on selection.

Here are some general guidelines for selecting camels for breeding or purchase.

- **Choose strong, healthy animals**, without obvious faults (▷*How to examine a camel*). Camels sold in markets are often inferior animals, so it may be better to go out to the herd where it is grazing. As a rule, valuable (milking) animals are not used to carry loads, so there should be no signs that the animal has been used in this way.
- **Temperament** Handle the camel to check this.
- **Head** Check for blindness or defects in both eyes. Check the teeth to determine the animal's age (▷*Estimating a camel's weight and age*). Press your hand on the animal's cheek to make sure that all the teeth are present. Check whether the jaw is under- or over-shot. 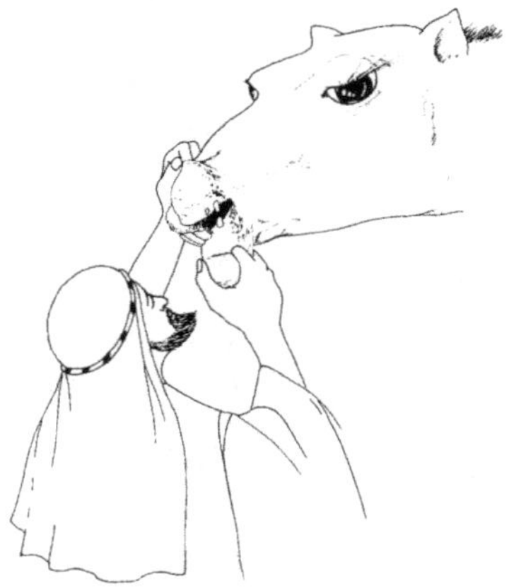
- **Legs** These should be straight. Check for limping or other problems when the camel is walking, sitting down or getting up.
- **Front legs** There should be ample space (wide enough to put your hand in) between the chest and the front legs. The legs should not rub against the chest-pad, and the knees should not rub against each other. The fetlocks should be straight. Check under the knees for sores or scars: they show that the camel has been restrained with a rope around its front legs. This may indicate that it was not considered valuable during the rut, and was used for work instead.
- **Back legs** The hock joints should not be too close to each other when the camel is standing, and should not touch when it walks. Check also that the Achilles tendon on the hock is not swollen or painful (this may show that the camel has been used too early and too much as a pack animal).
- **Feet** Check the soles of the feet for wounds or bruises.
- **Chest** A narrow chest can show that the camel was malnourished as a young calf. There should be no sores or abnormal growths on the chest-pad.
- **Hump** The hump should not be very big. A very large hump is a sign that a male is a poor breeder (no rut) and that a female is sterile.
- **Brand marks** Often a good indication of the diseases a camel has been treated for in the past. Brand marks on a joint may show the camel has had joint problems or lameness. As a rule, only tribal brand marks should be present.
- **Scars** Check for scars and old wounds, especially on the short ribs and shoulders; these heal with difficulty and show that the camel has been used as a pack

animal (▷*Saddle sores*). A tuft of white hair on the hump or shoulder indicates a wound caused by use as a pack animal.

- **Females** If a breeding, pregnant or lactating female is being sold, it has problems (this is why it is being sold). Remember also that a female may still be a heifer because it is sterile. All four quarters of the udder should be well developed, distinct, and evenly spaced. The teats should be large. If the animal is lactating, ask the owner to milk it. Check whether the female is pregnant (if it lifts its tail when approached by a bull or a man, it is pregnant). Ask how many calves a female has delivered, and check against the animal's age.
- **Males** The penis should be very long and the scrotum should be well developed. The penis and testicles should not be injured or swollen. Ask to see any offspring the bull has sired.
- **Calves** Ask to see the mother and father if possible.

References

Evans et al. (1995) p. 4:1–2; Manefield and Tinson (1997) p. 66–7; Rathore (1986) p. 50–3; Schwartz and Dioli (1992) p. 69–72.

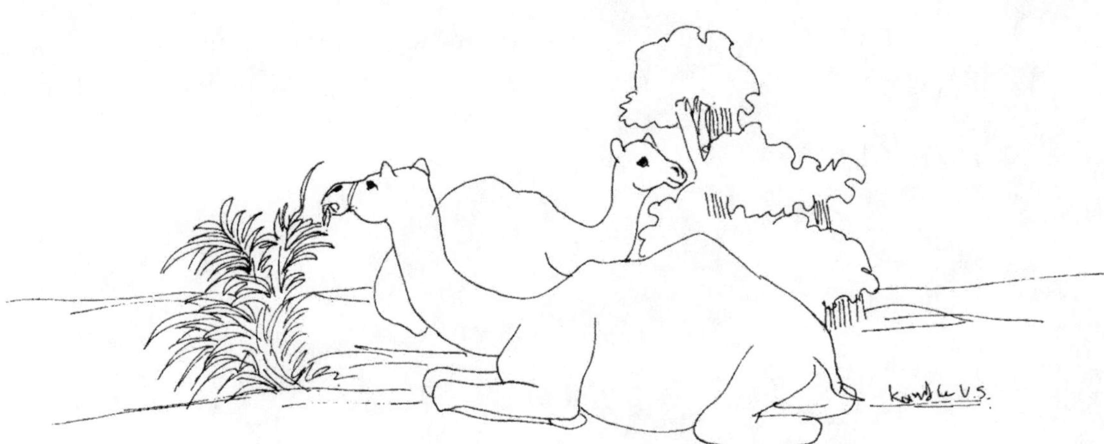

2 Skin problems

Camels suffer from a wide variety of skin ailments: diseases such as ▷*Orf* and ▷*Pox*, mites (▷*Mange*), bites and wounds caused by insects (▷*Bites and stings*), ill-fitting saddles (▷*Saddle sores*), careless handlers, and many other causes.

Use the tables below to identify the cause of the problem, then check the relevant section for the treatment.

Diseases covered in this chapter

Type of swelling or sore	Location	Course	Cause	Disease
First small bumps, later hair loss, then thickening of skin, severe itching	All over body, except hump. Starts in armpits and groin	Spreads throughout herd	Parasite	▷*Mange*
Crusts on skin, open sores exuding fluid	Neck, shoulders, withers, sides, quarters; rarely on lower legs	More frequently in young animals	Bacteria	▷*Contagious skin necrosis*
Hairless spots, beginning 1–2 cm across, with thick, grey-whitish crust	Head, neck, shoulder, legs and flanks	Only in young animals; heals by itself	Fungus	▷*Ringworm*
Small blisters; then crusts and scabs	Starts around mouth, nose and eyelids, may spread to whole body	Spreads rapidly among young animals	Virus	▷*Pox*
Like pox, but only on the head; swelling of head	Lips, head	Spreads rapidly among young animals	Virus	▷*Orf*
Ticks attached, itchiness and irritation	Base of tail, anus, groin, armpit, ears, nostrils	Ticks drop off after a few days, but new ones can attach	Ticks	▷*Ticks*

Type of swelling or sore	Location	Course	Cause	Disease
Hair loss, irritation, itchiness	Especially on flanks and shoulders		Lice, fleas	▷*Lice and fleas*
Matted hair, crusts with thick, bloody fluid underneath	Base of neck, flanks and sometimes legs	Mainly young camels; heals by itself	Fungus-like bacteria	▷*Dermato-philosis*
Localized swelling	Anywhere on body		Insects, spiders, naked mole-rats, scorpions	▷*Bites and stings, Snake bite*
Bites, cuts, bleeding or infected wounds	Anywhere, especially on chest-pad, saddle area and feet		Bites, accidents, castration, surgery	▷*Wounds and burns*
Abscesses (pus surrounded by inflamed tissue)	Anywhere on body, mostly on head, neck, chest-pad, saddle, feet	Usually isolated but may spread	Bacteria, thorns, sharp stones on ground	▷*Skin abscesses, Chest-pad abscess*
Abscesses (pus surrounded by inflamed tissue)	Lymph nodes, often at base of neck, between front legs	Very common; spreads slowly from one lymph node to another	Bacteria	▷*Abscesses on the lymph nodes*
Raw or dry and cold skin, then a sore that drains pus	Where the saddle presses on the body	In draught camels	Ill-fitting saddle	▷*Saddle sores*
Painless growth	Ears, neck	Not contagious		▷*Dermoids*

Diseases covered in other chapters

Type of swelling or sore	Location	Course	Cause	Disease
No sweat	Whole body	Especially in draught animals	Unknown. Lack of salt?	▷*Dry coat*
Soft, painless swellings	Face, jaws, belly, lower limbs, udder		Various causes	▷*Oedema*
Raised skin patches, loss of hair, irritation	Anywhere on body		Allergy-causing substance	▷*Allergy*
Localized swelling (can be pushed back by hand)	Belly		Gap in belly muscles where organs inside push through	Hernia or rupture (not covered in this book)

Mange

Sarcoptic mange, scabies
***Chitto* (Borana, Gabbra), *khaj, khujli, paam, paanv, pom* (India), *gerrab* (Kordofan), *haddo* (Rendille), *ilbebedo, lpepedo* (Samburu), *addha, addo, chitto* (Somali), *gerab* (Sudan), *ametina, ekoikoi, emitina* (Turkana)**

Mange is a widespread and highly contagious skin disease which causes severe itchiness, poor growth, low milk production, and even death. It is one of the most common and important diseases in camels, especially in temperate regions with cold winters or areas with long wet seasons. Mange is caused by a mite which prefers areas of the body that have little hair. The disease is more severe during the cold part of the year and in the rainy season; it often declines during the summer.

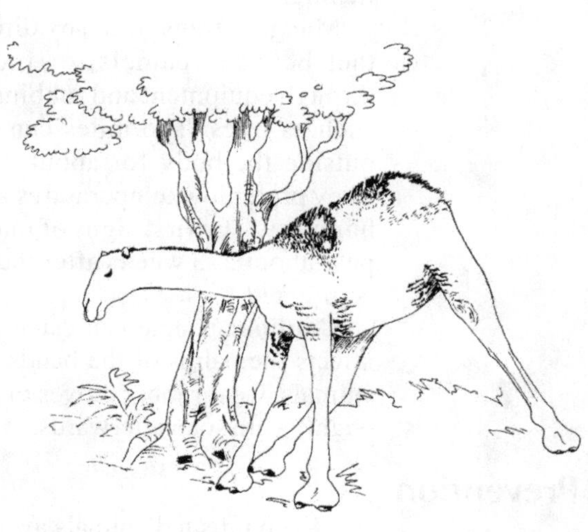

Signs

- Mange usually starts in the armpit and groin, and spreads from there to the rest of the body.
- One of the first signs is that the animal rubs and scratches the affected area with its teeth or against trees, so spreading the disease to new areas.
- In the early stages, the skin is covered with small bumps. Hairless patches develop, and the skin becomes raw from scratching, and begins to weep.
- Scabs develop, and in serious cases, the skin becomes grey, thickens, becomes wrinkled and cracked, like dried mud.
- The camel spends its time scratching itself rather than eating or resting. It loses weight and becomes weak and anaemic.
- If the disease is not treated, secondary bacterial infections may develop and the camel may become more susceptible to trypanosomiasis and other diseases, such as pneumonia.
- Many camels in the herd may be affected at the same time.

You can usually tell if a camel has mange if you see the signs above. Mange can be confused with ▷*Pox, Ringworm* and *Contagious skin necrosis*.

If in doubt, take a skin sample from the edge of the scabs (▷*How to collect samples for testing*). Take samples from three different places on the skin, and check for the mites and eggs using a microscope. You may have to look at a lot of different skin samples before you see even a single mite (▷*Checking for diseases in the laboratory*).

Cause

A burrowing mite known as *Sarcoptes scabiei* var *cameli*. This is about 0.3–0.5 mm long and can barely be seen by the naked eye. The mites dig tunnels into the upper layer of the skin and lay their eggs there. This causes an allergic reaction, leading to intense itching.

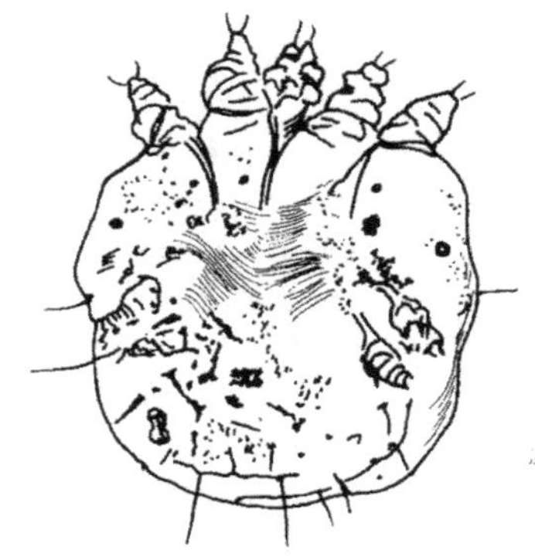

Enlarged mange mite, as seen under a microscope

Mange is transmitted by direct contact between camels, or indirectly through equipment and rubbing places such as trees. The mites can survive outside the body for about 2 weeks. They prefer low temperatures and high humidity. The first signs of mange appear about 2–3 weeks after the animal is infected.

Caution: people can catch mange from camels (though this is rare). It often affects the palms of the hands and between the fingers. When handling infected animals, wear rubber gloves or plastic bags on your hands. Wash your hands thoroughly with soap afterwards.

Prevention

- Keep infected animals away from healthy ones. Avoid infected herds, and do not touch equipment or rubbing spots they may have come into contact with. TRAD+SCI
- Mange is very common in baggage or pack camels. Avoid contact with such animals. TRAD+SCI
- Make camels wade in shallow sea water and pour sea water over the whole body for several hours. BEJA (SUDAN)
- Allow camels to roll in salt pans, or plaster their skin with salty mud. GABBRA, RENDILLE

Treatment

Once a camel herd has become infected with mange, it is very difficult and expensive to eradicate the disease. Identify and treat mange early, before it has spread to many animals. Diligent and repeated brushing of acaricide into the skin will be necessary. Try to eradicate the disease completely, rather than trying merely to control it.

Treat all the animals at the same time, to avoid the disease re-infecting animals that have been cured. Treat both infected and healthy animals, as the mites can already be hiding in apparently healthy animals.

It is not enough just to treat the animals. Move them away from the area where they are kept (for example, their night enclosures) and any rubbing spots. If you are using an acaricide spray (see under *Modern treatments*), spray these places too.

It may be helpful to deworm the animals before using one of the treatments below (▷*Internal parasites [worms]*). This makes sure the animal is strong enough to fight the mange disease.

Traditional treatments

Since mange is an important disease, many traditional remedies exist. These often work quite well, but take a long time and a lot of work to make and use. Many use a thick tar-like liquid to suffocate the mites in their tunnels in the camel's skin. For a fuller summary and bibliography of traditional remedies, see Bizimana (1994).

Tie the animal down so you can reach all parts of its body. Shear the animal, for example by rubbing ash from *Acacia mellifera* (known as *kitir* in Sudan) on the skin, and pulling the hair out. Then, using a stiff brush, a piece of coarse sacking or a sharp stone, vigorously scrub away the crusts on the affected areas until the skin bleeds. Then use one of the treatments below.

- Allow the camels to roll in salt pans, or plaster them with salty mud. GABBRA, RENDILLE
- Rub a thick layer of wet pond mud vigorously into the skin, and allow it to dry. Repeat this twice a week for 4 weeks. W RAJASTHAN
- Apply used engine oil (from a car's oil sump) in a thin layer all over the affected parts of the animal's skin. The animal should recover within 2–4 weeks. ERITREA, KENYA, SOMALIA
- Apply kerosene on the skin during the cool of the night. Leave for 2 hours, then wash the camel with mud and water. Then apply cooking oil to the skin. INDIA
  Caution: Use engine oil or kerosene only if you have no other treatment available. Engine oil can cause cancer. Wear plastic bags on your hands as gloves, and avoid getting it on your skin (▷*Handling medicines and pesticides*).
- Make a paste of 5 g of sulphur, 50 ml of cooking oil and 1 g of camphor. Wash the affected part of the animal, scrub it smooth with a brush, and apply the paste twice a day for 10–12 days. TRAD+SCI
- Chop a root of desert rose (*Adenium obesum*) into pieces, and leave in a basin overnight. Use the fluid that oozes out to wash the affected parts of the animal once. (**Caution:** desert rose is poisonous. Handle with care.) TURKANA
- Boil young neem (*Azadirachta indica*) leaves in water for about 30 minutes. Allow to cool, and then spray the liquid on the affected part. TRAD+SCI
- Grind the seeds of *Citrullus colocynthis* (bitter apple, *handal*) and heat them until they form a liquid tar (called *gutran* in Arabic). Rub the tar into the affected area. Repeat this treatment at 2-day intervals until the animal is cured. Instead of the colocynth seeds, a mixture of sesame or cottonseed oil with table salt (sodium chloride) can be used at 7–10 day intervals until the sores disappear. LAHAWIYIN, RASHAIDA, SHUKRIYA
- Make tar from *Juniperus phoenicea* or *Thuja articulata*, mix with 1–2 parts of warm water, and rub this on the affected area. About 4–6 litres of this mixture are needed for one animal. ARABS
- Light a smoky fire under trees where *Agnosceles versicolor* bugs (known as *andad*) congregate. These insects are a common pest of sorghum; they are black with yellow spots. Collect the insects on a sheet as they fall. Crush them and squeeze the liquid out through a cloth, or heat them in water to obtain the oil they contain. You can crush several litres of the insects at one time. Apply the liquid directly to the affected part of the camel. Repeat the treatment once a week if necessary. SHUKRIA
- Rub the white juice of *Euphorbia* sp. (*E. robecchii* [*dharkeyn*], *E. somalensis* [*falanfalho*], or *E. gossypina* [*cinjir*]) into the affected area. The juice can also be mixed with water or urine. **Caution**: the juice can burn your skin, so wear gloves or plastic bags on your hands when using it. SOMALI

- Make bone-marrow by crushing animal bones in a large mortar and heating them over the fire. Rub the marrow onto the affected area. The crushed fruits of the *aborak* tree (*Balanites aegyptiaca*) can also be used. TUAREG
- Boil *habagar* (the gum of a *Commiphora* sp.) with water and smear it on all affected body parts. Usually one application is sufficient. GARI SOMALI
- Apply *taramira* oil (made from *Eruca sativa*) or sesame (*Sesamum indicum*) oil all over the camel's body with a rag. Keep the camel in the shade while the oil is on its body because exposure to the sun will cause it to blister. The oiling causes the camel's temperature to rise 1–2 degrees, and may cause swelling under the belly. After 48 hours, take the camel to the bank of a stream and cover it all over with mud. Leave this on for 3 days before removing it. PUNJAB
- During the cool time of the morning or evening, rub the oil of *Derris indica* (known as *karanji-ka-tel* in Rajasthan) all over the camel's body. Repeat the treatment 2–3 times at 7–10-day intervals. Do not use this with a pregnant camel, since it causes the animal to become 'hot'. S RAJASTHAN, TRAD+SCI
- Shear the animal and scrub away the crusts on the skin (see above under *Traditional treatments*). Treat the infected area with Ectosep or Charmil once a day until cured. AYURVEDIC
- Other plants used in Africa to treat mange include:
  - *Acacia laeta*
  - *Avicennia africana*
  - *Calligonum comosum*
  - *Calotropis procera* (whole plant)
  - *Capparis spinosa* (leaf)
  - *Commiphora africana* (gum)
  - *Cucumis colocynthis*
  - *Cucurbita maxima*
  - *Cymbopogon schoenanthus* (whole plant)
  - *Euphorbia balsamifera* (latex)
  - *Ricinus communis* (grain)
  - *Tamarix aphylla*

  Caution: Be careful when using some of these plants: they may be poisonous.

Modern treatments

- Shear the animal and scrub away the crusts, then spray the whole body with one of the following acaricides 2–3 times at 7–10-day intervals, and brush the acaricide into the skin. It is important to scrub the whole body, as the mange mites may be hiding in apparently healthy skin. These acaricides are also available in a form that can be poured on the animals instead of being sprayed.

  Severe cases may require more than 3 treatments, especially if they recur. Continue treatment until the signs have disappeared.
  - Amitraz 250 mg/litre (e.g., Taktic, 2 ml/litre of water).
  - Quintiophos 0.02% (e.g., Bacdip, 10 ml in 18 litres of water).
  - Deltamethrin 1% (e.g., Butox solution, 2–4 ml/litre of water).
  - Diazinon (Bremer dip, Neocidol) as 0.05–0.1% solution.
  - Gamma benzene hexachloride or gamma BHC 0.025–0.05% (Gammatox, 8 g sachet in 4 litres of water).

  Caution: acaricides are poisonous. Wear rubber gloves or plastic bags on your hands, and wash your hands thoroughly afterwards. Store poisons safely away from animals and children. Do not pour them away, and make sure they do not get into the drinking-water supply (▷*Handling medicines and pesticides*).

  In some countries, gamma BHC (Gammatox) is banned for use with animals because the body absorbs it and it can get into the milk. Never use it with animals giving milk.

- Inject ivermectin (Ivomec) at a dose of 0.2 mg/kg body weight under the camel's skin (i.e., 1 ml of Ivomec for every 50 kg of the camel's body weight) (▷*Estimating a camel's weight and age* and *Using the right amount of medicine*). Repeat the injection after 2 weeks. This treatment is expensive, but it is nearly always successful. Ivermectin may lose its effectiveness very quickly if it is underdosed or not stored correctly.

References

Bizimana (1994) p. 327–31; Evans et al. (1995) p. 7:9–10, 7:30; FAO (1994) p. 189, 256; Forse (1999) p. 154–6, 339–45; Higgins (1986) p. 73–6; ITDG and IIRR (1996) p. 96–7; Köhler-Rollefson (1996) p. 130–2; Projet Cameline (1999) p.15–18; Rathore (1986) p. 178–81; Schwartz and Dioli (1992) p. 173–5, 203–5; Sewell and Brocklesby (1990) p. 2–3, 28–32; Wanyama (1997) vol. 2, p. 84; Wilson (1998) p. 105–6.

Contagious skin necrosis

Staphylococcal dermatitis

***Dulla* (Borana), *dula, kharfat, garfat, hilaliit* (Gabbra), *jooling* (India), *phoda* (Rajasthan), *garfat, kharfat* (Rendille), *lomgoi, ngamanyeni* (Samburu), *dalleham, dhaleeco, dulla, garfat, ma'ah, maha* (Somali), *al ni'aita, na'eita* (Sudan), *lelebunai* (Turkana)**

Camels frequently suffer from skin necrosis (the death of living skin tissue), especially if they are kept in crowded conditions. The disease affects camels of all ages, although young animals seem to be more susceptible. Calves may die from the disease.

Signs

- Painful skin sores, on which the hair falls out. The sores are usually found on the neck, shoulders, withers, sides and quarters, and rarely on the lower legs.
- A circular sore, a few centimetres in diameter appears on the skin. It begins to weep fluid. The dead skin falls off, leaving a circular ulcer that does not heal, and may form a thick scab. The camel tries to rub and bite the sore. Lymph glands nearby may become swollen.
- After 7–14 days, the dead skin comes off, and the sore opens into a wound. An ulcer may form in the centre of the sore.
- Rarely, the camel may develop septicaemia (blood poisoning).
- When the sore heals, it leaves a star-shaped scar.

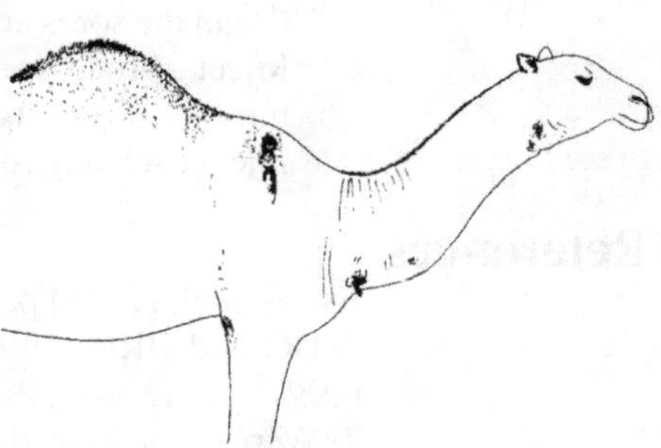

Contagious skin necrosis can be confused with ▷*Dermatophilosis*, *Mange*, *Ringworm*, or individual abscesses or diseases that can cause them (▷*Skin abscesses* and *Abscesses on the lymph nodes*).

Cause

Contagious skin necrosis was once thought to be due to lack of salt. It is now known to be caused by various bacteria and fungi that infect the skin, including *Actinomyces*, *Corynebacterium pyogenes*, *Staphylococcus aureus* and *Streptococcus*.

The disease is spread through physical contact and by the animals rubbing on contaminated trees and posts. Punjabi herders believe that grazing on *Acacia arabica* and tamarisk makes camels susceptible to the disease.

Prevention

- Separate infected camels from healthy ones.
- Disinfect pens and surroundings, or change the night enclosure.
- Add salt to the drinking water.
- Inject with a vaccine (specialized labs can make these).

Treatment

Traditional treatments

Herders know of no effective treatment against this disease. However, they say that changing the pasture may ease the condition, and they try the following treatments.

- In the early stage of the disease (where the skin swells), hold hot stones against the swelling to warm the skin.
- Brand the skin in a ring around the sores (▷*Branding*). GABBRA
- Brand the skin at the top of the base of the tail (▷*Branding*).
- Grind sorghum to flour and cook in water to make a paste. Allow this to cool overnight. Remove the dead tissue, and put the paste on the open sores. Leave it for several days, or repeat the treatment each day if needed. E SUDAN
- Rub the sap of *Caralluma socotrana* (*gowracata*) onto the sores. SOMALI
- Apply the sap of *Euphorbia*, sheep's fat or oil onto the sores. RENDILLE

Modern treatments

- Mix 100 g of sulphur powder with 900 g of Vaseline to make a paste. Remove the dead tissue and put the paste on the sores.
- Remove the dead tissue, then clean and disinfect the wound with a mild antiseptic such as acriflavine, potassium permanganate, tincture of iodine, or a 50:50 mixture of tincture of iodine and glycerine.
- Clean the sores and apply antibiotic ointment.
- Inject a broad-spectrum antibiotic such as long-acting oxytetracycline into the muscle. If you use a long-acting injection, repeat after 3–5 days. Otherwise, inject each day for about a week. Spray the sore with a topical antibiotic.

References

Evans et al. (1995) p. 7:12–13; Forse (1999) p. 169–70; Higgins (1986) p. 100–2; ITDG and IIRR (1996) p. 76; Kaufmann (1998) p. 189; Manefield and Tinson (1997) p. 242, 247; Rathore (1986) p. 168; Schwartz and Dioli (1992) p. 176, 206–7; Wernery and Kaaden (1995) p. 65–7.

Ringworm

Dermatophytosis, dermatomycosis
***Robbi, ropi* (Borana, Gabbra), *daad, taat* (India), *ngamunyeni, nkamunyani* (Samburu), *ambarr, robi* (Somali), *gara'a, goub* (Sudan), *akiserit, akisorit, epara, ekithariit* (Turkana)**

This skin disease mainly affects camels less than 3 years old, peaking between 3 and 12 months. As many as 80% of young camels in a herd may be affected.

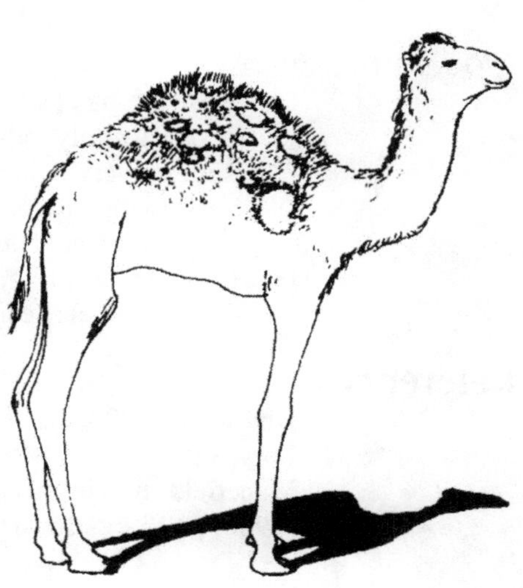

Ringworm reduces the animal's value, but not its performance. It usually heals by itself. It is probably worth treating only if you want to sell the animal.

Warning: People can catch ringworm from camels, though it is not a dangerous disease. Do not touch the infected parts with your skin. Put plastic bags on your hands like gloves, or use a rag to apply medicine. Wash your hands well after handling the animal (▷*Diseases that people can catch from camels*).

Signs

- Dry, hairless, circular patches, with a thick, scaly, grey-whitish encrustation. The patches occur mostly on the head, neck, shoulder, legs and flanks.
- The patches begin small, about 1–2 cm in diameter. They gradually get bigger, and may merge.
- The patches do not itch. In time, the camels normally recover without treatment.

You can usually tell if a camel has ringworm if you see the signs above. If you are not sure, take scrapings of the skin and hair from the edges of the hairless patches (not from the middle) and check for the fungus spores under a microscope (▷*Checking for diseases in the laboratory*). If ringworm affects the whole body, it can easily be confused with ▷*Mange*. It is also often confused with ▷*Contagious skin necrosis*.

Cause

Fungus (*Trichophyton* and *Microsporum*). Ringworm spreads slowly by direct contact or by contact with infected materials. The fungus spores may survive for months outside the animal, especially in rugs, blankets and saddles.

Prevention

- Separate affected animals from healthy ones.
- Vaccinate the camels at 30 days of age using a cattle vaccine. Repeat the vaccination after 2–3 weeks. FORMER SOVIET UNION, SCI

Treatment

It is not normally necessary to treat ringworm, since it usually heals by itself as the calf gets older.

Traditional treatments

- Add 100 g of table salt (sodium chloride) to 1 litre of vegetable cooking oil. Use a nylon brush to scrub the affected area thoroughly with the mixture every day until the patches disappear.
- Scrub the patches thoroughly with a dry brush. Smear tar or camel colostrum (the thick, first milk) on the patches once a day until they disappear.
- Make a paste of henna and water and use it to cover the affected area. INDIA
- Treat the infected area with Ectosep or Charmil once a day until cured. AYURVEDIC

Modern treatments

- Wash the patches with soap and water to remove the crusts. Allow the skin to dry, then apply iodine solution or a 50:50 tincture of iodine–glycerine mixture. Repeat every 2 days until the patches disappear.
- Spray with enilconazole 0.2% (Imaverol) 2–3 times at 3-day intervals.
- Apply a topical antimycotic agent such as Mycostatin.

Caution: Griseofulvin, used in other animals for treating ringworm, is not recommended for camels because it may have side-effects.

References

Bizimana (1994) p. 15; Evans et al. (1995) p. 7:8–9; FAO (1994) p. 190, 258; Forse (1999) p. 180–2; Higgins (1986) p. 107–8; ITDG and IIRR (1996) p. 82–3; Manefield and Tinson (1997) p. 220–1; Projet Cameline (1999) p. 15, 19–20; Rathore (1986) p. 159; Schwartz and Dioli (1992) p. 175, 205–6; Wilson (1998) p. 106.

Pox

***Abdarra, aftara, baga?, irgo* (Gabbra), *chechak, mata* (India), *mokoyon* (Pokot), *afturro, afturu* (Rendille), *afturro, abituro* (Samburu), *afrur, furuk* (Somali), *jedari* (Sudan), *ettune, ngiborwok* (Turkana)**

Pox is a contagious skin disease that mostly affects calves, but sometimes also adult camels. Outbreaks usually occur during the winter and early rainy season. The disease can be either mild or severe, and kills up to 30% of infected animals. The mild course is usually confined to the head. The severe form affects the whole body. The sores can become infected, worsening the animal's condition. Animals that recover are immune from the disease for life.

Signs

- Before any skin signs can be seen, the animals seem depressed, have fever and refuse to eat.
- Pimples begin around the mouth, nostrils and eyelids. They develop into blisters and eventually may form scabs. They may be found on the entire body.
- The hair falls out on the affected body parts.
- The lips and head may swell. In calves the head may be so swollen that they

cannot open their eyes or feed and suckle.

- Lymph nodes (particularly under the jaw) are swollen.
- The sores can attract flies, leading to maggot wounds.
- In the severest form, sores in the windpipe and lungs cause coughing.
- If the sores become infected, the animals may not eat enough, become weak and perhaps die.

Camel pox is easily confused with ▷*Orf*. Other diseases causing similar signs are ▷*Contagious skin necrosis*, *Ringworm* and *Mange*.

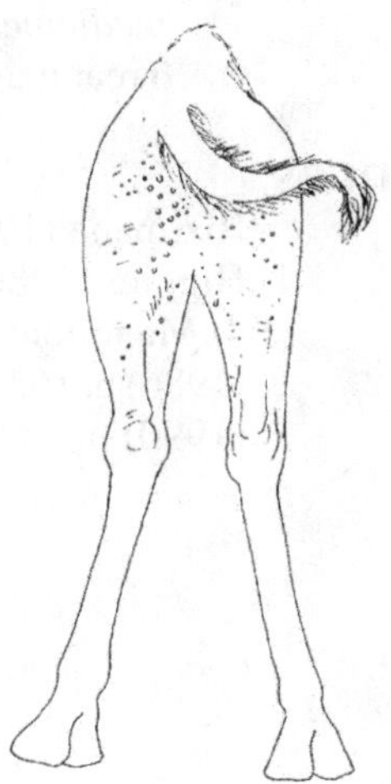

Cause

Orthopox virus. Pox is transmitted by direct contact with infected animals or by contaminated objects. Animals are immune after they recover from the disease.

Prevention

- Separate infected camels from healthy ones.
- Vaccinate camels against pox. A vaccine from South Africa is available. SCI
- Traditional vaccination: collect scabs from infected animals, and keep them in a coloured bottle in a cool place. Early in the dry season, grind the scabs and dissolve them in milk. Prick the lips or nose of healthy calves and rub the milk mixture into the scratches. RAIKA, REBARI, GARI SOMALI

Treatment

Because pox is caused by a virus, you can treat only the symptoms and prevent the sores from becoming infected. Make sure the animal eats and drinks enough so it can recover by itself. If calves are in good condition and are encouraged to suckle, they usually survive.

Traditional treatments

- Apply fine mud on the sores.
- Grind the seeds of bitter apple (*Citrullus colocynthis*), and heat them until they form a liquid tar (called *gutran* in Arabic). Rub the tar into the affected area. Repeat this treatment at 2-day intervals until the animal is cured. Instead of the bitter apple seeds, a mixture of sesame or cottonseed oil with table salt (sodium chloride) can be used at 7–10 day intervals until the sores disappear. LAHAWIYIN, RASHAIDA, SHUKRIYA
- Apply sheep-tail fat or goat fat onto the sores. RENDILLE, GABBRA
- Apply camel urine on the sores. RENDILLE
- Apply fresh camel milk twice daily on the sores. GARI SOMALI

Modern treatments

- Spray the affected body parts with a mild, non-irritant antiseptic, such as potassium permanganate. Inject antihistamines such as pheniramine maleate (e.g.,

5–10 ml Avil) into the muscle to control the severe irritation and itching.

- If the sores become infected, inject a broad-spectrum antibiotic (▷*Common medicines*), and spray the sores with a topical antibiotic.
- Treat maggot wounds (▷*Wounds and burns*).

References

Bizimana (1994) p. 324–6; Evans et al. (1995) p. 7:7–8; Forse (1999) p. 177–80; Higgins (1986) p. 93–5; ITDG and IIRR (1996) p. 80–1; Kaufmann (1998) p. 193–4; Manefield and Tinson (1997) p. 240; Projet Cameline (1999) p. 21–2; Rathore (1986) p. 167–8; Schwartz and Dioli (1992) p. 155–6, 163–4; Sewell and Brocklesby (1990) p. 283–4; Wernery and Kaaden (1995) p. 81–5; Wilson (1998) p. 99.

Orf

Camel contagious ecthyma, contagious pustular dermatitis, scabby mouth, parapox cameli

humbururu, mburur **(Borana, Gabbra),** ***moomri*** **(India),** ***auzdik*** **(Kazakhstan),** ***ngirimen*** **(Pokot),** ***non-kutukie, lopedo*** **(Samburu),** ***ambarrur, mburur*** **(Somali),** ***kulait, abu shalamboo*** **(Sudan),** ***ngiborwok, mburuwok*** **(Turkana)**

Orf is an acute pox-like disease that mostly infects calves, although adult animals can also be affected. Diseased animals lose condition and have pustules on the lips and face. Orf does not usually kill camels, but if they are not able to eat, they may die. The local names for orf are often the same as for ▷*Pox*.

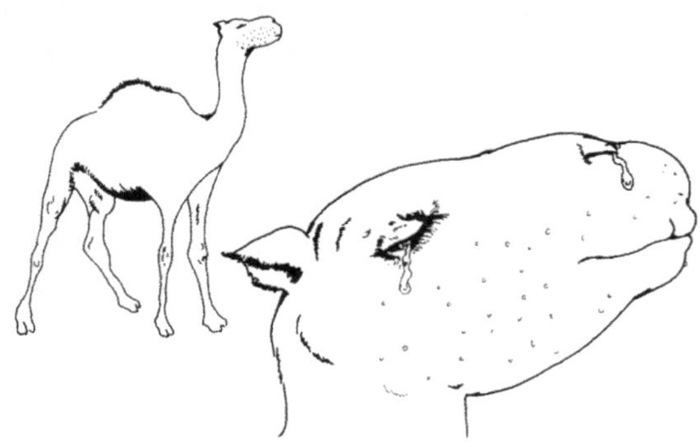

Signs

- Fever and depression.
- Watery eyes.
- Nodules develop on the lips. They quickly change into small blisters that contain fluid. These break open, forming scabs and then cracked crusts, which may bleed if you try to remove them.
- More blisters may form on the lips and sometimes inside the mouth and nose.
- The whole head may swell, possibly making the animal blind.
- The sores may become infected by bacteria or attract flies (▷*Pox*).

Orf is easy to confuse with ▷*Pox*. It usually occurs at the start of the rainy season, when camels are browsing on thorny trees. The sores are usually only on the lips and head. An electron microscope is necessary to distinguish the orf virus from that of pox. In the field it is often difficult to tell the two diseases apart.

Other diseases that may be confused with orf are ▷*Contagious skin necrosis, Ringworm* and *Mange.*

Orf can occasionally be transmitted to humans.

Cause

Parapox virus. The disease occurs mainly during the rainy season. It is highly contagious, transmitted through body contact and contaminated objects. Small injuries on the lips from browsing on thorny trees make it easy for the disease to infect animals. Animals that recover seem to be immune.

Prevention

No orf vaccine specifically for camels is yet available. Some specialists say they have used sheep vaccine successfully, but others say this is not effective. Scientists are developing a vaccine against both camel pox and orf.

- **Traditional vaccination**: early in the dry season, collect scabs from infected animals during an outbreak of the disease. Store these until needed in a plastic bag. Crush the scabs and mix with a little milk. Rub a rough stone on the lips of young camels (3–4 months old) until they begin to bleed, then smear on the milk mixture. Do this during the dry season, as then the disease will be mild. The animals recover in a few days, and their feeding is not disturbed. RAJASTHAN, TRAD+SCI

Treatment

Because orf is caused by a virus, you can treat only the symptoms. Treat the sores and prevent them from becoming infected. Watch the animal and make sure it eats and drinks enough so it can recover by itself.

Traditional treatments

- Make tar from the seeds of bitter apple (colocynth, *Citrullus colocynthis*) and apply this on the sores.
- Boil the fruits of *Ximenia americana* to make a paste. Smear this on the affected parts. KENYA
- Apply sheep-tail fat or goat fat on the sores. RENDILLE, GABBRA
- Apply camel urine on the sores. RENDILLE
- Firing on the lymph glands under the back of the jaw. This is said to activate the animal's defence mechanism (▷*Branding*). SHUKRIYA

Modern treatments

- Rub antiseptic ointment onto the sores. Inject a broad-spectrum antibiotic to avoid secondary bacterial complications (▷*Common medicines*).
- Since calves have difficulties feeding, watch them closely to make sure they eat and drink enough.

References

Bizimana (1994) p. 327; Evans et al. (1995) p. 7:8; Forse (1999) p. 167–8; ITDG and IIRR (1996) p. 79; Kaufmann (1998) p. 193–4; Manefield and Tinson (1997) p. 241; Schwartz and Dioli (1992) p. 156, 165; Sewell and Brocklesby (1990) p. 337–40; Wernery and Kaaden (1995) p. 85–7; Wilson (1998) p. 99–100.

Ticks

***Shelem, shini* (Borana), *chilim, shilmi, yagar, yakhal* (Gabbra), *gudad* (Kordofan), *shilim, chillim, turdach* (Rendille), *ilmangeri, lmanjeri, lmansher, ltunturi* (Samburu), *shilin, yakhal* (Somali), *gurad* (Sudan), *emadang, ngimadang* (Turkana)**

Ticks are external parasites that attach themselves to the animal's skin and suck blood. They occur throughout the year, though their numbers are highest after the rainy season and decrease towards the end of the dry season. They are much more common in East Africa than in India. In Kenya, a camel can have 50–100 ticks or more.

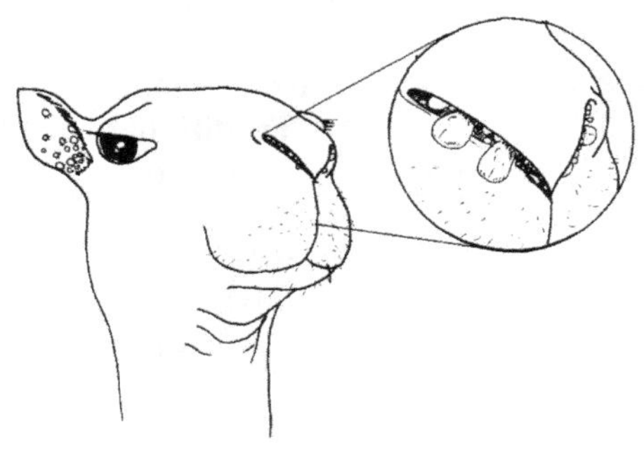

Ticks may play a role in causing ▷*Haemorrhagic septicaemia*, but the main harm they cause is by sucking blood, which may lead to anaemia in camel calves. In Kenya, anaemia caused by ticks is an important cause of calf deaths. Ticks can also cause paralysis in calves.

Ticks carry several diseases that cause no signs of illness in camels, but which may be serious in people. These include Crimean-Congo haemorrhagic fever and Q-fever (▷*Diseases that people can catch from camels*).

Signs

- Ticks on the body: most often around the base of the tail and the anus, in the groin and armpit, and around the ears and eyes.
- Itchiness and irritation where ticks are attached.
- The bites may become infected.
- Sometimes extensive bleeding and anaemia if there are large numbers of ticks.
- Pale colour on the gums and under the tongue (anaemia).
- Weakness and loss of weight.
- Ticks around the eye can cause conjunctivitis (▷*Eye problems*).
- If there are many ticks on the body, the animal may become paralysed (see below).
- Ticks on the udder (especially *Amblyomma*) can cause deep wounds (▷*Wounds and burns*) or ▷*Mastitis*.

Cause

The most common ticks affecting camels belong to the genera *Amblyomma, Hyalomma, Dermacentor* and *Rhipicephalus* (all hard ticks) or the family Argasidae (soft ticks). The life cycle of ticks is quite complex.

- ***Hyalomma*** tick larvae wait on vegetation until an animal or bird passes by.

They attach themselves to the host's skin, suck blood, develop into nymphs, and then drop off. They develop into adults on the ground, then attach themselves to another host animal (such as a camel), where they breed and the females suck more blood. The females then drop off again and lay their eggs on the ground.

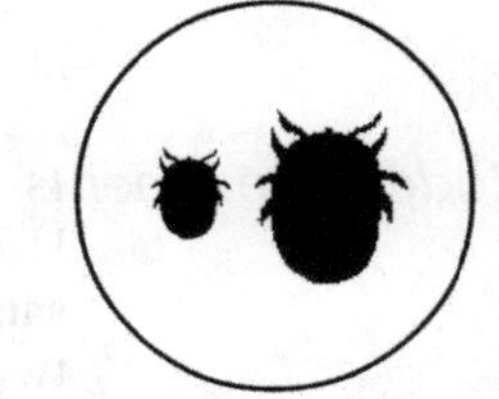

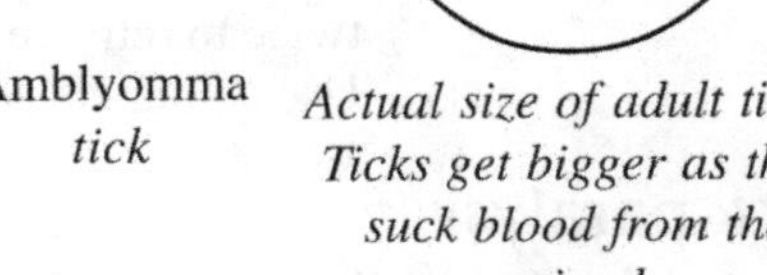

Amblyomma *tick*

Actual size of adult ticks. Ticks get bigger as they suck blood from the animal.

- ***Amblyomma, Dermacentor*** **and** ***Rhipicephalus*** ticks have a similar life cycle, except that they have three hosts instead of two.
- **Argasidae**, or soft ticks, can have many host animals. They suck blood from one host for up to 90 minutes, then drop off to develop into the next stage in their life cycle. They then attach to another host, suck some more blood, and drop off again. They may do this many times during their life cycle.

Prevention

- Avoid tick-infested pastures.
- Avoid overcrowding at watering sites and in enclosures.
- If there are too many ticks, move the enclosure site.
- Regularly remove ticks from calves.
- Routinely smear the places on the camel's body preferred by ticks with acaricidal (anti-tick) grease or ointment.

Treatment

- **Removing ticks by hand** If you pull hard on a tick to remove it, the mouth parts may stay embedded in the camel's skin, causing an infection. Instead, gently pull on its body and turn it around several times. Collect the ticks and burn them or drop them in a can containing mineral oil.

Traditional treatments

- Carefully pull ticks off the animal and burn them. Apply oil or warm ash to treat wounds that may occur. TURKANA, TRAD+SCI
- Graze the camels on young (20–30 cm high) *Cymbopogon nerrvalus(?)* (*nal*) plants. This will remove all the ticks. SUDAN
- Allow the camels to wallow in shallow, muddy pools. SAMBURU, TURKANA
- Make the camels wade in sea water, or pour sea water on them for several hours. This will get rid of adult ticks and those that have sucked blood. The ticks dry out in place, or they drop off.
- Boil 0.25 kg of tobacco leaves in 4 litres of water. Add 1 litre of soapy water. Use this liquid to wash the animal. TRAD+SCI
- Crush 1 handful of *Aloe broomii* leaves, mix with 1 litre of water, and brush on infested parts of the animal's body.
- Mix 1 litre of camel urine with a handful of gum resin of *hagar* (*Commiphora erythraea*) or *damaji* (*Commiphora incisa*). Heat and stir to make a paste.

Apply on parts where the ticks attach. They die and other ticks are repelled for 1 week. SOMALI

- Dry 5 kg of *eteteleit (Acalypha fruticosa)* leaves and crush them to powder. Soak one handful of the powder in 250 ml of water for 1 hour. Pour off the water and smear the sediment onto the tick-infested ears. TURKANA

Modern treatments

- Use commercial acaricides such as Gammatox, Bremer dip and Triatix with the same dilutions prescribed for mange (▷*Mange*). Repeat the treatments at least twice to remove all the ticks.
- Use a pour-on acaricide such as flumethrin (Bayticol) every 3–4 weeks.

Tick paralysis

Very large numbers of ticks on a camel's body can cause paralysis and death. Tick paralysis particularly affects camel calves. The animal recovers rapidly (in 1–3 days) if the ticks are removed in time.

Young ticks (nymphs) can be hard to see because they attach themselves in areas with long hair, such as the shoulders and hump. You have to touch these places to detect the ticks. This is one reason that calves are often sheared around the shoulder and hump.

Signs

- Hundreds of ticks all over the camel's body.
- High temperature, marked dullness and anaemia.
- Stiff legs, stiffness when walking.
- These signs get stronger and spread to other parts of the body within a few hours.
- The animal cannot get up, sit or move its legs.
- The animal does not suckle or feed.
- It has difficulty in breathing, chewing and swallowing.
- The animal loses consciousness and dies because it cannot breathe.

Treatment

- Remove the ticks (see above). Shear the fur and use an acaricide (anti-tick medicine) if there are too many ticks to remove by hand (see *Modern treatments* above). SCI
- Give glucose solution or sugary water to the animal to drink if it is already weak. SCI

References

Bizimana (1994) p. 24–8; Evans et al. (1995) p. 7:10–11; FAO (1994) p. 189–90; Forse (1999) p. 105–8, 339–45; Higgins (1986) p. 76–81; ITDG and IIRR (1996) p. 101–3; Kaufmann (1998) p. 194; Manefield and Tinson (1997) p. 260–2; Projet Cameline (1999) p. 23; Rathore (1986) p. 181; Schwartz and Dioli (1992) p. 177–8, 207–8; Sewell and Brocklesby (1990) p. 3–12; 28–32; Wilson (1998) p. 104–5.

Lice and fleas

Lice: injirre (Gabbra), lache (Samburu), injir (Somali Kenya), elachit, ng'ilach (Turkana), jehun, khosa (India)
Fleas: Tuffi njiraa (Gabbra), losusu (Samburu), injit (Somali Kenya), ng'ikorobotio (Turkana)

Lice and fleas can be a problem especially in areas with cold winters where camels grow long hair.

Signs

- Irritation and itchiness.
- Hair loss, especially at flanks and shoulder, from rubbing and biting.
- Loss of weight.
- Decrease in milk yield.
- Lice (about 4 mm long and greyish) can be seen when parting the skin; their greyish-yellow eggs (nits) are attached to the base of the hairs.
- Fleas can sometimes be seen jumping from the camel.

Cause

The scientific name of the camel louse is *Haematopinus cameli.* The flea that infects camels is *Vermipsylla* spp. Lice spend all their life on the camel, reproduce there, and suck the camel's blood. Fleas lay their eggs off the camel, e.g., in the grass where the camel rests. The eggs hatch and develop into larvae and then into mature adults. The adults jump on and off camels and feed on their blood.

Prevention

Keep resting places and all things that come into contact with the camels (e.g., harness, saddles, blankets) clean.

Treatment

Traditional treatments

- Cut the camel's hair short. Mix salty soil with enough water or camel's urine to make a creamy mixture. Dip a cloth into the mixture and rub it over the camel's body. Make sure the mixture does not enter the eyes. The lice will fall off and die. Repeat as often as necessary. GABBRA
- Wash the camel with naturally salty water. GABBRA, SOMALI

Modern treatments

- Spray with cypermethrin, permethrin, or deltamethrin (▷*Common medicines*). Treat the whole herd. Repeat after 2 weeks. Also spray the harness, saddles and blankets.
- Inject with ivermectin at a dose of 0.2 mg/kg body weight under the skin (e.g., 1 ml of Ivomec for every 50 kg of the camel's body weight). Repeat after 2 months.

References

ITDG and IIRR (1996) p. 93–5; Leese (1927) p. 349; Manefield and Tinson (1997) p. 98, 149; Rathore (1986) p. 181.

Dermatophilosis

Mycotic dermatitis, streptothricosis

A skin disease mainly of young camels. The hair becomes matted and encrusted. Adults are rarely infected. People can catch the disease if they come into contact with infected animals.

Signs

- The skin becomes swollen and red, and begins to weep fluid.
- The fluid dries, forming a characteristic crust. If the crust is removed, you can see a wet, reddish area that weeps a thick, bloody fluid.
- The base of the neck, flanks and sometimes the legs are most often affected.

Other diseases producing similar signs are ▷*Ringworm, Mange* and *Contagious skin necrosis*.

Cause

A fungus-like bacterium (*Dermatophilus congolensis*). Camels become infected by rubbing against infected animals or objects, through the bites of insects and ticks, and through scratches from acacia thorns. The disease is found in rainy areas.

Prevention

- Isolate and treat infected animals.
- Control ticks (▷*Ticks*).

Treatment

The disease can usually be left untreated, as it will disappear as the camel grows. If you do treat an animal, the sores take about 4 weeks to heal fully.

- Remove the scabs and hair, then hand-spray the sores with an antiseptic such as Dermaclens, Otoderm, or a 5% solution of Lotagen once a day for 10 days. SCI
- Inject long-acting tetracycline into the muscle twice (wait for 3 days before giving the second injection). SCI
- Apply 1% potassium aluminium sulphate solution on the affected areas, and inject procaine penicillin and streptomycin (▷*Common medicines*). SCI
- Wash the sores with iodine solution once a day for 7 days to help the skin to heal. SCI

References

Forse (1999) p. 170–1; Manefield and Tinson (1997) p. 72–3; Sewell and Brocklesby (1990) p. 68–72; Wanyama (1997) vol. 2, p. 25–9, 61–2; Wernery and Kaaden (1995) p. 67–70.

Bites and stings

Biting flies: *lajuigani* (Samburu), *ng'ichuchu* (Turkana)
Camel flies (*Hippobosca camelina*): *takar* (Somali)
Mosquitoes: *binni* (Gabbra), *nkajing'ani* (Samburu), *kanea* (Somali), *ng'isuru* (Turkana)
Tsetse flies: *dug, duga* (Gabbra), *gendi* (Somali), *lopodokong'or* (Turkana)
Tanganids and tsetse: *lpupoi* (Samburu)

Camels can be bitten or stung by various types of flies, spiders, scorpions and naked mole-rats. These cause irritation and localized swelling. Some insects can spread diseases such as trypanosomiasis.

The Samburu, Rendille and Gabbra in Kenya attribute sudden, unexplained deaths to bites of hunting spiders and even naked mole-rats. Although scorpion stings are very painful and sometimes can kill people, they do not seem to have the same effect on camels.

For information on bites caused by dogs, predators and snakes, ▷*Wounds and burns* and *Snake bites*.

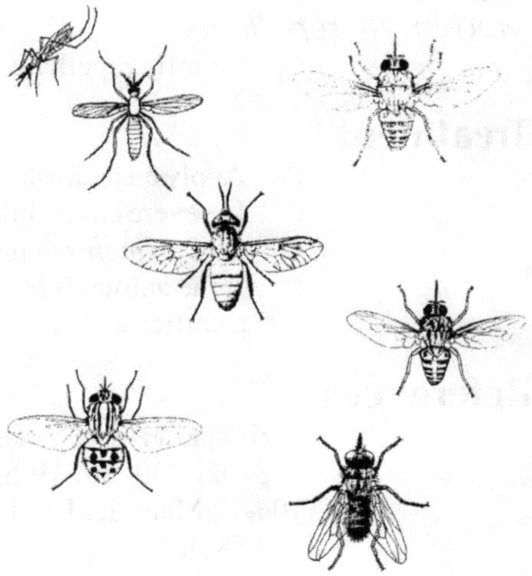

Signs

- Camel does not feed properly.
- Camel runs away.
- Localized swelling.
- Blood stains on the belly.

Cause

- Most biting animals introduce a toxin, to which the camel has a mild (or occasionally severe) localized allergic reaction.

Prevention

- Avoid areas with biting flies, especially thick bush or woodland. TRAD
- Move animals to watering places when few flies are active – i.e., in the middle of the day. TRAD
- Avoid building enclosures where scorpion holes or naked mole-rat mounds occur. TRAD
- Move to a windy area where there are fewer flies. TRAD

Smoke to drive away flies and mosquitoes

- Burn dung or green wood upwind so the smoke drives away the flies.
- Burn *Commiphora erythraea* (*hagar*) gum upwind of the animals. SOMALI
- Burn the dry leaves of *Boscia coriacea* (*edung*), *Salvadora persica* (*esokon*), *Cadaba rotundifolia* (*epuu*) and *Calotropis procera* (*etesuro*) upwind of the animals. TURKANA
- Burn *Eucalyptus* (*bahra-saf*) upwind of the animals. SOMALI

Traditional fly repellents

- Apply mud all over the camel's body. Useful against mosquitoes if done at night.
- Remove the outer coat of fresh neem (*Azadirachta indica*) seeds and pound the seeds until the kernels turn brown and slightly sticky. Add a little water to make a kneadable paste. Knead and squeeze the paste until no more oil comes out. You can get about 100–150 ml of oil per kg of neem seed. Collect the oil and smear on the animal's skin. Ready-made neem oil is also sold commercially in some places.
- Break off a small branch of *Euphorbia balsamifera*, peel the bark off, and collect the latex in a bowl. Smear the latex on the animal's body.
- Pound fresh leaves of *Sesbania sesban* in a container. Add water and rub the mixture on the animal's body.
- Pound the roots of *Cissus producta* and add enough water to make an emulsion. Apply the emulsion to the animal's body.
- Pound 1 kg of fresh root of *anthatha*. Mix with 1 litre of water and let it stand overnight. Apply to the animal's body. GABBRA

Modern fly repellents

- Pour fly repellents such as permethrin and cypermethrin on the animals' backs.

Treatment

- Apply an antihistamine for painful local swellings (▷*Common medicines*). SCI
- In severe cases, inject an antibiotic to prevent the bites from becoming infected (▷*Common medicines*). SCI
- If the animal is in shock (for example, calves after a scorpion sting), inject with a corticosteroid. SCI

References

Bizimana (1994) p. 18–20; Evans (1995) p. 7:9, 11–12; Forse (1999) p. 103–5, 158–62, 339–45; Higgins (1986) p. 85–8; ITDG and IIRR (1996) p. 88–9, 98, 104–5; Manefield and Tinson (1997) p. 99–100; Rathore (1986) p. 181; Schwartz and Dioli (1992) p. 179–80, 209; Sewell and Brocklesby (1990) p. 13–32.

Snake bite

***Onyoto la surai* (Samburu), *akanyyat* (Turkana)**

Snakes can bite on the legs, udder, lips, and any part of the body while the camel is sitting or browsing. It can be hard to see the bite site if it is on a hairy part of the body.

Signs

The signs depend on the type of snake and the body part bitten.

- The animal bellows loudly and for a long time.
- It stops grazing.

- It becomes restless and loses co-ordination.
- Swelling at the site of the bite.
- Foaming from the mouth, protruding tongue.
- The bite wound bleeds if the animal is bitten by certain snakes, such as a brownish snake called *enum bokirimu* in Turkana.
- Sloughing off of the udder quarter affected (if the bite is on the udder).
- Death, especially when bitten in the throat.

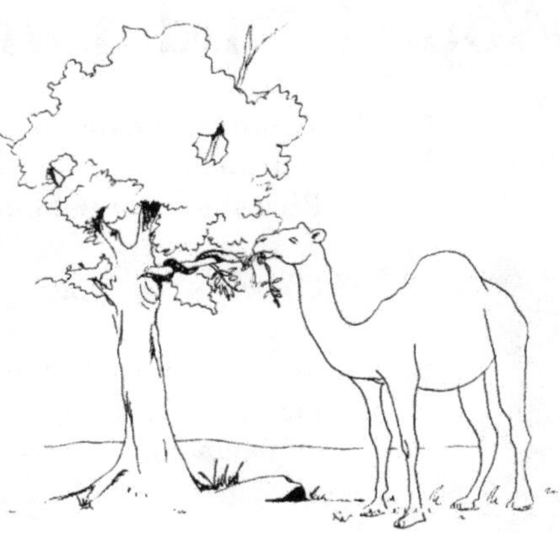

Prevention

- Clear the bush around the enclosure.
- Pour salty water around places where snakes are found. TRAD

Treatment

Traditional treatments

- Tie a tourniquet (a tight rope or bandage) above the bite. Using a knife, widen the location of the bite, and allow it to bleed. The poison flows out together with the blood. SCI+TRAD
- After making the site of the bite bleed (see above), press a black, volcanic stone, 2–3 cm in diameter, on the fresh wound. If the snake is poisonous, the stone sticks to the wound. It falls off after a few hours or days. After the stone falls off, soak it in milk overnight and then rinse it with water. Stick it on the wound again. Press it on the wound for 5 minutes. It will fall off again if all the poison has been removed. In Kenya, the stones are obtained from Tanzania. Treat the wound like any other wound (▷*Wounds and burns*). LAMU, KENYA
- Drench with 2–4 kg of cow ghee, mixed with 150–250 g of powdered black pepper. INDIA
- Drench with 2–3 litres of human urine, and repeat 2 hours later with another 2 litres. INDIA

Modern treatments

- Electric shock treatment for snake bites: as soon as possible after the animal is bitten, put the affected area (usually a leg) on the ground (to earth it electrically). Use a cattle prod or a lead from a car spark plug to apply an electric shock to the bite for 1–2 seconds. Repeat 4–5 times at intervals of 5–10 seconds. If treated soon enough (within 30 minutes of the bite), all pain disappears in 10–15 minutes.
- If available, inject antihistamines and antivenin (i.e., the medicine that counteracts the poison).

References

Bizimana (1994) p. 381; Evans et al. (1995) p. 7:32, 7:36; FAO (1994) p. 227; Forse (1999) p. 307; ITDG and IIRR (1996) p. 37; Manefield and Tinson (1997) p. 243–4; Rathore (1986) p. 190–1.

Wounds and burns

Wounds: *madaa* (Gabbra), *ngoldonyot* (Samburu), *boog* (Somali), *ngajemei* (Turkana)
Burns: *gubatu* (Gabbra), *gubush* (Somali), *nganoman* (Turkana)

Camels are very prone to wounds. Wounds may be shallow (such as scratches caused by thorns) or deep (such as a spear wound). Wounds are injuries that cause breaks in the skin. The type of wound depends on what caused it. Burns damage the skin and, like wounds, can result in infection.

Wounds often heal slowly, especially if they are infected by maggots. The wounds presented to the veterinarian are often old ones. For more information on infected wounds, ▻*Skin abscesses*. For how to sew fresh wounds closed, ▻*Surgery*.

Signs

- Broken skin.
- Bleeding in fresh wounds.
- Wounds attract flies.
- Pus, crust or maggots in older wounds.
- Dead flesh in older wounds.
- Dirt in the wound, especially in puncture wounds and if the wound touches the ground.
- Possibly a bad smell from older wounds.
- Lameness, in foot wounds (▻*Foot problems*).
- Grunting while rising or sitting down, in chest-pad wounds (▻*Chest-pad abscess*).

Causes

- Injury by thorns during grazing.
- Ill-fitting saddles, poor tethering or tying.
- Whipping or beating the animal too hard with a stick.
- Bites by male camels or wild animals.
- Injury to the feet or chest-pad by sharp stones or thorns.
- Castration.

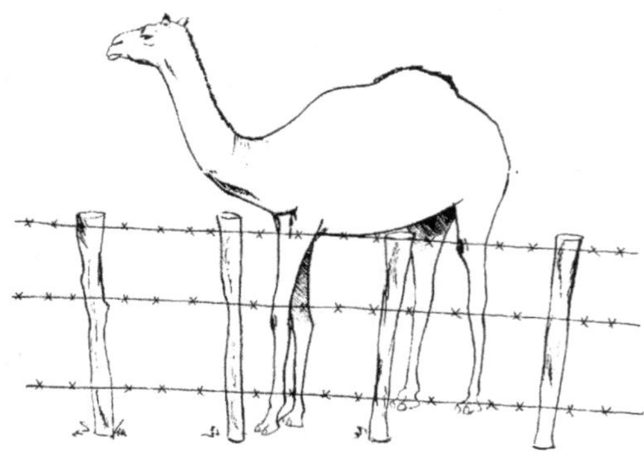

Prevention

- Use thick rope to tie animals so the rope does not cut into the skin. Do not tie the rope too tightly.
- Make sure that saddles fit well and have enough padding.
- Avoid herding on stony ground.
- Prevent fights among males and attacks by wild animals.
- Treat any skin infections promptly.

- Sterilize knives used for castration or surgery by holding them over a flame until they are red-hot. Cool them before using, but do not put them on the ground.

Treatment

Wounds can easily become infested with fly maggots, so many of the treatments given here are used to repel flies. See ▷*Bites and stings* for other fly repellents. There are many traditional treatments for wounds. Some are listed below.

Basic wound treatments

- Clean the wound with salt water (mix 2 teaspoons of common salt with a bottle of clean, boiled water), or with diluted vinegar or sodium bicarbonate (dilute in the same way as the salt). TRAD
- Clean the wound with Ectosep, Charmil or Himax. Renew the dressing once a day until the wound heals. AYURVEDIC
- Clean the wound (see above). Mix a little very clean, fine white wood-ash with the salty water to make a paste, and put this on the wound. TRAD
- Clean the wound with an antiseptic (▷*Common medicines*) and dress with tetracycline spray, antibiotic cream, sulphanilamide or Negasunt. Renew the dressing once a day until the wound heals. You can also use this for older wounds that are slightly infected (contain pus). SCI
- It may be necessary to sew closed a fresh wound, such as an incision made during surgery. Clean the wound with an antiseptic, cut out any dead flesh, and sew the skin closed with a needle and strong thread (▷*Surgery*). Do not sew closed any old or infected wounds.
- To stop bleeding, apply the juice or flesh of *Aloe* leaves or a 10% solution of alum.

See also the list of traditional wound dressings below.

Traditional wound dressings

- Grind or chew a 7 cm root of *hamboy* (*Aerva* spp.). Add a little water if necessary to make a paste. Apply the paste to the bleeding wound. SOMALI
- Pound 10 seeds of *seketet* (*Myrsine africana*) into powder. Apply the powder directly to the wound to dry it. SAMBURU
- Grind a handful of *habak cadad* (gum arabic, from *Acacia senegal*) and add a glass of water. Boil the mixture to make a paste. Apply the paste to the wound surface once a day. Isolate the animal for close observation and nursing. The sticky gum dries the wound and repels flies. SOMALI
- Crush a handful of fresh *habak hagar* (gum from *Commiphora erythraea*) or *malmal* (myrrh, from *Commiphora myrrha*) in a mortar. Add a glass of warm water and stir to make a paste. Apply the paste to the wound once a day until the wound heals. This repels flies. SOMALI
- Crush a handful of fresh gum from *habak hagar* (gum from *Commiphora erythraea*) in a mortar to make a powder. Dust the powder onto the wound to control bleeding. SOMALI
- Crush the inner layer of *Acacia bussei* bark and mix in 1 litre of water. Pour the liquid drop by drop into the wound until it is covered. SOMALI ETHIOPIA
- Uproot a whole *qorsa worana* plant and burn it to charcoal. Crush to powder. Apply a handful of this onto the wound. GABBRA
- Grind 1 kg of *eteteleit (Acalypha fruticosa)* into powder. Apply the powder onto the wound. Repeat treatment after every 2 days until the wound heals. TURKANA

- Apply juice from *lokurusio* (*Caralluma* sp.) onto the wound every 2 days until it heals. TURKANA
- Puncture the stem or leaves of *lparaa* (*Euphorbia* sp.), collect the latex and smear it on the wound. SAMBURU
- Crush the terminal root of the *balan baal* (*Ficus populifolia*) tree and apply the sap on the wound. SOMALI ETHIOPIA
- Crush seeds of *Ricinus communis* and boil them to make an oil. Apply this on the wound. NIGERIA
- Make oil from the seeds of *Balanites aegyptiaca* and apply it on the wound. NIGERIA
- Burn the roots and root-bark of *Calotropis procera* to make charcoal, and mix with a little liquid to make an ointment. Apply this on the wound. NIGERIA
- Grind the leaves of *Solenostemma argel* into a powder and apply on the wound. NIGERIA
- Grind the bark of *Acacia nilotica* or *Adansonia digitata* into a powder and apply on the wound. DOSSO
- Crush 0.25 kg of dried seeds of *seketet (Myrsine africana)* and boil in sheep fat. Allow to cool. Pour the fat while it is still liquid onto the wound. This treatment is especially used for deep wounds. Repeat if the wound has not healed. Alternatively, apply the dry powered seeds directly. SAMBURU

Burns

- Wash the burn with a lot of clean, cold water as soon as possible. Wash it with a mild antiseptic, then put on a wound dressing (see above). If the burn is large and severe, inject with an antibiotic. SCI
- Apply the clear, gel-like pulp from aloe (*Aloe vera*) to the burn. TRAD
- Smear cow dung or goat dung onto the wound and leave it for 2 days. Then treat with *eteteleit* (*Acalypha fruticosa*) or *lokurusio* (*Caralluma* sp.). TURKANA

Infected wounds

For minor infections, see *Basic wound treatments* and *Traditional wound dressings* above. For more serious infections (with pus and possibly maggots), use one of the treatments below.

- Clean the wound with hydrogen peroxide and put brown sugar or honey on it.
- For wounds with maggots, dip a swab of cotton wool in Maggacite and pack into the wound for at least one day. Next day, clean the wound and remove the dead maggots. AYURVEDIC
- Cut off the hair around the wound. Pick out any maggots, either with a forceps or by applying a ball of cotton wool soaked with a medicine that kills maggots, such as phenyl or turpentine oil, for 10 minutes. Make sure any pus can drain out by cutting a slot into the skin. Remove dead tissue from the edge of the wound with a scalpel or clean, sharp knife. Clean the wound by flushing it with an antiseptic. Apply an antibiotic dressing. If the animal is valuable, consider injecting it against tetanus. SCI
- Treat deep wounds with an antibiotic used against mastitis. These antibiotics come in a syringe with a blunt point instead of a needle. Use this syringe to squirt the antibiotic into the wound. SCI
- If the wound is deep and produces pus, use the treatment above, and flush it out with an antiseptic once a day for several days (▷*Common medicines*). SCI

References

Bizimana (1994) p. 365–6; Evans et al. (1995) p. 7:33; FAO (1994) p. 215–18, 254; Forse (1999) p. 69–73; Gahlot and Chouhan (1992) p. 148–9; Higgins (1986) p. 124–5; ITDG and IIRR (1996) p. 69–72; Leese (1927) p. 161–4; Projet Cameline (1999) p. 23; Rathore (1986) p. 204; Schwartz and Dioli (1992) p. 186–90, 213–14; Wanyama (1997) vol. 2, p. 47–52, 85–90.

Skin abscesses

***Mala, malah* (Gabbra, Rendille), *ngemek, ntubui* (Samburu), *mal, mala, malah, bahtin, waglal* (Somali), *adjumei, abus, ngubuthien, lobus* (Turkana)**

An abscess is a collection of pus, surrounded by inflamed tissue. Abscesses can occur anywhere on the body, but they are most common on the lymph nodes (▷*Abscesses on the lymph nodes*), the head and neck, chest-pad, saddle region and feet.

Signs

- Painful, inflamed swelling, often hot.
- The abscess may break open, releasing yellow, creamy pus.

A swollen area on the left flank of the body may be a hernia (where the a loop of the intestine has pushed its way through the muscle around the body cavity). Press on this swelling with your hand. If it is a hernia or rupture, you should be able to reduce the swelling completely by pushing the intestine back into the body. Do not cut a hernia open.

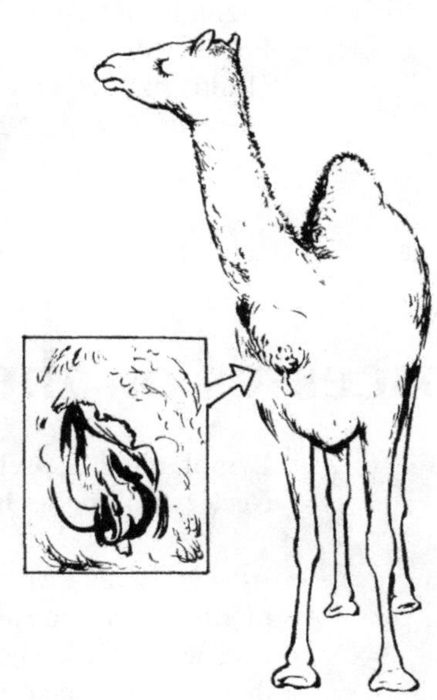

Cause

Abscesses may be caused by infection of scratches and wounds, as well as by various diseases (▷*Contagious skin necrosis, Abscesses on the lymph nodes* and *Wounds and burns*). For abscesses under the saddle and on the chest-pad, ▷*Saddle sores* and *Chest-pad abscess*.

Prevention

- Avoid injuring camels, for example with tools.
- Treat wounds early to avoid infection.
- Use clean needles for injections.

Treatment

Small abscesses often heal by themselves and require no treatment. Treat larger abscesses using the methods below.

Traditional treatments

Traditional healers often treat abscesses by ▷*Branding*.

The following treatments are used after the abscess has burst (or been opened).

- Burn an entire *qorsa worana* plant to make charcoal. Grind the charcoal to powder and apply to the wound once every 3 days until it heals. GABBRA
- Boil a handful of gum from *hagar* (*Commiphora erythraea*) in 50 ml of water. Cool and apply once onto the abscess wound. SOMALI

Modern treatments

- If the abscess is ripe, use a sterile scalpel blade, or heat a sharp knife in the fire to sterilize it. Cut the bottom of the abscess open so the pus can drain out. Make a big cut, so it continues to drain and does not close and seal the infection inside. Wash the wound with warm water to remove all the pus and debris, and then flush with an antiseptic (e.g., sterile water, saline solution, or 0.2–0.3% hydrogen peroxide). Apply a dressing such as tetracycline spray, antibiotic cream or sulphanilamide powder. If the camel has fever, inject an antibiotic such as penicillin or tetracycline (▷*Common medicines*).

References

Bizimana (1994) p. 356–7, 364; Evans et al. (1995) p. 7:13; FAO (1994) p. 223–4; Forse (1999) p. 252–3; Gahlot and Chouhan (1992) p. 41–2, 82, 109–10; Higgins (1986) p. 125; ITDG and IIRR (1996) p. 73–4; Kaufmann (1998) p. 188; Projet Cameline (1999) p. 25; Rathore (1986) p. 204; Schwartz and Dioli (1992) p. 212–13.

Abscesses on the lymph nodes

Lymphadenitis, pseudotuberculosis
Neck lymph nodes only: *Habis* (Sudan)

Abscesses may form in the lymph nodes of camels. The lymph nodes most commonly affected are at the bottom of the base of the neck, around the jaws, and on the back leg above the hock. Abscesses most frequently form in the lymph nodes, though they can also occur on other parts of the body (▷*Skin abscesses, Saddle sores* and *Chest-pad abscess*).

Signs

- The affected lymph nodes gradually increase in size, up to the size of an orange or larger.
- The lymph nodes are warm and can be painful.
- Small abscesses may disappear by themselves.
- Large abscesses burst open and discharge a creamy-yellowish pus.

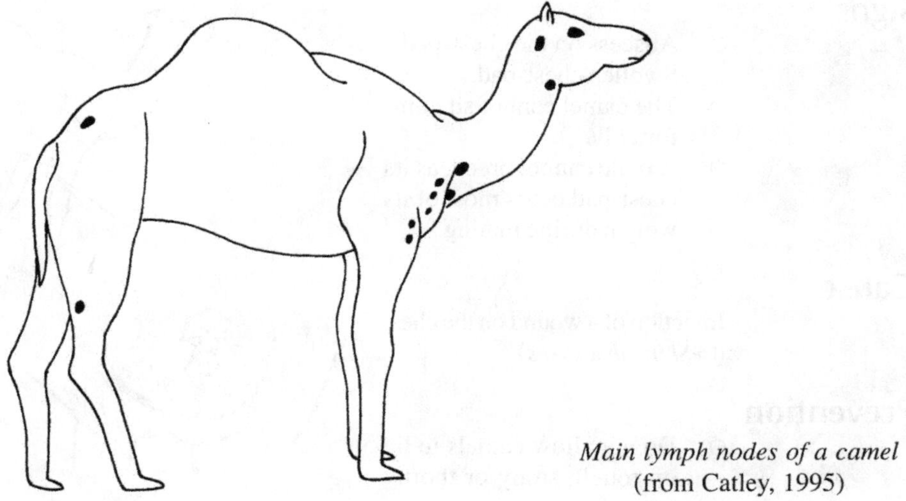

Main lymph nodes of a camel
(from Catley, 1995)

Some diseases make the lymph nodes swell without an abscess being present. Do not cut these lymph nodes open. Identify and treat the underlying disease instead (▷*Swollen glands, khanid*).

Cause

Bacteria, frequently *Corynebacterium pseudotuberculosis* (in adults) and *Staphylococcus* and *Streptococcus* in calves.

Prevention

- Keep healthy animals away from infected ones.

Treatment

See ▷*Skin abscesses* for treatments.

References

Catley (1995); Evans et al. (1995) p. 7:13; FAO (1994) p.223–4; Forse (1999) p. 186–7; Manefield and Tinson (1997) p. 240; Projet Cameline (1999) p. 25; Schwartz and Dioli (1992) p. 181–3, 212–13.

Chest-pad abscess

Pedestal abscess, sternal pad abscess
***Adder, adder badhana, adder ki chot* (India)**

The chest-pad of a camel touches the ground when the animal is sitting, so it can be injured easily by gravel or sharp objects on the ground. An abscess may form, and if untreated, this may cause the chest-pad to become swollen.

Signs

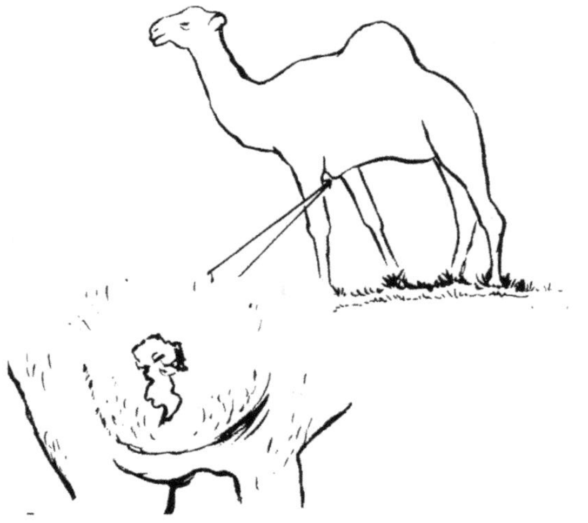

- Abscess on the chest-pad.
- Swollen chest-pad.
- The camel cannot sit comfortably.
- A male cannot breed, as its chest-pad bears most of its weight during mating.

Cause

Infection of a wound on the chest (▷*Skin abscesses*).

Prevention

- Do not allow camels to lie on rough, stony or thorny ground.
- Remove thorns from the night enclosure.

Treatment

Traditional treatments

- Apply turmeric (*Curcuma longa*) powder to the abscess.
- Apply kerosene or burnt engine oil on the abscess.

Modern treatments

- Restrain the animal and if possible, sedate it. Then treat as for ▷*Skin abscesses*. Tie a gunny bag over the dressing to protect the wound. Inject a broad-spectrum antibiotic into the muscle for 7–10 days (▷*Common medicines*).
- After opening and treating the abscess (see above), fix a doughnut-shaped dressing over the chest-pad to take the weight off the pad and prevent it from touching the ground when the camel is sitting.
- If the chest-pad is left untreated for a long time, it may grow very large, and it may be necessary to cut out the excess tissue. This is a major operation, difficult to do in the field. Anaesthetize the camel and lie it on its side (▷*Sedation and anaesthesia* and *Surgery*). Cut off the enlarged chest-pad with a sterilized scalpel and hacksaw. The wound will bleed profusely: stop this by cauterizing the wound with potassium permanganate or a red-hot iron (▷*Branding*). Then put on a clean dressing and protect the wound (see above).

References

Bizimana (1994) p. 359; Gahlot and Chouhan (1992) p. 124–5; Higgins (1986) p. 126; Leese (1927) p. 186; Manefield and Tinson (1997) p. 184; Rathore (1986) p. 214; Schwartz and Dioli (1992) p. 186–7, 214.

Saddle sores

Saddle gall
***Chandi, palan ka ghaw* (India)**

Saddle sores affect camels used for riding or carrying loads.

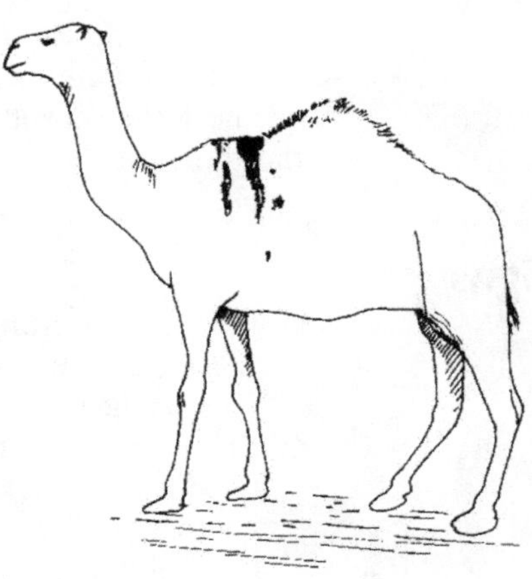

Signs

- ○ The animal feels pain when the saddle is put on.
- ○ The skin where the saddle presses becomes raw, or dry and cold.
- ○ Abscesses may develop (▷*Skin abscesses*).

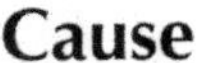

Cause

Continuous rubbing and pressure from the saddle damages the skin and tissue underneath. Pecking by birds may keep the sore open.

Prevention

- ○ Use a well-fitted and well-padded saddle.
- ○ Do not overload the animal.

Treatment

Traditional treatments

- ○ Cut open the sore and allow the pus to drain out. TUAREG AJJER
- ○ Dress the wound with the pounded bark of *Acacia nilotica* or *Adansonia digitata*. DOSSO
- ○ Dress the wound with dried, pounded *Khaya senegalensis*. NIGERIA
- ○ Cover the wound to protect it from birds.

Modern treatments

- ○ Restrain the animal, and if possible, sedate it. Using a scalpel, open the sore to drain out the pus and remove the dead tissue. Put magnesium sulphate powder in the hole. Flush each day for 3–4 days with 0.1% solution of potassium permanganate, then put in some more magnesium sulphate powder. Once the wound begins to heal, apply an antiseptic, fly repellent ointment. Cover it to protect it from birds. Inject a broad-spectrum antibiotic for 1 week (▷*Common medicines*). Do not put the saddle back on until the sores have healed (this may take weeks).

References

Bizimana (1994) p. 365–6; Forse (1999) p. 165; Gahlot and Chouhan (1992) p. 117–18; Higgins (1986) p. 125–6; Leese (1927) p. 164; Manefield and Tinson (1997) p. 227–8; Rathore (1986) p. 204.

Dermoids

Dermoid cysts
***Foda, maid* (India)**

Dermoids are egg-shaped growths on the skin, up to the size of an orange. They are found on the ears (firmly attached) and neck (loosely attached). They spoil the looks of the camel and lower its value.

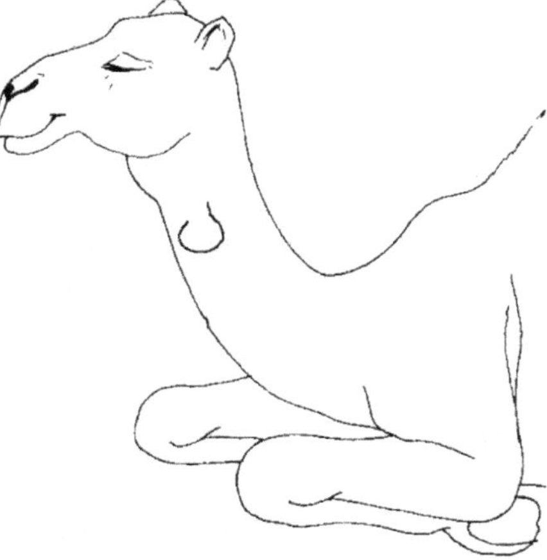

Signs

- Painless swellings (usually a pair) on the ears, or a single, large swelling on the neck.
- If you puncture the swelling with a needle, a black, odourless fluid comes out.

Dermoids may sometimes be confused with ▻*Skin abscesses*.

Treatment

Dermoids are harmless, and it is not normally necessary to remove them. If desired, the operation can be done by a skilled surgeon.

References

Gahlot and Chouhan (1992) p. 37–8; Manefield and Tinson (1997) p. 73.

3 Problems of the head and neck

This chapter covers problems of the eyes, ears, nose, mouth, teeth and neck. Many of the diseases covered in other chapters may also show signs in the camel's head and neck. See the tables below for details.

Problems affecting the eyes

Signs	Location	Cause	Disease
Partly or totally closed eye	Eyes	Pox, orf, other infections	▷*Eye problems, Pox, Orf*
Pimples on eyelids	Eyes	Pox, orf	▷*Pox, Orf*
Watery eyes, pus in eye	Eyes	Orf, saam, eye worms, nose or lung infection	▷*Orf, Eye problems, Problems of the nose and lungs, Saam*
Bloodshot eye	Eyes	Foreign body in eye, ticks, eye injury, sunstroke, eye worms	▷*Eye problems, Sunstroke, Ticks*
Animal bumps into objects	One or both eyes	Blindness, vitamin A deficiency	▷*Eye problems*
Whitish film on the eye ball (corneal opacity)	One or both eyes	Foreign body in eye, age	▷*Eye problems*
White of the eye seems to grow across eyeball	One eye	Third eyelid carcinoma	▷*Eye problems*
Membrane appears across eye	Eyes	Tetanus	▷*Tetanus*

Problems affecting the eyes, mouth and ears

Signs	Location	Cause	Disease
Pale mucous membranes in the eyes and mouth	Eyes, mouth	Anaemia (lack of red blood cells), loss of blood	▷*Trypanosomiasis, Internal parasites (worms), Saam, Ticks, Wounds and burns*
Dark red mucous membranes in the eyes and mouth	Eyes, mouth	Bacteria	▷*Haemorrhagic septicaemia*
Pus in ear	Ear	Ear infection, ticks in ear	▷*Ear infection*

Problems affecting the nose and mouth

Signs	Location	Cause	Disease
Wounded nostrils	Nose	Torn nostrils	▷*Torn nostrils*
Blisters	Mouth	Infection, vitamin B deficiency	▷*Blisters in the mouth*
Dulaa hangs out	Mouth	Injured *dulaa*	▷*Injured dulaa*
Poor chewing	Mouth	Molars irregular or too long	▷*Teeth problems*
Bad breath	Mouth	Normal in camels. Also, one cheek tooth too long, lungworms	▷*Teeth problems, Lungworms, Indigestion*
Lower jaw hangs down	Mouth	Broken jaw	▷*Broken jaw*
Coughing, difficulty breathing	Nose, mouth	Various	▷*Problems of the nose and lungs*

Problems affecting the neck

Signs	Location	Cause	Disease
Neck in S-shape	Neck	Injury, other causes	▷*Wry neck*
Swelling under jaw (enlarged thyroid gland)	Neck	Lack of iodine	▷*Goitre*

Eye problems

***Dhaasi* (Gabbra), *moyian yoonkouyek* (Samburu), *itwaren* (Somali), *edeke ankonyen* (Turkana)**
Corneal opacity: *fula* (Hindi)

Camels are prone to eye problems, because their eyes protrude and because they graze on thorny vegetation. If something (such as a thorn or piece of straw) gets stuck in the eye, the cornea may become cloudy ('corneal opacity'). Older animals also sometimes suffer from a cloudy cornea.

Inflammation of the transparent part of the eyeball (the 'cornea') is called 'keratitis'. Inflammation of the membranes around the eyeball is called 'conjunctivitis'.

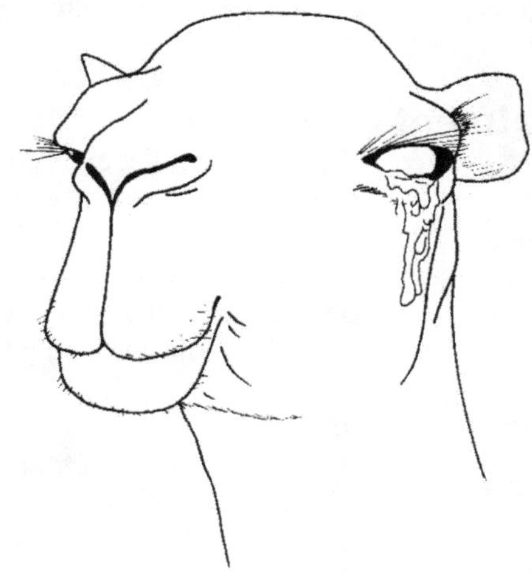

It is reported from India that a lack of vitamin A (due to not enough green fodder during dry periods) can cause night-blindness or complete blindness. The camel walks into trees and walls.

The camel eye worm is a parasite carried by flies. It normally causes few problems.

Blind or partly blind animals can lose condition quite quickly because they cannot graze properly; they may also be attacked by predators.

Signs

Depending on the cause of the problem, the camel may have the following signs:

- Swollen eye.
- Partially or totally closed eye.
- Whitish film on the eye ball ('corneal opacity').
- Reddish or pink eye.
- Watery (or yellowish) discharge from the eye.
- The animal seeks shade (fever also causes camels to do this).
- It holds its head tilted.
- It rubs the eye.
- It walks uncertainly and bumps into objects.

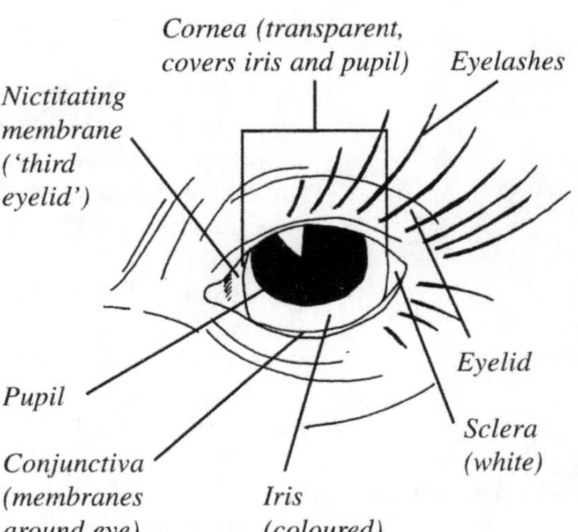

Parts of a camel's left eye

Cause

- Foreign bodies: thorns, sand or feed can get lodged under the eyelids.
- Injuries, especially from thorns or herders' sticks, or irritating juices, seeds or pollen of certain plants.
- Ticks and insect bites (▷*Ticks* and *Bites and stings*).
- Infectious diseases, especially ▷*Pox* and *Orf*.
- Eye worms.
- Tetanus: membrane appears across the eye (▷*Tetanus*).
- Possibly vitamin A deficiency.
- Conjunctivitis (virus or bacterial infection of the membranes around the eye).

Prevention

- Provide green fodder when possible.
- Keep the animal free from ticks (▷*Ticks*).
- Do not hit the animal around the eyes.
- Control pox (▷*Pox*).

Treatment

The treatment depends on what causes the problem. To examine the eye, you must restrain the animal properly and you may have to sedate it. If the eye is painful, use a painkiller; e.g., inject Novalgin into the muscle.

Feed and water an animal with eye problems separately from others to prevent other animals from taking its feed. Put it in a separate enclosure at night to reduce the risk of injuries, and guard it carefully against predators.

Traditional treatments

- Crush a stem of *dharkeyn* (*Euphorbia robecchii*) to make a brush, and apply the sap to the eye. SOMALI
- Soak roots of *Withania somnifera* in water and apply the liquid to the eye.
- Pound turmeric and alum into powder, sift, and put into the eye once a day for 4–5 days. RAIKA
- Chew a mouthful of *marer* (*Cordia sinensis*) bark. Hold the animal's eye open and spit the juice into the eye. Then hold the eyelid closed for 2 minutes. SOMALI
- Crush 10 g of chewing tobacco. Add 1 tablespoon (15 ml) of water and put several drops into the eye. Apply to only one eye at a time because the treatment may cause temporary blindness. Repeat as necessary. SOMALI, TURKANA
- Spit the juice of *kif* (pipe tobacco) into the injured eye. TUAREG
- Soak the cloth used when smoking a pipe in water and apply the water to the eye. RAIKA
- Grind a handful of dried *ebei (Balanites rotundifolia)* leaves, dry *edung* (*Boscia coriacea*) seeds or dried crow's meat and blood into powder. Put a pinch of powder in the eye twice a day until it heals. TURKANA
- Grind dried *iti* (*Acacia mellifera*) leaves into powder. Clean the eye with warm water. Apply a pinch of powder into the eye. SAMBURU

Modern treatments

- **Vitamin A deficiency:** Inject 2 400 000 international units of vitamin A into the muscle twice a week for 2–3 weeks.
- **Foreign body:** Remove it and flush with salty water.

- **Conjunctivitis:** Apply eye ointment containing antibiotics (chloramphenicol, tetracycline or penicillin).
- **Keratitis:** Inject an antibiotic into the membrane around the eye.
- **Injury of the cornea** ('corneal ulcer'): dip a small piece of cotton wool in 2.5% tincture of iodine or 1% silver nitrate solution and touch it onto the injury. Immediately flush the eyeball with normal saline solution. Cover the eye with sterile gauze and give antibacterial eye drops for 2–3 weeks until the ulcer heals. **Caution:** silver nitrate may cause a deeper ulcer, so use it only if you are experienced.
- **Injured eye:** flush with salty water and apply an antibiotic eye ointment. Sometimes stitching is required.
- **Eye worm:** Squeeze the juice from three or four tobacco leaves. Put three drops into the eye once a day for 3 days.
- In the case of cancerous growth or if the eyeball is ruptured, it may be necessary to remove the eyeball by surgery.

References

Bizimana (1994) p. 361–3; Evans et al. (1995) p. 7:29; FAO (1994) p. 211–14, 258; Forse (1999) p.147–51, 349; Gahlot (2000) p. 367; Gahlot and Chouhan (1992) p. 42–7; Higgins (1986) p. 69; ITDG and IIRR (1996) p. 84–6; Manefield and Tinson (1997) p. 98; Projet Cameline (1999) p. 43–4; Rathore (1986) p. 154–5, 186; Schwartz and Dioli (1992) p. 223–4; Sewell and Brocklesby (1990) p. 147–8; Wanyama (1997) vol. 2, p. 34–9, 74–8.

Ear infection

Otitis externa
***Kaan bahana* (India)**

Ear infections are seen occasionally in camels.

Signs

- A thick, sticky fluid comes out of the ear canal.
- The camel shakes its head vigorously, many times a day.
- It tries to rub its ear against hard objects.
- It keeps its head tilted with the affected ear down (this is a sign that the ear is infected deep inside).
- Loss of balance (another sign of a deeper ear infection).

Cause

- Bacterial infection, possibly due to water getting into the ear canal.
- Mites or ticks in the ear.

Prevention

- Avoid water entering the ear during bathing.
- Remove ticks regularly.

Treatment

Remove any ticks and use one of the following treatments.

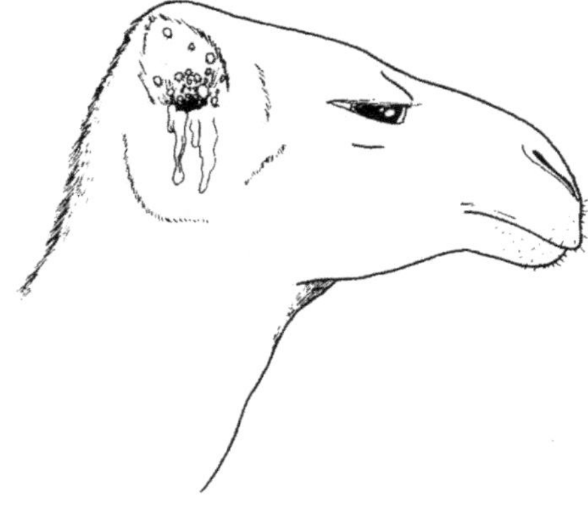

Traditional treatment

- Put lukewarm mustard oil in the ear once a day.

Modern treatments

- Clean the ear with an antiseptic (e.g., Dermaclens) and put in an antibiotic and antifungal ointment (e.g., Panalog). Repeat if necessary.
- Flush the ear canal with 5% solution of hydrogen peroxide or warm saline solution. Remove the ear wax and sticky fluid with cotton wool. Put ear drops containing chloramphenicol or gentamicin into the ear.
- If the problem is caused by mites, inject ivermectin (0.2 mg/kg body weight) under the skin.
- If the ear seems to be infected deep inside (see *Signs* above), do the above, and inject into the muscle 10 mg/kg body weight of ampicillin twice a day, and 8–10 mg/kg of phenylbutazone once a day for 3 days.

References

Bizimana (1994) p. 363; Evans et al. (1995) p. 7:26; FAO (1994) p. 258; Forse (1999) p. 152–349; Gahlot and Chouhan (1992) p. 39; Manefield and Tinson (1997) p. 179; Rathore (1986) p. 157.

Torn nostrils

***Naas phatna* (India)**

Camels often are led by nose halters attached to pegs in the nose. If the halter is pulled too hard, or if the camel is startled and jerks its head, the pegs can tear out. The resulting wound can become infected. Even after the skin has healed, it is still weak, so nose-pegs cannot be used.

Signs

- Torn, bleeding skin in the nose.
- The wound heals but leaves behind a long, open slit where the nose-pegs were embedded.
- The wound can become infested with maggots.

Cause

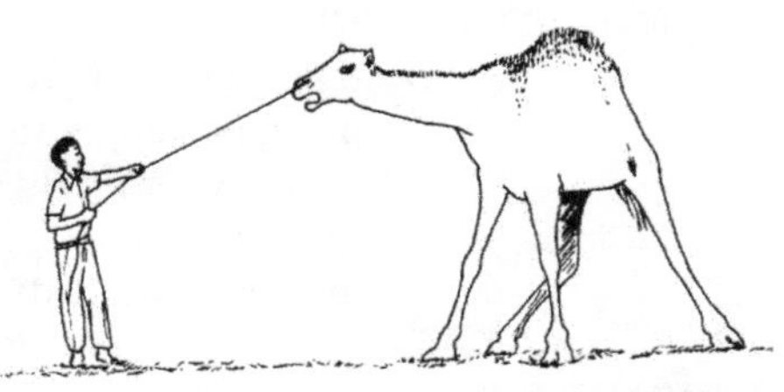

- The nose-peg is torn out.
- Some herders in Kenya slit the nostrils of a calf deliberately to wean it.

Prevention

- Do not pull the animal too tightly by the nose-rope.
- Tether the animal by the neck rather than by the nose-peg.

Treatment

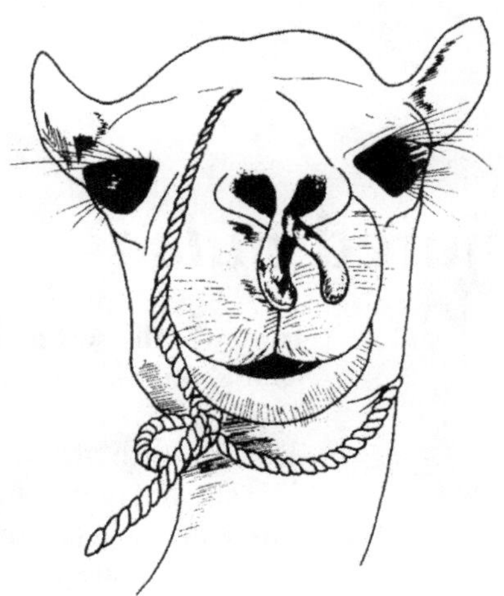

Calf with nostrils slit deliberately for weaning.

- Sedate the animal and apply a local anaesthetic. Clean the wound with a sterile scalpel or sharp knife. Stitch the wound together and smear on a fly repellent ointment (▷*Surgery* and *Bites and stings*). Inject a broad-spectrum antibiotic for 3–5 days (e.g., oxytetracycline at a dosage of 50 mg/10 kg body weight). Remove the stitches after 10–15 days. SCI

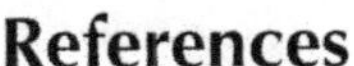

References

Gahlot and Chouhan (1992) p. 34–5; Manefield and Tinson (1997) p. 171.

Blisters in the mouth

Vesicular stomatitis
Mooh upadana, mooh ke chhale **(Rajasthan)**

Cause

Infection, vitamin B deficiency, injury to the mouth.

Signs

- Sores inside the mouth, swelling in the mouth.
- Loss of appetite, reduced chewing.
- Increased salivation.
- Loss in condition.

Treatment

Traditional treatment

- Apply honey mixed with ginger extract to the affected parts of the mouth.

Modern treatments

- Dip a cloth or piece of cotton wool in a 0.1% solution of potassium permanganate, and apply to the sores. Repeat this every day until the blisters disappear.
- Inject vitamin B complex into the muscle once a day for 3–5 days.
- In serious cases, inject 50 mg/10 kg body weight of oxytetracycline into the muscle, once a day for 3–5 days.

References

FAO (1994) p. 205–6, 252; Rathore (1986) p. 126.

Injured *dulaa*

Injury to the soft palate
***Gulla phansa, ghayal hona* (India)**

This problem affects only male camels in the 'rut' or mating season (▷*Rutting*). The excited male camel balloons out its soft palate (called the '*dulaa*' in Arabic) and makes a gurgling sound. The *dulaa* can become injured by the teeth, in fights with other males, or through accidents. The injured *dulaa* can be stuck inside the mouth, or may hang out and become swollen.

Signs

- The male is unable to balloon out its *dulaa*, or the *dulaa* stays hanging out, becomes infected, and swells.
- If the *dulaa* is hanging out, the animal does not eat or drink.
- If the *dulaa* is trapped inside, the animal will drink but not eat. If you squeeze the throat, the *dulaa* may balloon slightly inside the mouth but does not come out.
- If untreated, the animal dies of starvation.

Cause

- Bites on the *dulaa*, either in fights with other males, or by the animal itself, for example when it is restrained for an injection.
- Accidents.

Prevention

- Prevent male camels from fighting.

Treatment

Traditional treatments

- Push the *dulaa* back into the mouth and tie a piece of cloth around the mouth to keep it there.
- If the *dulaa* is too swollen, release some of the fluid in it by stabbing it in several places with a sterilized, sharp knife or razor blade. Then push it back into the mouth, as above.

Modern treatment

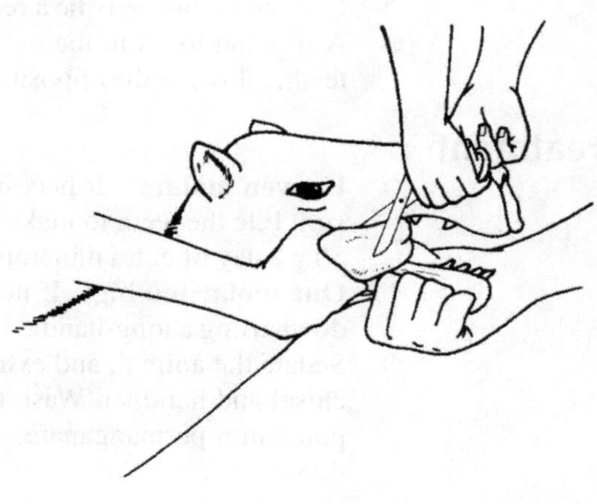

1. Restrain and sedate the animal with xylazine (▷*Sedation and anaesthesia*).
2. If the *dulaa* is trapped inside the mouth, squeeze the throat to balloon it into the mouth, then stick a sharp hook into it to hold it firm. Hold the *dulaa* with a piece of towel and pull it out.
3. Cut the *dulaa* off at its base with a pair of surgical scissors. There will be only a little bleeding.
4. Flush the mouth out with 5 litres of a 0.1% solution of potassium permanganate once a day for 1 week after feeding.
5. Inject a broad-spectrum antibiotic into the muscle for 5–7 days (▷*Common medicines*). If the animal is valuable, consider injecting with tetanus antitoxin.
6. Give the normal feed to the animal after the operation.

References

Bizimana (1994) p. 337–8; Gahlot and Chouhan (1992) p. 47–52; Leese (1927) p. 296; Manefield and Tinson (1997) p. 78–80.

Teeth problems

***Dant bhadhana, daadh badhana, ubad-khabad dhadh* (India)**

The cheek teeth (molars) may develop an irregular surface, which prevents the camel from chewing properly. If there is a cheek tooth missing in either the upper or lower jaw, the tooth above or below it can grow too big. This also interferes with eating. ▷*Estimating a camel's weight and age* for more information on camels' teeth.

Signs

- The animal does not chew properly: it chews on one side only.
- Worsening body condition.
- Bad smell from the mouth.
- The animal grinds its teeth even without feed in its mouth. (*Note*: males normally do this during the rut.)
- The teeth are worn unevenly.
- One cheek tooth is longer than the others.
- A swelling may appear in the cheek if feed accumulates in the space where a tooth is missing.

Cause

- Uneven molars may be a result of poor health or under-nourishment.
- A missing tooth in the upper or lower jaw, or too large a space between the teeth, allowing the opposite tooth to grow too large.

Treatment

- **Uneven molars** If necessary, sedate the animal (▷*Sedation and anaesthesia*). File the teeth to make them even and to smooth out sharp edges. Provide 50 g a day of extra minerals and vitamins in powder form for 3 months. SCI
- **One molar too big** If necessary, sedate the animal. File the enlarged tooth down using a long-handled tooth rasp. TRAD+SCI
- Sedate the animal, and extract the enlarged tooth using a molar extractor or a chisel and hammer. Wash the mouth daily for 7 days with a light solution of potassium permanganate. This operation is difficult to do under field conditions. SCI

References

Bizimana (1994) p. 338; Gahlot and Chouhan (1992) p. 38–9; Manefield and Tinson (1997) p. 254; Rathore (1986) p. 90, 206.

Broken jaw

Mandibular fracture
***Jabadi tutana, jadi tutana* (India)**

Broken jaws are common in male camels, especially during the breeding season (▷*Rutting*). The camel's lower jaw is inherently weak, making it easily broken during fights between males. The jaw may be broken on one side only, but often both sides are broken in several places. A broken jaw prevents the camel from eating; unless treated, the animal will starve to death.

If the jaw is broken in only one place, there is some hope of recovery. If there are several breaks, it is best to kill the animal.

Signs

- Lower jaw hangs down and moves loosely.
- The camel is unable to eat or drink.
- Often wounds inside the mouth.
- Little feeling in the lower jaw.

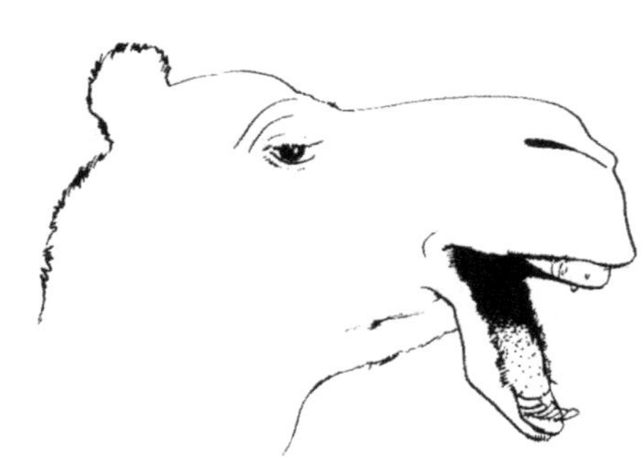

Cause

- Inherently weak lower jaw of camels.
- Fighting between males.
- Biting on hard objects, such as trees.

- Owner hitting the camel.
- Road accidents.

Prevention

- Muzzle males during the breeding season.
- Keep male camels away from each other.
- Do not tie an animal to a post or tree using a rope tied to the lower jaw. If the animal jerks its head, it may break its jaw (▷*Restraining*).

Treatment

After applying any of the treatments below, keep the camel muzzled and away from other animals and fixed objects while it recovers. Give it soft feed for 2 weeks.

Traditional treatments

- **First aid:** Put a wide cloth (20 cm × 50 cm) under the jaw and tie the two ends together firmly above the bridge of the nose to hold the lower jaw in place.
- Punch holes in the four corners of a piece of metal (30 cm × 45 cm). Put string through the holes, and bend the metal to a 'U' shape so it fits underneath the lower jaw. Tie the strings over the bridge of the nose to support the lower jaw. Remove the device once a day to give liquid feed to the camel.
- Fix a wooden splint under the jaw, using two lengths of copper wire passing through the mouth: one wire just behind the front teeth, and the other just in front of the cheek teeth. Put pieces of cloth or some other padding under the wire and the wooden splint to protect the gums and skin. Leave the splint in place for 3–4 months.

Modern treatments

Treating a broken jaw is difficult to do successfully in the field. It may be better to kill the animal immediately.

If the jaw is broken in the same place on both sides:

1. Make sure all the equipment you will use is clean and sterile. Restrain the animal in a sitting position and sedate it by injecting 5 ml of xylazine into the vein.
2. Use a hand drill to drill a hole through the gums between the first two cheek teeth on each side of the jaw.
3. Push a copper or stainless steel wire (2 mm in diameter) through the hole on one side, bring the end to the front of the mouth, and put it through the space between the two front teeth.

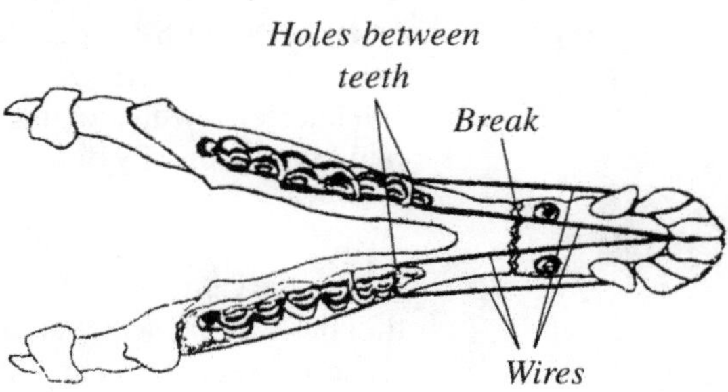

Jawbone of camel showing wires to hold bone together

4. Tie a piece of thin rope around the front of the jaw and pull on it to make sure the jaw is positioned correctly.
5. Tie the two ends of the wire together to hold the jaw in place.
6. Do the same with the wire on the other side of the mouth.
7. Inject a broad-spectrum antibiotic such as long-acting oxytetracycline into the muscle every 2–3 days for 7–10 days.
8. Wash the mouth out with a 0.1% solution of potassium permanganate every day for 10 days.
9. If an abscess develops under the jaw, open it with a sharp knife to drain the pus out, wash it out with potassium permanganate solution, and dress with a fly repellent ointment.
10. Remove the wires after 8–10 weeks.

If the jaw is broken in several places, or at different places on each side, it is probably better to kill the animal, as there is only a small chance it will recover. An experienced vet may be able to treat the animal.

References

Gahlot and Chouhan (1992) p. 54–63; Leese (1927) p. 173; Manefield and Tinson (1997) p. 150–2; Rathore (1986) p. 207–9.

Wry neck

Kinked neck, bent neck, torticollis, cold struck
***Simpiro, chachabsa* (Gabbra), *wadi* (Hindi), *kasara* (Kordofan), *dahasi* (Rendille), *shimper, gudanki, simpiro, gusam* (Somali), *haboub* (Sudan)**

Wry neck syndrome is fairly frequent but poorly understood. It may interfere with feeding and grazing, so the animal loses condition. Sometimes the animal recovers by itself in several months.

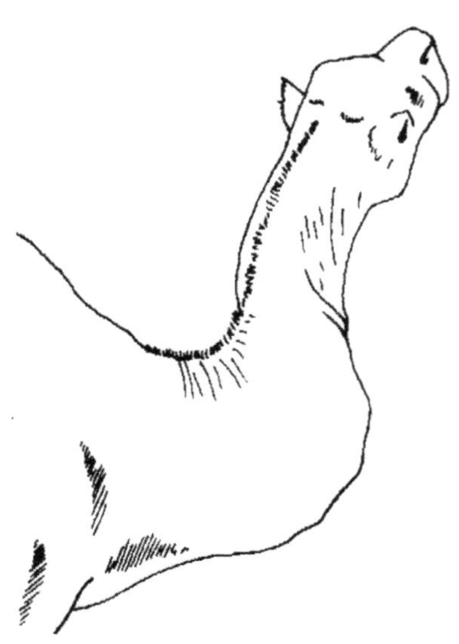

Signs

- The neck becomes bent to the side or takes on an S-shape. This happens very suddenly.
- If it interferes with grazing, the animal may eventually die.

Cause

- Injury: the camel falls, breaking the thin parts of the neck bones.
- Genetic: seems to run in certain families.

- Shortage of vitamin B in the feed.
- When there is a lot of lush forage at the beginning of rainy season.
- After the animal has been sedated or anaesthetized for surgery.
- Plant poisoning, suspected in northern Kenya (▷*Plant poisoning*).

Prevention

- Keep the neck in a natural position during sedation or anaesthesia. Afterwards, take care that the camel does not injure itself when it wakes and struggles to get up.
- If you suspect that the defect is inherited, do not use the animal for breeding.

Treatment

Traditional treatments

- Mix up brew of yeast with sugar or molasses and drench 2–3 times per day.
- Drench with a soup made from sheep's head, put boiled sheep-tail fat into the nostrils, and rub hot sheep-tail fat onto the head. Drench with milk and salt.
- Mix clay with hot water to make a compress, and apply it to the paralysed area.
- Bleed from the jugular vein (the large vein in the neck).
- Chop up the root of *adeh* (*Salvadora persica*) and the leaves of a plant called *odha*, mix with water and drench. GABBRA
- Pastoralists usually brand on both sides of the neck (▷*Branding*).

Modern treatments

- Inject vitamin B6 or vitamin B complex into the muscle.
- Drench with 1.5 kg of Epsom salts immediately after the disease appears.

References

Bizimana (1994) p. 359; Gahlot and Chouhan (1992) p. 63; Kaufmann (1998) p. 191–2; Leese (1927) p. 327; Manefield and Tinson (1997) p. 143–4; Rathore (1986) p. 149–50; Schwartz and Dioli (1992) p. 191–2, 219.

Goitre

Colloid goitre, iodine deficiency

The mineral iodine is necessary for the thyroid gland to function properly. The thyroid is an important gland located in the angle between the camel's neck and its jaw. It is vital for keeping the animal healthy and making it grow properly. Goitre occurs in areas where the soil and plants contain too little iodine, such as the Darfur area of Sudan.

Signs

- Swelling in the front of the neck due to the enlarged thyroid gland: just below the jaw, either on one side or on both sides.

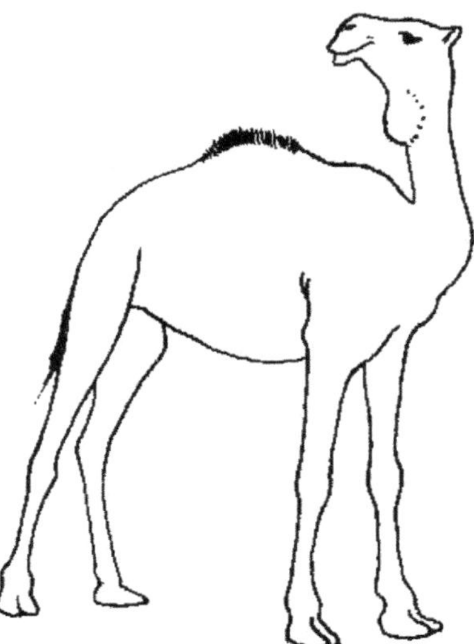

- Abortion or poor reproductive performance.
- Calves born with enlarged thyroid.
- Infertility or lack of heat in females.
- In the dead animal, the thyroid gland is swollen up to 30 times its normal weight.

To check for iodine deficiency, take a blood sample and have it analysed for the content of thyroxine (the hormone produced by the thyroid gland) (▷*How to collect samples for testing*).

Be careful not to confuse goitre with an abscess or oedema (swelling) of the neck (▷*Skin abscesses, Oedema*).

Cause

Lack of iodine in the feed and water.

Prevention and treatment

- In areas known or thought to be deficient in iodine, regularly add iodized salt to the feed or water. SCI
- Water at places with adequate mineral content in the water (pastoralists often know of such places). SCI

References

Manefield and Tinson (1997) p. 113.

4 Problems of the legs, feet and tail

The table below shows the main signs of diseases affecting the legs, feet and tail.

Signs	Location	Cause	Disease
Limping, lameness	Legs	Various	▷*Broken bones, Arthritis, Dislocated kneecap, Foot problems, Blackquarter, Haemorrhagic septicaemia*
Animal in pain and cannot get up	Legs	Broken leg	▷*Broken bones*
Animal cannot get up, but not in pain		Various	▷*Downer, Sunstroke, Infectious diseases, Non-infectious diseases*
Cracking sound when walking	Hind leg	Dislocated kneecap	▷*Dislocated kneecap*
Hind leg shakes	Hind leg	Myopathy, tetanus	▷*Myopathy, Tetanus*
Front legs stiff	Front legs	Chest sprain	▷*Chest sprain, Tetanus*
Growth of flesh in foot	Foot	Elephant foot	▷*Foot problems*
Tip of tail hairless, cold and without feeling	Tail	Infection in the tail	▷*Tail gangrene*
Dark skin on leg, swellings, crackling sound when touched	Leg	Blackquarter	▷*Blackquarter*
Standing with legs splayed, stiff tail	Legs, tail	Tetanus	▷*Tetanus*

Broken bones

Fractures
***Chachaba* (Gabbra), *ngilata e loito* (Samburu), *jab* (Somali Ethiopia), *abila* (Turkana)**
Broken foot: *pag tutana, pagtali kanne tutfut* (Rajasthan)
Broken leg: *nali ka tutuna, far ka tutuna, larle kulhe ki haddi ka tutana* (Rajasthan)

Camels frequently suffer from broken bones, or 'fractures', in the legs. There are several different types of fractures:

- An 'open' fracture is where the bones break through the skin. A 'closed' fracture is where the bones remain inside the skin.
- Bones can break in the middle or at the joints.
- Bones may break in several places. This is called a 'multiple fracture'.

Signs

- Swelling of the area around the break.
- The animal is in pain.
- Reduced appetite.
- You may be able to hear a cracking sound of bones rubbing together when the affected bones are moved.
- Broken long bones: the animal cannot get up.
- Broken foot: the animal limps and carries the foot, or puts its weight on its toes while standing.

Cause

- Falls on slippery ground or steep slopes.
- Road accidents.
- Leg trapped in a pit.

Prevention

- Avoid keeping animals in slippery or steep areas.
- Herd animals away from public roads.

Treatment

Broken bones are difficult to treat, especially in adult animals. Recovery takes a long time (if the animal recovers), and the animal will need special care. You should consider killing the animal rather than trying to treat it. The chances of recovery are better for calves.

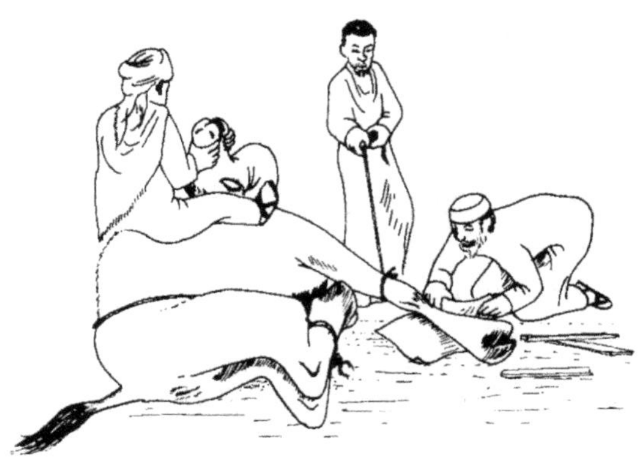

Open fractures, broken joints, and multiple fractures are difficult to treat. Breaks above the knee or hock also heal with difficulty. Such animals are unlikely to recover, and should probably be killed. Breaks in the lower leg and foot have a better chance of recovery (▷*Parts of a camel*).

Traditional treatment

1. Restrain the animal by tying it firmly on the ground.
2. Find the broken area by feeling carefully along the limb with your hands.
3. Hold the broken bones straight and still.
4. If the broken area is swollen, dip a cloth in warm water mixed with salt or sugar and press the cloth against the swelling. Keep it there for 0.5–1 hour to reduce the swelling.
5. Put soft material such as a cloth or animal skin around the affected area.
6. Place two or more strong pieces of wood or bark around the broken area to keep the bones in place. These pieces of wood are called 'splints'. They should be long enough to stop the joints above and below the break from moving.
7. Tie the ends of the splints tightly (but not *too* tightly) to the leg with a strip of cloth, skin, or rope. Do not tie directly over the broken area.
8. Confine the animal until it starts to walk. Provide high quality feed and water. Make sure the pen is not too crowded with other animals.
9. After 1 week, untie the splints and check for healing. If the fracture has not healed, straighten it again if necessary and fix it for 2 weeks. The best time to change the dressing or untie the splints depends on the wound. GABBRA, TURKANA

Modern treatments

If the bones in the foot are broken:

- Cover the foot with a reasonably thick layer of cotton and start wrapping a cotton cloth bandage around it. Lay wooden splints between the layers of the bandage. Finally, apply three or four plaster-of-Paris bandages over the foot. Leave in place for 8 weeks. Check regularly and remove or replace the bandages if there is a bad smell or discharge.

If one of the long bones in the leg below the elbow or stifle (knee) is broken :

1. Sedate the animal and restrain it on its side, keeping the affected leg uppermost.
2. Straighten the broken bones by pulling the broken foot gently but firmly away from the body, and pull the leg in the opposite direction.
3. Wrap cotton wool around the injured part.
4. Soak a gauze bandage in lukewarm water and wrap it around the cotton wool.
5. Place two metal splints against the bandage to hold the broken bone in place: one in front of the limb, and the other behind. Tie them firmly in place with a bandage.
6. Soak five 15 × 180 cm plaster-of-Paris bandages in lukewarm water and wrap them around the limb and splints. Allow the plaster to dry and harden.
8. Remove the plaster cast after 6–8 weeks (the length of time depends on whether the animal puts its weight on the injured foot).
9. Keep the camel confined for at least 3 months after the injury.

References

Bizimana (1994) p. 353; FAO (1994) p. 219–21; Forse (1999) p. 73–4; Gahlot and Chouhan (1992) p. 72–7, 90–6; Higgins (1986) p. 126–30; ITDG and IIRR (1996) p. 66–8; Manefield and Tinson (1997) p. 107–9; Projet Cameline (1999) p. 53; Rathore (1986) p. 212, 216–17; Wanyama (1997) vol. 2, p. 30–3.

Arthritis

***Ras bharna* (India)**

Draught camels can suffer from lameness due to arthritis in one or both hind legs. This dramatically reduces the amount of work the camel can do, as well as its value.

Usually the hock (the middle joint on the back leg) is affected; the stifle (top) and fetlock (ankle) are less frequently affected.

Signs

- The camel limps in its back legs.
- The camel does not bend one or both of its hocks as much as usual when walking. Its stride is shorter than usual, and it drags its toe.
- It bends the hock only partly when sitting.
- The hock joint may be swollen, or the 'hock bone' may become bigger.

Cause

Old age, overwork.

Treatment

After treating the disease, allow the camel to rest for several weeks before working or exercising it. If there have been changes in the bone, chances of recovery are not good.

Traditional treatment

- Point-fire on the hock joint (on the inside and the outside) with an iron rod (▷*Branding*).

Modern treatment

- Inject 5 ml/100 kg body weight of Dexa-Tomanol into the vein once a day for 2–3 days, and apply an anti-inflammatory cream such as DMSO–Flucort onto the affected joint twice a day. Make the animal rest for at least 3 weeks.

Caution: do not give a corticosteroid such as Dexa-Tomanol to a female camel during the last 4 months of a pregnancy because it can cause an abortion.

References

Bizimana (1994) p. 354; Evans et al. (1995) p. 7:26; Forse (1999) p. 250–1; Gahlot and Chouhan (1992) p. 97–100; Higgins (1986) p. 128–9; Leese (1927) p. 214; Manefield and Tinson (1997) p. 137–41; Rathore (1986) p. 156–7, 211–12, 217.

Dislocated kneecap

Upward fixation of the patella, luxation of the patella
Chitki, chatkan, saran **(India)**

Dislocated kneecap occurs occasionally in draught camels. In the hind leg, the kneecap (the 'patella') becomes dislocated, reducing the camel's ability to work. If untreated, the disease makes the camel unfit for work for the rest of its life. It is common in weak animals, such as those with chronic trypanosomiasis (▷*Trypanosomiasis*). This problem is sometimes incorrectly called 'stringhalt'.

Signs

- Limping with the affected hind leg. The animal keeps this leg straight and drags it forward, then bends it with a jerk.
- A cracking sound while walking.
- The camel limps after getting up or when moving after a long rest; the limping disappears once the camel warms up but reappears after rest.

Cause

Unknown.

Treatment

Traditional treatments

Note: branding is of dubious value to treat dislocated kneecap.

- Branding on the inside and outside of the stifle (the 'knee' in the back leg) (▷*Branding*).
- Branding on the backbone above the hips.
- Branding on the outside of the thigh.

Modern treatment

- Inject 20–30 ml of an irritant, such as equal amounts of chloroform and turpentine oil or Lugol's iodine on the inside of the stifle. Rest the animal for 4 weeks. A swelling may develop at the injection site, and the animal may go partially lame. The swelling usually disappears after 7–10 days.

References

Gahlot and Chouhan (1992) p. 87–9; Higgins (1986) p. 130; Manefield and Tinson (1997) p. 139–40; Rathore (1986) p. 160–1, 216–17.

Myopathy

***Makiola* (Arabic), *kumri* (India)**

Myopathy is a disease of the muscles. It occurs mainly in unconditioned racing camels which have been raced over long distances, in animals that are tied down for too long (e.g., when transporting them on a lorry), animals recovering from a long period of anaesthesia, and where there are nutritional deficiencies in the feed.

In Rajasthan, a similar disease, known as *kumri*, causes a peculiar shivering of the back legs when the animal tries to sit. It affects male animals. Owners usually abandon such camels, although otherwise the animals seem normal.

Signs

- Difficulty in standing up and walking: the hind legs shake from side to side.

The following are signs of *kumri:*

- Shivering of the hindquarters when camel attempts to sit. When it has reached the half sitting position, it falls down.
- The hindquarters appear weak, and the camel is not able to pull heavy loads.

Myopathy affects both hind legs, while ▷*Dislocated kneecap* (the hind leg hesitates before it is placed on the ground) is usually in one leg only.

Cause

Various causes: over-exertion, prolonged lack of movement followed by vigorous work, plant poisoning, vitamin E or selenium deficiency, calcium/phosphorus imbalance, or genetic defects.

Prevention

- Do not overwork unconditioned camels.
- Do not force animals to sit immediately after hard work.
- Do not tie animals down for more than 5 hours at a time.
- Watch as a camel wakes from anaesthesia, and treat immediately if needed.
- Supplement the feed with vitamin E and selenium.
- Ensure the correct balance between calcium and phosphorus in the feed.
- Do not breed from parents that have the disease.
- Avoid grazing in areas that you suspect may cause the disease.

Treatment

Treat the animal promptly.

- Inject an anti-inflammatory medicine such as 5 ml/100 kg body weight of Tomanol or Dexa-Tomanol slowly into the vein, and possibly also 5–10 ml of Dexone-5. In severe cases, administer intravenous fluids such as Hartman's solution. SCI
- Supplement the feed with vitamin E and selenium (Selevite-E). SCI
- Inject prednisolone (200 mg) into the muscle for 5–7 days against *kumri*. SCI

Caution: do not give corticosteroids such as Dexa-Tomanol, Dexone-5 or prednisolone to a female camel during the last 4 months of a pregnancy because they can cause an abortion.

References

Higgins (1986) p. 161; Manefield and Tinson (1997) p. 161–4; Rathore (1986) p. 152.

Chest sprain

***Maachijana, maachhijgaya* (India)**

Draught camels can sprain the muscles in their chest, making it difficult for them to walk with their front legs.

Signs

- Stiff gait in the forelimbs.
- The stride in the forelimbs is shorter.
- The camel feels pain if you press on its chest.
- It sits and gets up with difficulty.
- It is reluctant to walk.

Cause

Sprain or injury to the muscles in the chest that help move the forelegs. Such injuries can occur if the animal slips on slippery ground or if it is waking up from sedation or anaesthesia. Chest sprains are common in racing camels that slip during a race.

Prevention

- Avoid slippery surfaces.
- Keep the animal tied down until it is completely awake after an operation (▷*Sedation and anaesthesia*).

Treatment

Traditional treatment

- Drench with vegetable ghee and turmeric powder.

Modern treatments

- Massage with A.B.C. liniment.
- Inject into the muscle 40 mg of dexamethasone and 8–10 mg per kg body weight of phenylbutazone for 3 days. Keep the animal confined for 1 week or more.

Caution: do not give dexamethasone or other corticosteroids to a female camel during the last 4 months of a pregnancy because they can cause an abortion.

References

Manefield and Tinson (1997) p. 162; Rathore (1986) p. 210.

Foot problems

Infected toes: *suul* (Somali)

Camels have soft feet, best suited to dry, sandy ground. They are easily injured by thorns and other sharp objects. Their feet can be bruised and damaged on rocky or hard ground, especially if they are not accustomed to such areas. Foot wounds are more likely during rainy periods when the foot-pads become soft.

Some breeds of camels naturally have tougher feet than others. Young camels have particularly soft feet. Camels' feet can be hardened gradually to make them used to rougher ground. For information on broken foot, ▷*Broken bones.*

Signs

- Lameness, difficulty in walking. The type and severity of the lameness depends on the cause of the problem. For specific signs, see below.

Cause

Wounds caused by thorns or stones.

Prevention

- Avoid walking camels over hard ground or sharp rocks.
- Accustom the animals to the hard ground gradually.
- Tie a boot on the animal's foot.
- Trim broken toenails so they do not catch on things.
- Give food supplements containing biotin (Biopad or Biocare) to harden the foot-pads. SCI

General treatment

- Rest the camel from walking or working.
- For foot wounds, keep the foot as clean as possible. Wash the foot with salty water and dry the foot.
- Cover the foot with a boot made of leather or sacking, three times the diameter of the foot. Make holes around the edge and thread a string through them. Tie the boot tightly on the foot so dirt cannot get in. Remove and clean the boot frequently, especially when wet.

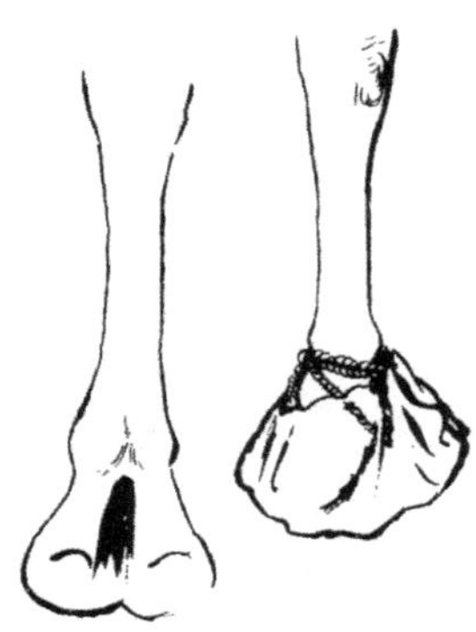

Sore feet

Signs

- The camel is lame and has a shortened stride.
- The affected foot or feet are raw, hot and swollen ('congested').

Cause

Rocky, stony or hard ground leads to bruising or abrasions on soles.

Treatment

- If the surface layers are intact, the animal usually recovers with rest and a mild topical dressing (▷*Wounds and burns*). SCI

Cracked or worn pads

***Talhas* (North and West Africa)**

Treatments

- Cauterize with a hot iron. N AND W AFRICA
- Treat holes and crevices with a mixture of sheep grease and salt from the Adrar region, or with a mixture of ash, date pulp and salty earth; then brand with a hot iron. N AND W AFRICA
- Tie a leather boot on the foot. TRAD+SCI
- Trim off any loose flaps in the pad. Allow the camel to rest on a sandy surface. Apply 4% Lotagen or another commerical astringent (Pad Paint, Copperox) twice a day for 1 week to harden the affected pad. SCI
- Apply 10% solution of copper sulphate followed by Charmil gel. AYURVEDIC

Ulcers on the sole

Ulcerative dermatitis, *makales* (Tuareg)

Signs

- Seen mainly in racing camels or camels that are introduced to new ground.
- The skin on the sole of the foot becomes thin and flaky, and dirt becomes trapped in the skin.
- On the parts of the sole the skin is worn away, leaving raw, sore areas that make the camel lame.
- In severe cases, the foot becomes infected, and abscesses may develop.

Treatments

- Remove the infected tissue, apply a topical antibiotic, dress the wound, and tie a boot over the foot. SCI
- Incise the abscess and release the pus. Apply heated butter on the wound. TUAREG
- Puncture the abscess and cauterize around it with a hot iron (▷*Branding*). MALI

Foot wounds

Punctured foot, traumatic pododermatitis

***Ragat* (Somalia)**

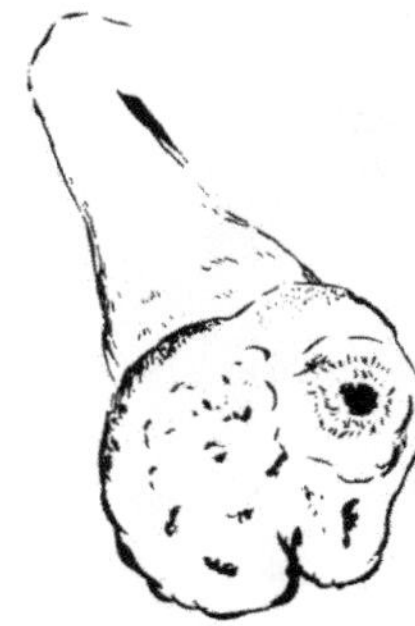

Signs

- Severe lameness.
- Foot is very swollen and painful.
- If a wound is visible, there may be pus running from it.

Cause

A thorn or nail in the sole of the foot. It can track deep inside, severely damaging the bone and other parts of the foot.

Traditional treatments

- Chew tobacco and mix it with coal dust. Apply as a dressing to the wound. TUAREG
- Pound together the still-green fruits of *Boscia senegalensis*, the bark of *Maerua crassifolia* and millet. Apply as a dressing to the wound. TUAREG

Modern treatment

- Surgery by a skilled practitioner. Restrain and sedate the camel. Clean the wound, remove the infected tissue and thorn or nail, and drain the wound. Pack it with sulphanilamide powder or nitrofurazone powder. Plug it with cotton wool and tie a bandage over it. Tie a leather boot over the foot. Inject with systemic antibiotics and 3000 international units of tetanus antitoxin. Change the dressing weekly until the wound has healed.

Elephant foot

Signs

- A wild growth of flesh in the foot. Usually affects only one foot.

Cause

Not certain. May result from sand-fly bites.

Treatments

- Treat with a long-acting cortisone. For example, inject 200 mg of methylprednisolone (e.g., Depo Medrol) into the muscle.
- Rub a corticosteroid cream (e.g., Dermobion) into the affected area.

Caution: do not give corticosteroids to a female camel during the last 4 months of a pregnancy because they can cause an abortion.

- It may be necessary to cut off the affected toe.

References

Bizimana (1994) p. 355–7; Evans et al. (1995) 6:12–13, 7:29; FAO (1994) p. 191–2; Forse (1999) p. 252–3; Gahlot and Chouhan (1992) p. 107–9; Higgins (1986) p. 126–7; Manefield and Tinson (1997) p. 84, 101–5, 242; Rathore (1986) p. 210; Schwartz and Dioli (1992) p. 186, 189, 213–14.

Tail gangrene

***Leathery, poonchh sookna, ponchh mein, keeda lagna* (India)**

The saddle rope tied around the camel's tail may restrict the flow of blood, eventually killing the tissue in the tail. This reduces the value of the animal, and may kill an otherwise healthy animal.

Signs

- No hair at the tip of the tail.
- The tip of the tail is cold and insensitive.
- The skin at the tip of the tail turns blue and dry.
- An apparently healthy animal may die suddenly.

Cause

Injury of the tail due to the pressure of the saddle rope tied around it. This causes gangrene at the tip of the tail, which may spread up the tail if it is not treated. It may kill the animal if it is not treated.

Prevention

- Adjust the saddle rope so it does not injure the tail.

Treatment

Traditional treatments

- Line-fire over the base of the tail (▻*Branding*).
- Dip the tail in boiling edible oil.

Modern treatment

- Give an epidural anaesthetic (▻*Sedation and anaesthesia*). Tie a bandage tightly around the base of the tail to reduce the blood flow. Make two semicircular cuts in the healthy skin, one on the top of the tail and one underneath, to make two flaps of skin. Tie off the blood vessels to stop the bleeding. Cut off the diseased part of the tail by cutting between the tail bones. Sew the two flaps of skin together. Keep the tail stump covered for 2 weeks before removing the stitches (▻*Surgery*).

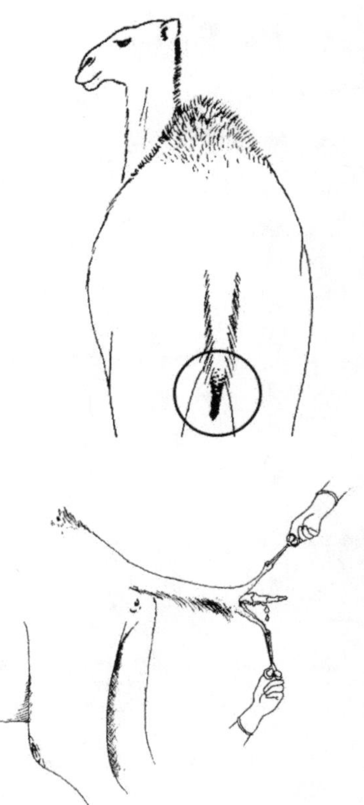

References

Gahlot and Chouhan (1992) p. 147–8; Leese (1927) p. 189; Rathore (1986) p. 215.

5 Problems of the nose and lungs

Coughing, colds, runny nose, difficulty in breathing and other respiratory problems can be caused by many different things. It can be difficult to identify the problem and select the correct treatment.

It is important to find out what is causing the problem before treating it. Look carefully for other, more specific, signs of disease (such as the pimples typical of ▻*Pox*) before deciding what the problem is and how to treat it. In field conditions, one rarely knows the cause of the disease for sure. In any case, respiratory infections are often caused by a mix of viruses and bacteria. It may be necessary to test the blood or discharge from the nose to identify the disease for certain (▻*Checking for diseases in the laboratory*).

Some of these diseases can spread rapidly and kill many animals. Some, such as tuberculosis, can affect people (▻*Diseases that people can catch from camels*). The tables below list some, but not all, of the causes of coughing, runny nose and breathing problems in camels. See the relevant sections in this book for other signs of these diseases and how to prevent and treat them.

Problems covered in this chapter

Signs	Causal organisms	Disease	See section
Rapid breathing		Typical of fever and acute infections of the nose and lungs; many possible causes	
Cough, runny nose, difficulty breathing, swollen tonsils, rapid breathing	Virus, bacteria	Cough, cold, bronchitis, pneumonia, pleuropneumonia, tuberculosis	▻*Coughs, colds and pneumonia*
Cough, gagging	Parasite	Leeches in mouth and nose, lungworms	▻*Leeches, Lungworms*

Signs	Causal organisms	Disease	See section
Sneezing	Parasite	Ticks in the nostrils, nasal bots (maggots in the back of the nose and mouth)	▷*Ticks, Nasal bots*
Discharge from a single nostril	Parasite	Nasal bots, foreign body	▷*Nasal bots*
Runny nose, tears in eyes, drooling from mouth, yellowish-white discharge from nose	Parasite	Lungworms	▷*Lungworms*
Cysts found in lungs of dead camel	Parasite	Cysts of hydatid tapeworm	▷*Hydatid disease*

Problems covered in other chapters

Signs	Causal organisms	Disease	See section
Choking, coughing	Foreign body	Object caught in throat	▷*Swallowed objects*
Choking, coughing during sedation or while drenching	Liquid in lungs	Medicines going into lungs, vomit going into lungs during sedation	▷*Administering medicines, Sedation and anaesthesia*
Difficulty in breathing	Bacteria, parasite	Salmonellosis, dipetalonemiasis	▷*Salmonellosis, Dipetalonemiasis*
Cough, pimples on skin	Virus	Pox	▷*Pox*
Dark red mucous membranes in eyes and mouth, weak cough, rapid, shallow breathing	Bacteria	Haemorrhagic septicaemia	▷*Haemorrhagic septicaemia*
Dry cough	Bacteria	Haemorrhagic disease	▷*Haemorrhagic disease*

Coughs, colds and pneumonia

Kharoo* (Afar, Ethiopia), *nahaz* (Arabic), *kufa', qufa* (Gabbra), *khassi* (India), *ghudda, al fahada, habub* (Kordofan), *n'haz* (Moorish), *psosoi, songoghowio, erukum, arrkum* (Pokot), *yaharr, dahassi* (Rendille), *nkorroget, loroget, lchama, lbus bus (literally, 'lungs') **(Samburu), *ah, dhugato, dugub, erghib, kharid dugub, oof, laxawgal* (Somali), *abunzhur, torza* (Tuareg), *loukoi, lotai* (Turkana), *qufaa* (Yaa Galba, Kenya)**
'Autumn pneumonia': *rnaze* (Algeria)
Respiratory diseases in general: *dougouda, ene kouffa* (Borana)
Cold, influenza: *furri* (Gabbra)

Respiratory diseases are very important health problems in camels. They lower production and can kill the animal.

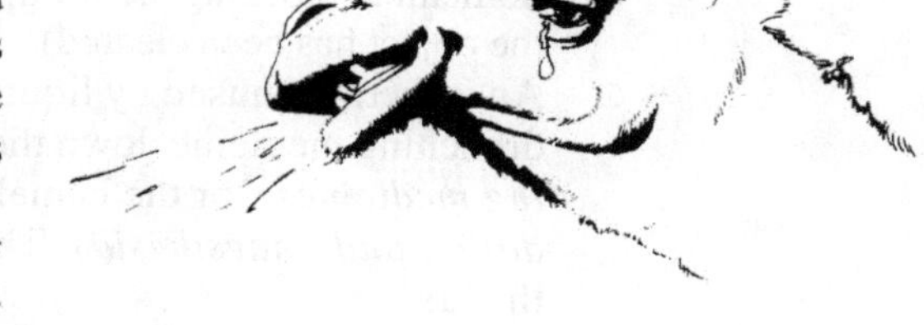

Coughing, runny nose and difficulty in breathing are signs of a problem somewhere in the respiratory tract. This consists of two main parts:

- The **'upper respiratory tract'**: nose, larynx (voice-box), trachea (windpipe) and bronchi (air passages leading to the lungs).
- The **'lower respiratory tract'**: lungs and pleura (the membrane that lines the chest cavity).

Camel **cough** has a characteristic sound and seems to come from deep in the chest.

Inflammation of the **nose** is called 'rhinitis'.

Inflammation of the **airway** is called 'bronchitis'.

Inflammation of the **lungs** is called 'pneumonia'. There are many different types of pneumonia, depending on the cause of the disease and the parts of the lungs infected.

Infections occur more frequently at the beginning of the rainy season. If animals are weakened (due to lack of food), stressed (due to work or transport), being weaned, or crowded together, they are more likely to become sick. Although usually not many camels die from such diseases, it takes them a long time to recover and production will be affected.

Signs

- Coughing, sneezing.
- Difficulty in breathing or drinking.
- Rapid breathing (over 10–15 times a minute).
- Dilated (widened) nostrils.
- Runny nose, tears in the eyes, drooling from the mouth.
- Poor appetite.
- Fever.

- Pregnant camels may abort, and milking animals may stop giving milk (▷*Abortion*).

There may be other signs, depending on the cause of the disease. Watch out for signs in other parts of the body (such as ▷*Diarrhoea* or *Abortion*) or unusual behaviour.

Cause

Coughing and runny nose in camels can be caused by many different things, including worms and other parasites, viruses and bacteria (▷*Problems of the nose and lungs*).

- Infection with viruses and bacteria. These can specifically affect the respiratory tract (for instance the influenza viruses) or the respiratory tract can be affected together with other parts of the body (as is the case with ▷*Haemorrhagic septicaemia*). An illness may begin as a virus infection but later turn into a bacterial infection. This often happens if the camel is not allowed to rest enough during the first few days of illness.
- Parasites such as ▷*Lungworms* that live in the respiratory tract and block the passage of air.
- Something blocking the windpipe or throat (the choking or coughing stops after the object has been cleared).
- An infection caused by liquid mistakenly put in the lungs: for example, by drenching medicine down the windpipe instead of the gullet (▷*Administering medicines*), or the camel breathing in vomit while it is sedated (▷*Sedation and anaesthesia*). These can quickly lead to serious infections of the lungs.

Pneumonia is rare is camels, but is hard to diagnose. A camel with pneumonia has fever and difficulty in breathing. Check for signs of an underlying disease, such as ▷*Haemorrhagic enteritis* or *Colibacillosis*.

Diseases of the nose and lungs can be transmitted in different ways. Some diseases spread from sick camels to healthy ones when they are close together during watering or in pens at night. Bacteria and viruses are spread by coughing and sneezing. Larger parasites such as lungworms are spread through contaminated pasture. Nasal bot flies lay their larvae in the camels' nostrils.

Prevention

- Keep sick camels away from healthy ones. Feed and water them separately, and build a separate pen for the sick animals. TRAD+SCI
- Give camels warm, salty water to drink.
- If the weather is cold, water in the middle of the day.
- Reduce stress.
- Shelter animals from the wind with a thick enclosure fence.
- Build the enclosure on a gentle slope so water drains away easily.
- Avoid building enclosures on valley bottoms or hilltops, as they are both prone to cold.
- Provide extra shelter for calves, especially if the mother has died or has rejected the calf.
- When drenching medicines, make sure that the liquid goes into the gullet rather than the windpipe (▷*Administering medicines*).
- To avoid a camel choking on its vomit during sedation, do not allow it to eat for 12 hours beforehand, and keep its head down during the sedation (▷*Sedation and anaesthesia*).

Treatment

If the camel has high fever, breathes rapidly, and its condition deteriorates quickly, treat with antibiotics. Allow the sick camel to rest for 7–10 days.

Use great care when giving liquid medicines to sick and coughing camels. The medicine should be given slowly so that the camel can swallow the medicine properly. If the medicine is given too quickly, some of the liquid may go into the camel's lungs and make the sickness worse.

Traditional treatments

Many of the treatments below aim to relieve the cough. They do not necessarily treat the underlying disease that causes it.

Herbal remedies

- Boil the resin of *galool* (*Acacia bussei*) in water and give the liquid as a drench. N SOMALIA
- Crush 0.5 kg of roots of *Adenia volkensii* (*loarakimak*) and soak in 2 litres of water for 12 hours. Drench with the liquid and repeat every 4 days until the camel recovers. TURKANA
- Give the roots of *Adenium aculeatum* (*dhalaandax*) to coughing camels to chew. SOMALI
- Drench with an infusion prepared from the roots of *Calotropis procera* (*etesuro*). TURKANA
- Pound the fibres of *Cissampelos pareira* (*malutyan*) and soak in water. Give the liquid as a drench. POKOT
- Mix the fruit of *Cucumis aculeatus* (*qalfoon*) with water and drench. SOMALI
- Crush the fruit of *Cucumis* sp. (*qaro*) in water and filter the liquid. Give as a drench. SOMALI
- Pound bark of *Cyperus alternifolius* (*sokwon*) and soak it in 0.5 litre of water. Give the liquid as a drench. POKOT
- Crush the tuberous root of *Entada leptostachya* (*gacmo-dheere*) in water and give the liquid as a drench. SOMALI
- Roast a branch of *Euphorbia robecchii* (*dharkeyn*) and give it to the camel to chew. SOMALI
- Crush the root of *Gutenbergia somalensis* (*nagaadh*), mix with ghee and force-feed it. SOMALI
- Soak fruits and bark of *Zanthoxylum chalybeum* in water. Give 0.5 litre of the liquid as a drench. POKOT
- Grind a handful of seeds of *Zanthoxylum chalybeum* (*loisuk*) into powder and drench with 0.5 litre of water. RENDILLE, SAMBURU

Ayurvedic remedies

- Mix 30–40 g of Caflon with *gur* (molasses) or treacle and put into the mouth 2–3 times per day. INDIA
- Put 25–30 g of Catcough into the mouth, 3 times a day. INDIA

Heat

- Isolate sick camels and surround the healthy animals with camel-dung fires in the evening. TUAREG
- Dry out weak animals near a fire after heavy rain.

Bleeding

- ○ Let blood from the angular vein of the eye and the superficial vein on the nose. Wash the inside of the nose with fresh goat's milk. MALI
- ○ Bleed the veins near the nostrils. TUAREG

Branding

- ○ Cauterize along the ribs with a hot iron, and wash the camel with a solution of soda ash (▷*Branding*). POKOT
- ○ Brand the ribcage and apply a paste of camel urine and faeces to the nostrils. N AND W AFRICA

Other

- ○ Put pepper, milk and butter into the nostrils. TUAREG
- ○ Wash the nostrils with warm water and throw pepper into them. MALI
- ○ Bung the nostrils with camel dung (used to treat *abanzhur*, a disease which causes a pus-like discharge from the nose). TUAREG
- ○ Make a soup or broth from the carcass of a wild animal. Feed the soup, called *maraq ugaadheed*, to the sick animal. N SOMALIA
- ○ Dissolve 0.25 kg of Magadi soda (*amakat*) in 2 litres of water and drench. Repeat every 4 days until the camel recovers. TURKANA

Modern treatments

Modern treatments depend on the cause of the disease. They include:

- ○ Antibiotics (usually injected) such as oxytetracycline for diseases caused by bacteria (▷*Common medicines*).
- ○ Anthelmintics (dewormers) for internal parasites (▷*Lungworms, Common medicines*).
- ○ Decongestants (medicines to clear mucus): e.g., 2 drops of 1% ephedrine sulphate every 3 hours into each nostril.
- ○ To loosen phlegm in the lungs, mix 2–4 g of ammonium carbonate in a ball of flour and give to the camel to eat.

References

Bizimana (1994) p. 343–6; Evans et al. (1995) p. 5:20; FAO (1994) p. 209–10; Forse (1999) p. 194–5, 350; ITDG and IIRR (1996) p. 130–2; Kaufmann (1998) p. 192; Leese (1927) p. 282; Manefield and Tinson (1997) p. 9, 190, 213–14; Projet Cameline (1999) p. 39; Rathore (1986) p. 127–34; Schwartz and Dioli (1992) p. 171–3, 199–202; Wernery and Kaaden (1995) p. 48–52; Wilson (1998) p. 106.

Leeches

***Lmolog* (Samburu), *calacuul* (Somali), *ngidike* (Turkana)**

Camels take in leeches when drinking infested water. The leeches attach on the back of the mouth and gums, and may disturb breathing.

Signs

- Coughing, gagging.
- Shaking of the head.
- Difficulty in eating.
- Blood from the mouth.

Other diseases causing similar signs are objects in the nose or mouth, and other mouth problems (▷*Problems of the nose and lungs, Problems of the head and neck*).

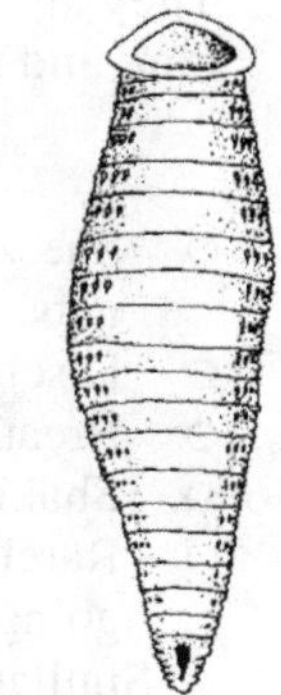

Leech (enlarged)

Cause

Drinking water infested with leeches.

Prevention

Preventing infestation by leeches is difficult.

- Avoid leech-infested water sources. Use water sources that are slightly salty rather than fresh, as freshwater leeches can survive only in fresh water.

Treatment

- Use a mouth gag to prevent the camel from biting, and detach the leeches by hand. To get a grip on the slippery leech, you can use a thin cloth or dip your fingers in dry soil or ash beforehand. TRAD
- Soak a handful of tobacco leaves in water and squeeze 50–100 ml of the juice into a cup. Very slowly pour this liquid into the mouth and nose. TRAD
- Give the camel chilli peppers (*Capsicum annuum*) to eat. TRAD
- Clean out the animal's mouth so you can see the leech. Then use a flattened stick to put a pinch of salt on the leech. TRAD
- Apply a hot object, such as a stick from the fire or a cigarette, on the leech. The leech will fall off. TRAD

References

Bizimana (1994) p. 343; Forse (1999) p. 175; ITDG and IIRR (1996) p. 91–2; Leese (1927) p. 299; 351; Manefield and Tinson (1997) p. 146; Wanyama (1997) vol. 2, p. 22–4.

Nasal bots

Nasal myiasis
***Al-naghaf* (Arabic), *rhamu* (Gabbra), *magaz ki kera* (India), *senghelel* (Rendille), *marsomwa* (Samburu), *sangaale* (Somali), *ekurrut* (Turkana)**

Nasal bots are fly maggots that live in the back of the camel's nose. They are very common under pastoral conditions, and can affect many animals in a herd. They are most common in the winter months. They are not an important problem, and rarely cause death.

Signs

- Sneezing, which may expel the maggots.
- Discharge from the nose.
- Breathing through the mouth.
- Shaking of the head.
- Rarely, unusual behaviour, such as going round in circles.

Similar signs can be caused by objects stuck in the nose or mouth, infections of the nose, windpipe and lungs (▷*Problems of the nose and lungs*), leeches in the nose (▷*Leeches*) and rabies (▷*Rabies*).

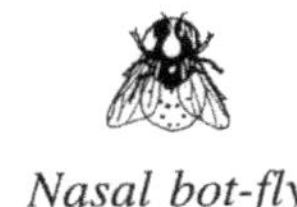

Nasal bot-fly

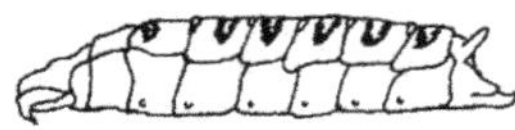

Maggot

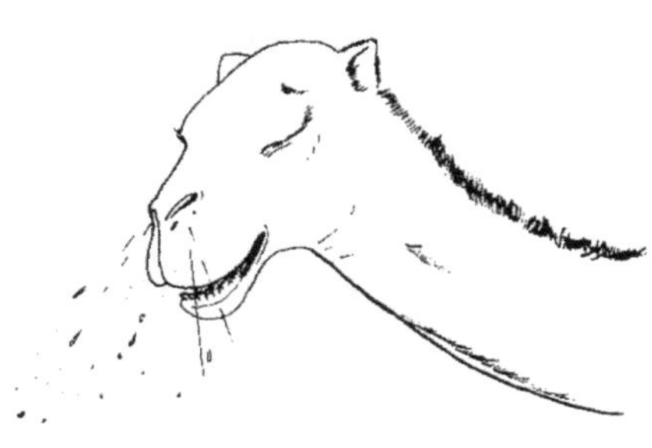

Cause

The nasal bot-fly (*Cephalopina titillator*) lays its larvae (maggots, or 'bots') in the camel's nostrils. The larvae crawl up the nose into the back of the nose and mouth. They can stay there for several months, causing irritation and making the animal sneeze. The maggots are white and about 35 mm long. The bot-flies themselves are rarely seen.

Prevention

- If nasal bots are an important disease, add trichlorfon (Neguvon) to the drinking water at a rate of 0.03–0.05% during the season when nasal bots occur. Do not give this to female camels in the last 6 weeks of pregnancy. SCI

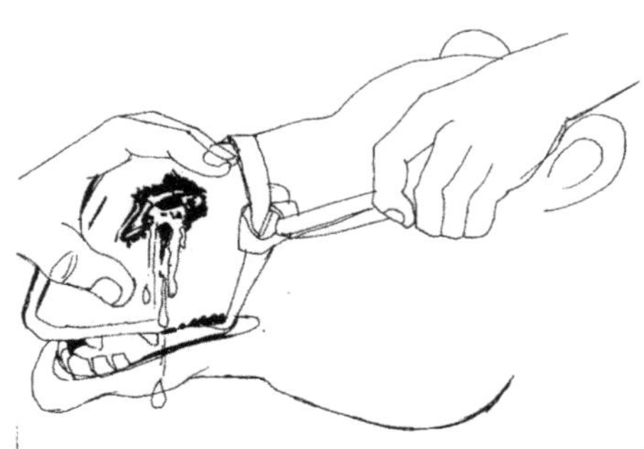

Treatment

Traditional treatments

- Apply a mixture of equal parts of turpentine and eucalyptus oil to the nostrils. This also repels flies. TRAD + SCI
- Soak tobacco leaves in water. **Very slowly** pour a small amount of the solution (less than 100 ml) into the nose.
- Lead the animal to a salty water source to drink. SOMALI KENYA
- Crush a 2.5 cm long piece of bark of *abach*, mix it with a glass of water, and let it stand for 12 hours. Draw about 20 ml of the fluid into a syringe, and squirt 10 ml into each nostril. This will make the animal sneeze several times. TURKANA

Modern treatments

Removing the larvae is impractical under field conditions, since it requires a special piece of equipment called an endoscope.

- Add trichlorfon (Neguvon) to the drinking water at a rate of 0.03–0.05%. Do not treat female camels in the last 6 weeks of pregnancy.

References

Evans et al. (1995) p. 7:30; Forse (1999) p. 202; Higgins (1986) p. 84–5; ITDG and IIRR (1996) p. 99–100; Leese (1927) p. 298; Manefield and Tinson (1997) p. 164; Rathore (1986) p. 189; Schwartz and Dioli (1992) p. 180, 209; Sewell and Brocklesby (1990) p. 20–1.

Lungworms

Verminous pneumonia
***Khurak* (India)**

This is a long-lasting disease of adult camels. The disease is common in the Indus and Nile deltas. It is more frequent after the rainy season from October to December. Many camels can be infected.

Signs

- Loss of appetite and general condition.
- Coughing.
- In later stages, the camel keeps its mouth open and tries to breathe through the mouth, with its head and nose stretched out.
- The camel is reluctant to move.
- Fever (38–40°C, 100–104°F) in the morning.
- Foul smell from the mouth.
- Yellowish-white discharge from both nostrils.
- The lips become itchy, and the camel rubs them on trees or walls. This leads to bloody sores on the lips.
- The camel may die after 15–20 days.

- After the animal has died and has been opened up, the worms can be seen in the lungs.
- The eggs and worm larvae can be seen through a microscope in the discharge from the nose and in dung samples.

The signs for lungworms are sometimes confused with ▷*Trypanosomiasis*.

Cause

Small, white roundworms (*Dictyocaulus filaria* and *D. viviparus*) that are 3–10 cm long and live in the air tubes (the 'bronchi') leading to and in the lungs. They infect camels, sheep and goats. Sick animals cough out the worm eggs onto pasture and into drinking water. Camels become infected by feeding on egg-infested pasture or drinking infested water.

Prevention

- Do not graze camels together with sheep and goats, and do not let them drink from the same water.

Treatment

Traditional treatments

- Drench with 1 litre of local alcohol or wine. INDIA
- Crush 500 g of *Albizia anthelmintica* (*ekapakiteng*) bark and soak in 2 litres of water for 6 hours. Stir, sieve and drench. TURKANA
- Crush 1 kg of *Diospyros scabra* (*eelim*) seeds. Soak in 4 litres of water for 6 hours. Sieve and drench with 2 litres of the liquid. TURKANA
- Soak about 250 g of *apetet* leaves in 2 litres of water and let stand for 6 hours. Stir, sieve and drench. TURKANA
- Soak about 250 g of *Trichilia emetica* (*ekuyen*) bark in 2 litres of water and let stand for 6 hours. Stir, sieve and drench. TURKANA
- Give 1 kg of salt lick the day after watering. Repeat each week. TURKANA

Modern treatments

- Inject once with ivermectin (0.2 mg/kg body weight) under the skin. Inject streptomycin and penicillin (e.g., 2–3 ml Penstrep per 50 kg body weight) into the muscle once a day for 7 days. Put 20 g of potassium iodide per day into the mouth, once a day for 7 days.
- Inject 22 mg/kg body weight of diethylcarbamazine citrate (e.g., 2.5 ml/50 kg body weight of Franocide) into the muscle, once a day for 3 days.

References

FAO (1994) p. 186–7; Forse (1999) p. 200–1; Higgins (1986) p. 69; ITDG and IIRR (1996) p. 114; Leese (1927) p. 287–9; Manefield and Tinson (1997) p. 150; Rathore (1986) p. 131–4; Sewell and Brocklesby (1990) p. 130–2.

Hydatid disease

Echinococcosis, hydatidosis

Hydatid disease is caused by a small tapeworm. The tapeworm itself infests dogs and hyenas, but camels, other livestock species and people can carry the immature forms of the tapeworms called cysts. Camels do not usually show any sign of the disease, but it is a serious problem in people, and can kill them.

Signs

- There are normally no signs in live camels, unless the cysts occur in the brain or heart (which is very rare).
- After the camel is slaughtered, the tapeworm cysts can be seen in the lungs and liver. They look like small ping-pong balls, but can be larger.

Cause

The small tapeworm *Echinococcus granulosus* infects the intestines of dogs and hyenas. The tapeworm eggs come out in the dog's faeces, and are eaten by browsing camels (and other animals such as cattle and sheep). The eggs hatch and form larvae, which move in the camel's body until they reach the lungs or liver, where they form cysts. Dogs that eat the offal of a dead camel take in the cysts, which then turn into adult tapeworms in the dog's intestines, so completing the life cycle.

People (especially small children) become infected because they come into close contact with dogs (and their faeces). If a person takes in the tapeworm eggs (for example, from dirty fingers), the cysts can develop in the person's lungs, liver or brain, causing serious illness or even death.

Prevention

- Do not allow dogs or hyenas to eat uncooked internal organs of camels.
- Deworm dogs with praziquantel (Droncit or Drontal Allwormer) every 3–12 months.

Treatment

- None.

References

Evans et al. (1995) p. 7:29; FAO (1994) p. 186–7, 234–5; Forse (1999) p. 7–8, 102; Higgins (1986) p. 70; ITDG and IIRR (1996) p. 111; Leese (1927) p. 291, 311, 331; Manefield and Tinson (1997) p. 82–3, 297; Rathore (1986) p. 136; Sewell and Brocklesby (1990) p. 117–19; Wilson (1998) p. 103.

6 Problems of the stomach and intestines

Problems in the stomach and intestines of camels can be caused by many different things: by what the camel has eaten, gut parasites, and general diseases that affect the whole body.

The tables below show the major diseases that can cause digestive problems in camels. See the relevant section for details on each disease.

Diarrhoea

For general diarrhoea treatments, ▷*Diarrhoea*.

Signs	Age group	Cause	See section
Loose faeces, normal colour	All ages	Intestinal worms, rut	▷*Internal parasites (worms), Rutting*
Various signs	Adults	Dietary changes, poisoning	▷*Diarrhoea, Plant poisoning*
Sudden, severe diarrhoea, with blood in faeces, often resulting in death	All ages	Clostridia (bacteria)	▷*Haemorrhagic enteritis*
Mild diarrhoea	All ages, especially calves after weaning	Trypanosomiasis (protozoan)	▷*Trypanosomiasis*
Black, soft faeces	All ages	Haemorrhagic septicaemia (bacteria)	▷*Haemorrhagic septicaemia*
White, liquid faeces	Calves	Drinking too much milk	▷*Calf diarrhoea*
Yellowish, watery faeces	Up to 4 weeks	Rotavirus, coronavirus	▷*Calf diarrhoea*

Signs	Age group	Cause	See section
Yellowish, often watery faeces; the animal becomes dehydrated	Calves	Colibacillosis (bacteria)	▷*Colibacillosis*
Yellow, greenish faeces, often blood	All ages	Salmonella (bacteria)	▷*Salmonellosis*

Constipation and other problems

Signs	Age group	Cause	See section
No faeces within 24 hours after birth	Newborns	Calf unable to pass first faeces	▷*Care of newborn calves*
Infrequent dung, large dung balls, straining when defecating	All ages	Lack of fibre in feed; low-quality roughage	▷*Constipation*
Few, black faeces, stained with mucus. Straining, but no dung. Belly swollen on the right side	All ages	Twisted intestine, intestinal worms, object in the gut	▷*Blocked intestines*
Black faeces or diarrhoea. Occasional bloat	All ages	Object blocking rumen	▷*Swallowed objects*
Belly pain, swollen on left side; little or no dung. Animal may die quickly	All ages	Gas: wrong feed	▷*Bloat*
Violent vomiting, bad breath	All ages	Acid rumen contents: wrong feed	▷*Indigestion*
Belly swollen on the right side, looks like abscess, but shrinks when you squeeze it. No signs of digestive disease	Especially pregnant females, but can also occur in males	Hernia (loop of intestine pushed through wall of abdomen)	Not covered in this manual (see Higgins (1986) p. 132–3)

Internal parasites (worms)

Tapeworms, roundworms, stomach worms, helminthiasis
***Kinyoot, ltuma, ltumai, ndumai* (Samburu), *bahala* (Somali), *ngirtan, nyiritan* (Turkana)**
Stomach worm (*Haemonchus longistipes*): *dud, hulaa, humar* (Sudan)

The camel is generally thought to be less prone to infection by internal parasites than are other livestock because it lives in dry areas and browses on trees rather than grazing close to the ground. Nevertheless, if camels are kept in areas with higher rainfall or in river valleys, then worm infestation can cause weakness, poor growth, low milk production, and even death.

The stomach worm is the most common type of parasitic worm. It is a serious blood-sucker, affecting between 25% and 75% of camels in some areas. It can kill camels, causing about 60% of deaths during the rainy season in Sudan.

Other roundworms and tapeworms can also grow in the camel's intestines.

Signs

The signs below are clearer during periods of stress, such as when feed is scarce or when the animals are moved frequently.

- General weakness and apathy.
- Drop of milk production in females.
- Diarrhoea, sometimes alternating with constipation.
- Pain in the belly.
- The animal may eat sand to get minerals (in stomach worm infestations).
- Anaemia.

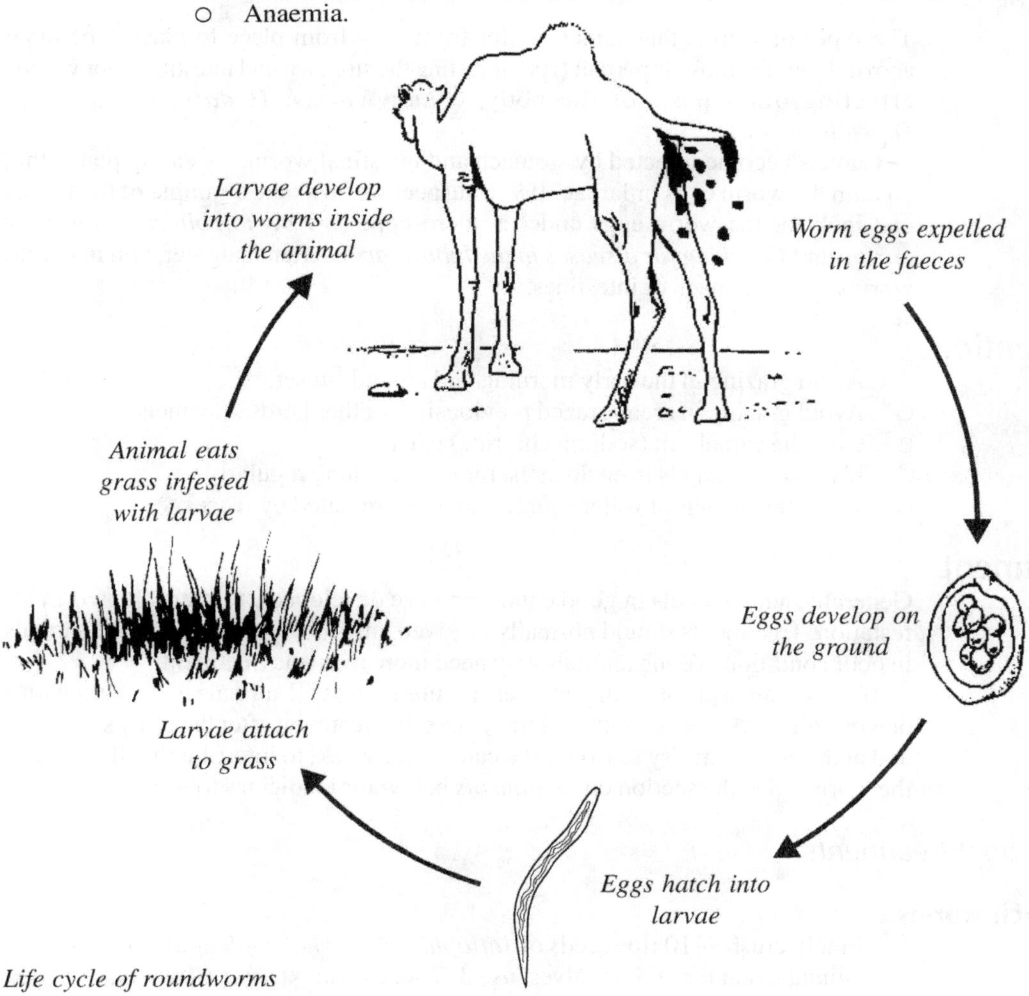

Larvae develop into worms inside the animal

Worm eggs expelled in the faeces

Eggs develop on the ground

Eggs hatch into larvae

Larvae attach to grass

Animal eats grass infested with larvae

Life cycle of roundworms

Type of worm	Worm species	Infects
Stomach worm (nematodes)	*Haemonchus longistipes*	Stomach
Other roundworms (nematodes)	*Cooperia pectinata* *Impalaia tuberculata* *Oesophagostomum columbianum* *Strongyloides papillosus* *Trichostrongylus probolurus*	Stomach, intestines
Tapeworms (cestodes)	*Moniezia expansa* *Stilesia vittata*	Intestines

- In severe cases, swelling above the eyes, on the sides of the chest-pad, and sometimes between the jaws.
- Lack of appetite, progressive wasting, and death after several weeks.

Causes

The types of worms that camels suffer from vary from place to place. The table above shows the most important types infesting the stomach and intestines. For worms affecting other parts of the body, ▷*Lungworms*, *Hydatid disease* and *Dipetalonemiasis*.

Camels become infected by stomach and intestinal worms by eating plants that contain the worm eggs or larvae. If you suspect worms, take a sample of the faeces and look for the worm eggs under a microscope (▷*How to collect samples for testing* and *Checking for diseases in the laboratory*). After slaughter, you may find worms in the stomach or intestines.

Prevention

- Avoid grazing in the early morning and around sunset.
- Avoid grazing in areas grazed previously by other herds of camels.
- Give the camel salt (sodium chloride) to eat.
- If you keep camels in enclosures, remove the dung regularly.
- Water the camels at water sources not contaminated by faeces.

Treatment

Generally, adult camels in good condition have developed a tolerance to worm infestation. Treatments should normally be given only to weaning calves and animals in poor condition. Young animals may need more than one treatment.

If worms are a problem in your area, regularly treat all animals in the herd with a deworming medicine or 'anthelmintic'. Give the treatment after the rainy season(s), and at the end of the dry season if the camels are weak, to interrupt the life cycle of the worms. See the section on *Treatments* below for medicines to use.

Traditional treatments

Stomach worms

- Finely crush 7–10 ripe seeds of *Jatropha curcas* (*habat almuluk*) and force the animal to eat these. For calves, use 3–7 seeds. SHUKRIYA, LAHAWIYIN, RASHAIDA

Roundworms

- Grind 1 *malwah* (2 kg) of seeds of *Acacia nilotica* (*garrad* in Arabic) into powder. Mix with water and drench early in the morning before grazing. Or soak the seeds in water overnight and drench. Repeat after 4 days.
  SHUKRIYA, LAHAWIYIN, RASHAIDA

Tapeworms

- Soak the bark of *Albizia anthelmintica* (*kamakiten*) for several hours in a little water overnight. Strain, then drench an adult animal with 100 ml of the liquid (only 10 ml for calves). POKOT
- Dry leaves of *Cassia senna* in the shade, then use them to make a soup or broth. Drench the animal with this liquid. The medicine will cause diarrhoea. The tapeworms will be expelled beginning about 1 hour later and throughout the whole day.

Other worm treatments

- Soak enough of the pods and bark of *Acacia mellifera* in water to make a thick liquid. Drench.
- Other formulations for worm infestations are sesame oil and table salt (sodium chloride).
- Soak 0.5 kg of the seeds of *Citrullus colocynthis* (bitter apple, *handal*) in 5 litres of water for about 12 hours. Drench the animal with this in the early morning. LAHAWIYIN, RASHAIDA, SHUKRIYA

Modern treatments

- Drench with 7.5 mg/kg body weight of albendazole (e.g., Valbazen).
- Mix 90 mg/kg of thiabendazole powder with water and drench, or put into the mouth as a bolus.
- Put oxfendazole paste or liquid into the mouth at a dose of 4.5–5 mg/kg body weight. (This also works against tapeworms.)
- Apply fenbendazole (Panacur) paste or liquid in the mouth at a dose of 5–7.5 mg/kg body weight.
- Inject ivermectin (Ivomec) under the skin at a dosage of 0.2 mg/kg of the camel's body weight.

Caution: Levamisole (sold as e.g., Nilverm) has been reported as ineffective, and may even be toxic in camels.

References

Bizimana (1994) p. 42–6; Evans et al. (1995) p. 5:20, 7:15–19; FAO (1994) p. 186–7; Forse (1999) p. 94–102, 218–20, 336–8; Higgins (1986) p. 60–6; ITDG and IIRR (1996) p. 115–17; Manefield and Tinson (1997) p. 119–23; Projet Cameline (1999) p. 27, 31–3; Rathore (1986) p. 182–9; Sewell and Brocklesby (1990) p. 108–9, 111–14, 130–2, 142–4, 149–55, 157; Wilson (1998) p. 102–3.

Diarrhoea

***Albati* (Borana, Gabbra), *dast* (Hindi), *ngorotit* (Samburu), *har, hardik* (Somali), *harr, diggheharr* (Rendille), *colera, loleo* (Turkana)**

Diarrhoea is common in calves and kills many of them. In adult animals, diarrhoea often occurs at the beginning of the rainy season. For information on diarrhoea in calves, ▷*Calf diarrhoea*, *Colibacillosis* and *Salmonellosis*.

Signs

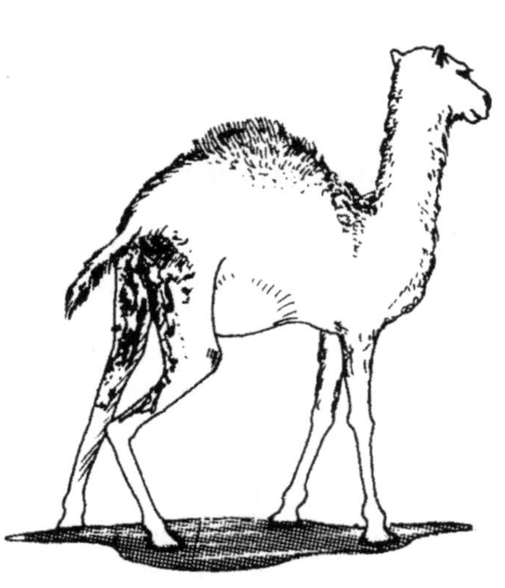

- ○ The faeces change colour and consistency, and often smell foul.
- ○ Weakness and loss of condition.
- ○ Fever (not always present).
- ○ Swollen belly.
- ○ Sunken eyes.
- ○ If the animal is a calf, it may stop suckling.

Causes

Many things can cause diarrhoea (▷*Problems of the stomach and intestines*):

- ○ Drinking too much milk (in calves).
- ○ Infection of the stomach or intestines with bacteria or viruses.
- ○ Sudden changes in the feed.
- ○ ▷*Internal parasites (worms)*.
- ○ ▷*Plant poisoning*.
- ○ Stress (for example, during transport by lorry, examination or treatment).
- ○ Rut (▷*Rutting*).
- ○ ▷*Trypanosomiasis*, *Haemorrhagic septicaemia* and other general infections.

Prevention

- ○ Keep sick animals away from healthy ones.
- ○ Manage grazing carefully: move animals away from infected ground and water holes contaminated with faeces.
- ○ Keep animals away from poisonous plants.
- ○ Control the milk intake of calves.

Treatments

It is important to find out what is causing the diarrhoea and, if necessary, to treat this underlying disease as well as the diarrhoea itself. ▷*Problems of the stomach and intestines* and the relevant sections of this manual for help on identifying and treating these diseases. Some additional treatments for diarrhoea are given below.

If the animal has high fever and heavy diarrhoea, and its condition is deteriorating rapidly, treat with antibiotics (▷*Common medicines*).

Traditional treatments

- Boil the bark of *Acacia nilotica* or *A. nubica* in water. Allow to cool, strain, then drench. KENYA
- Drench with tea.
- Soak the bark of *Boswellia hildebrandtii* (*sungululwa*) in 2 litres of water, then give as a drench. POKOT
- Boil the bark of *Ziziphus mauritiana* (*tilomwa*) in 1 litre of water. Allow to cool, then give the liquid as a drench. POKOT
- Provide boiled grains as additional feed. TRAD+SCI
- Crush 0.5 kg of *Zanthoxylum chalybeum* (*eusugu*) seeds, mix with 2 litres of water, stir thoroughly and drench. TURKANA
- Mix a 30 g sachet of Diaroak with five times the amount of water, shake well and drench. Repeat twice a day. Use half a sachet for calves. AYURVEDIC
- Mix 30–50 g of Neblon with curd or rice water and drench. Repeat 2–3 times a day. AYURVEDIC

Modern treatments

- Treat with oral rehydration liquid (▷*Calf diarrhoea*).
- Mix 200 ml kaolin (China clay) with about 1 litre of water and use this drench for an adult animal. For calves, use half these amounts.
- Give a commercial antidiarrhoea treatment by mouth, e.g., Antidiarrhoea Powder, Scourban or Biogent.
- Administer a long-acting antibiotic (▷*Common medicines*).

References

Bizimana (1994) p. 38–40; Evans et al. (1995) p. 5:20, 7:28; FAO (1994) p. 201–4, 257; Forse (1999) p. 211–12, 345–6; Higgins (1986) p. 160; ITDG and IIRR (1996) p. 145–8; Kaufmann (1998) p. 193; Manefield and Tinson (1997) p. 9, 73–4, 250, 287; Rathore (1986) p. 121–2; Schwartz and Dioli (1992) p. 169–71, 195–6; Wanyama (1997) vol. 2, p. 79–83; Wernery and Kaaden (1995) p. 37–45; Wilson (1998) p. 102–4.

Haemorrhagic enteritis

Enterotoxaemia

A severe disease, which often kills the animal very quickly.

Signs

- Shivering, sweating, staggering, aggressive behaviour, seizures.
- Enlarged lymph nodes.
- Sometimes acute diarrhoea; sometimes only unusual-coloured faeces.
- Abdominal pain.
- The animal is dull and listless.

- The animal may die only a few hours after the disease appears. In less severe cases, calves may survive for a few days and then recover.

After the animal has died, you may see the following:

- Bloody, blackened spots in the small intestine.
- Blood spots in the chest muscles, on the lungs and in the heart muscles.
- Large amount of yellowish fluid in the body cavities.
- Gas in the rumen (first compartment of the stomach).
- Under a microscope, large numbers of gram-positive, rod-shaped bacteria may be seen in the intestinal contents (▷*Checking for diseases in the laboratory*).

Haemorrhagic enteritis may be confused with ▷*Abscesses on the lymph nodes, Salmonellosis, Haemorrhagic septicaemia* and *Plant poisoning*.

Cause

Bacteria of the genus *Clostridium*, mostly *Clostridium perfringens* type A. These bacteria form spores which survive in the soil. The camel becomes infected by eating the soil. The disease may be triggered by another disease (such as ▷*Trypanosomiasis* or *Salmonellosis*), feeding the wrong feed (such as too much barley or milk), changes in the climate or pasture, or stress caused by transportation or weighing.

Prevention

- Vaccinate breeding females against haemorrhagic enteritis during late pregnancy, two times, 1 month apart. Then vaccinate the animals again once a year. SCI
- Make sure that calves drink as much colostrum (the mother's first milk) as possible. SCI
- Vaccinate calves during the first few months of life, and then once a year. SCI

Treatment

Treatment with antibiotics is usually not effective because the disease is too severe. To apply the antibiotic, it is necessary to put a tube down the animal's throat into the abomasum (the last of the camel's stomachs), so bypassing the rumen, and applying the antibiotic through this tube. Note: this is not practical in the field. SCI

References

Bizimana (1994) p. 41; Evans et al. (1995) 7:28; Forse (1999) p. 146; Higgins (1986) p. 104; Manefield and Tinson (1997) p. 88–9; Rathore (1986) p. 175–6; Sewell and Brocklesby (1990) p. 57–8; Wernery and Kaaden (1995) p. 6–12.

Constipation

***Udao dabab* (Gabbra), *pet band hona* (Hindi)**

Constipation is the delayed or infrequent passing of faeces. It can be a serious problem in calves. In adult animals it is more common among draught camels kept near towns, or with racing camels fed on concentrated feed.

Signs

- The camel stops eating, or eats less.
- The camel looks dull and lethargic.
- Dung balls become larger and longer.
- The camel strains when passing dung.

Other problems that cause similar signs are ▷*Blocked intestines, Bloat* and *Swallowed objects*.

Cause

- Pastoralists think that constipation in calves is caused by drinking too much milk.
- Lack of fibre in the feed (when camels are not allowed to browse by themselves).
- Feeding too much grain or pelleted food.
- Feeding low-quality roughage.

Prevention

- Make sure the camel gets plenty of green fodder.

Treatment

Traditional treatments

- For calves, pound a root called *saar* (from *Commiphora* sp.), mix it with water, boil it and allow it to cool, then drench with the liquid. GABBRA
- Pound *tambo* (a local tobacco plant) and mix with water and salt. Boil, cool, then drench. GABBRA
- Mix 1 kg of jaggery with plenty of water and drench. RAIKA
- Mix 10 g of *hing* (asafoetida) with *chach* (buttermilk) and drench. RAIKA
- Drench with 0.25 kg of Magadi soda dissolved in 2 litres of water. TURKANA

Other plants used for curing constipation include *Boscia senegalensis* (berries pounded in water) in West Africa, *Citrullus colocynthis* (fruits), and *Aerva tomentosa* in Nigeria.

Modern treatments

- Drench with 1–1.5 litres of cooking oil or liquid paraffin per day for 3 days.
- Drench with one or two bottles of molasses mixed with equal amount of water.
- Drench with 250g of Epsom salts (magnesium sulphate) in a large amount of water.
- Also inject with metamizole (e.g., 20–40 ml Novalgin) into the muscle or the vein as a supportive measure.
- Give 15–20 litres of fluid drip into the vein (▷*Administering medicines*).
- Force-feed with a faecal softener or laxative such as Tympanyl or Furlax paste.
- If the above treatment is unsuccessful, drench with a purgative such as Camelax mixed with water.
- Give an enema of soapy water.

References

Bizimana (1994) p. 35–8, 341; Evans et al. (1995) p. 7:28; FAO (1994) p. 201, 204, 258; Forse (1999) p. 212–13, 346–7; ITDG and IIRR (1996) p. 144; Manefield and Tinson (1997) p. 68–9; Rathore (1986) p. 118–19.

Blocked intestines

Intestinal obstruction
***Aant ka anta, ant ruk jana, ant ka but* (Rajasthan)**

If something blocks a camel's intestines, it cannot defecate. Unless the blockage is removed, the animal will die. Blocked intestines are very rare in camels.

Signs

- The belly is swollen on the camel's **right** side, and the swelling gradually increases.
- The animal stops eating, drinking or chewing the cud.
- At first there are a few black faeces, stained with mucus. Then there are no faeces at all, although the animal strains as if trying to defecate.
- The animal appears dull and depressed and is unwilling to move.
- The eyes are watery.
- The body temperature is below normal.
- The animal dies in about 10–12 days.
- If the animal is slaughtered, an obstruction in the intestine may be found: a twisting or telescoping of one part of the intestine into another.

Blocked intestines can be confused with ⊳*Bloat* (belly swollen on the left side of the animal), *Constipation*, or *Swallowed objects*.

Cause

- Twisting of the intestine, or telescoping of one part of the intestine into another (very rare in camels).
- Parasites, swallowed stones and other objects, hairballs, or balls of undigested vegetation in the intestine.
- Eating strange objects (⊳*Pica*).

Treatment

The obstruction will kill the animal if it is not treated adequately.

Traditional treatment

- Mix 1 kg of common salt with 1–2 litres of cooking oil or castor oil. Drench.

INDIA, AFRICA

Modern treatments

- Drench with castor oil or liquid paraffin.
- Give a drip of 10 to 15 litres of Ringer's lactate each day for 3 days (⊳*Administering medicines*). Inject into the muscle 1 mg per 50 kg body weight of neostigmine sulphate for 3 days. Drench a mixture of the following once a day for 3 days: 1 kg of salt, 1 kg of magnesium chloride and 1–2 litres of cooking oil. Give an enema of soapy water once a day. Stop the treatment if the obstruction clears.

See ⊳*Constipation* for other treatments. If the treatments fail, a skilled veterinarian may be able to perform surgery. However, the chances of success are small.

References

Forse (1999) p. 217–18; Manefield and Tinson (1997) p. 68, 111; Rathore (1986) p. 125–6.

Swallowed objects

Camels do not often swallow objects because they grasp their feed with their lips, but camels with mineral deficiency may eat strange objects. Feed concentrate sometimes contains stones or metal.

Signs

- Choking, coughing (object caught in throat).
- Occasional bloat.
- Black faeces or diarrhoea.
- Loss in condition.

Problems causing similar signs include ▷*Bloat* (belly swollen on the left side of the animal), *Blocked intestines*, and *Constipation*.

Cause

Objects in the feed, accidental swallowing of tools, hairballs in the stomach. Mineral deficiency (▷*Pica*) may make camels eat strange things, such as gravel.

Prevention

- Check that the camel is not eating strange things.
- Take care when operating on the mouth. Hold onto equipment like drenching tubes or balling guns tightly when using them.

Treatment

Object caught in the throat

Restrain the animal and sedate if necessary. Use a gag to hold the mouth open so you can remove the object.

Object in stomach (rumen)

Objects in the stomach can be removed by an operation. This should be done by a trained veterinarian.

References

Gahlot and Chouhan (1992) p. 129; Manefield and Tinson (1997) p. 110–11, 224–5.

Bloat

Rumen impaction, tympany
***Afra, pet jam hona, pet rukana* (Rajasthan)**

Bloat (the build-up of gases in the rumen) is not a common problem in camels, perhaps because (unlike some livestock) they are able to vomit.

Signs

- The belly is swollen on the camel's left side (the side where the rumen is).
- Mild signs of pain in the belly ('colic').
- The animal stops eating and drinking.
- The camel rolls on the ground on its left and right sides, but not on its back.
- The animal may die quickly – within 30 minutes!

Do not confuse bloat with ⊳*Blocked intestines* (belly swollen on the right side of the animal).

Cause

- Allowing the camel to drink soon after grazing certain types of fodder, such as groundnut leaves and roughage.
- Overfeeding on ghee, dates and alfalfa.

Prevention

- Do not allow camels to drink immediately after eating types of feed that cause bloat.
- Avoid overfeeding on ghee, dates and alfalfa.

Treatment

It is necessary to treat bloat very quickly, or the animal may die.

Traditional treatments

- Drench with 200 ml of kerosene or cooking oil, mixed with 800 ml of milk or water.
- Mix 500 g of *amakat* (Magadi soda) with 1 litre of water. Stir well and drench the animal with the mixture. For large camels, give 2 litres of the liquid.

TURKANA

Modern treatments

- Mild bloat: drench with 300–500 ml of Tympanyl.
- Inject into the vein by drip 10–15 litres of Ringer's lactate for 3 days. Drench with a mixture of 1 kg of salt, 1 kg of magnesium sulphate and 1–2 litres of cooking oil. Make the camel walk at least 500 m after giving the drench so that the liquid mixes well with the stomach contents and the intestines begin to work. Inject under the skin 1 mg/50 kg body weight of neostigmine sulphate per day for 3 days.
- In severe cases, make the animal lie on its chest. Put a stomach tube (a long rubber tube) through the animal's mouth and down into its stomach (⊳*Administering medicines*). Allow the gas in the stomach to come out gently. If necessary, pour 0.5–1 litre of Tympanyl or liquid paraffin down the tube to break up any froth.
- As a last resort, and only if the animal is going to die if you do not treat it immediately, pierce the abdomen with a trocar and cannula (a special, sharp, needle-like instrument with a tube attached), a sharp knife, or a long, thick needle, to release the gas from the rumen. Pierce the left side of the animal, 10 cm (about 1 hand's width) behind the last rib, and 7.5 cm below the ridge on the animal's side formed by the bones in the spine (see the picture on the next page). **Caution:** no smoking while doing this, as the gas is flammable!

References

Bizimana (1994) p. 34–5, 340–1; Evans et al. (1995) p. 7:26; FAO (1994) p. 257; Forse (1999) p. 215–17, 347; ITDG and IIRR (1996) p. 142–3; Manefield and Tinson (1997) p. 42; Rathore (1986) p. 119–20; Wanyama (1997) vol. 2, p. 44–6.

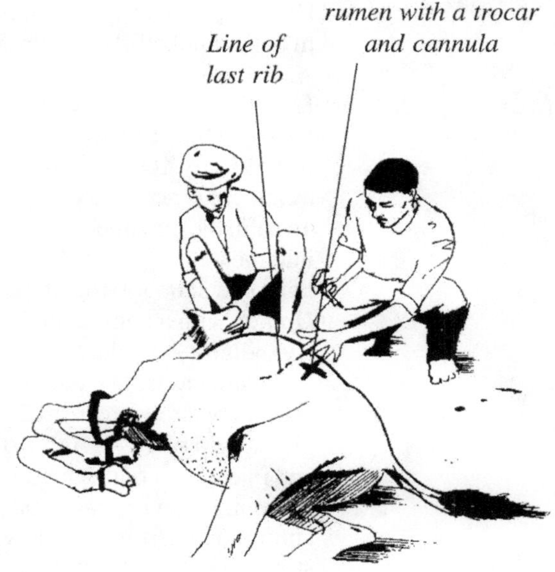

Indigestion

Rumen acidosis, overeating, ruminal overload
Apach, badi **(Rajasthan)**

Camels that are given feed concentrates and overeat may get indigestion. This is a problem in racing and working camels, not those kept by pastoralists.

Signs

- The camel vomits violently. The vomit is acidic.
- There is a foul, acidic smell from the mouth.
- The animal stops chewing the cud. It walks stiffly and is unwilling to move.

Cause

- Eating too much concentrate, wheat grain or flour, alfalfa, dates, jaggery (brown sugar), sugar or *gur* (molasses).

Prevention

- Prevent overeating of concentrates.
- Give a balanced diet with plenty of roughage.

Treatment

A camel will often immediately vomit up liquids given in a drench. To avoid this, have someone hold the animal's mouth up for at least 30 seconds after drenching the liquid (▷*Administering medicines*).

Traditional treatment

- Dissolve 0.5–1 kg of sodium bicarbonate (known as *meetha* soda in Rajasthan) in half a bucketful of water, and drench.

Modern treatments

- Dissolve 0.5–1 kg of sodium bicarbonate in water and drench on the first day, followed by 100 g per day for 2–3 days. If the disease is mild, then only this treatment is necessary.
- To calm the gut, inject with hyoscine (e.g., 20–30 ml of Buscopan Compositum) into the vein.
- Dissolve 250–500 mg of magnesium sulphate in 2.5–5 litres of water. Drench.
- Drench with a commercial anti-indigestion medicine such as Ruminodigest or Bykodigest Antacid.
- In severe cases, use one of the treatments above, and also inject 60–120 g of sodium bicarbonate in a 1.3–5% solution into the vein, once a day for 1–2 days; give a drip of 10–15 litres of 0.9% normal saline solution per day for 3 days; and inject with multivitamins.
- In the most severe cases, take 0.5–1 litre of the fluid from the rumen of another animal (e.g., from a healthy animal that has just been slaughtered, or using a stomach tube and pump), and drench the sick animal with this.

References

Manefield and Tinson (1997) p. 133–4; Rathore (1986) p. 118–19.

7 Infectious diseases

Camels suffer from many diseases that affect more than one part of their body. The major ones are listed in the table below.

Most of the diseases listed below cause fever and make the camel unwilling to eat. It loses weight and condition. Other signs include diarrhoea, bleeding in the mouth, nose or anus, and swollen lymph nodes.

It can be difficult to distinguish among these diseases. Check other sections of this book, remembering that the disease may not show the typical signs described here. If possible, take a sample and have it tested in the laboratory (▷*How to collect samples for testing* and *Checking for diseases in the laboratory*).

Several of these diseases can be transmitted to people. Be especially careful when handling or examining animals with these diseases (▷*Diseases that people can catch from camels*).

Diseases covered in this chapter

Major signs	Cause	Disease
Weight loss, fever, anaemia, oedema, abortion late in pregnancy	Blood parasite	▷*Trypanosomiasis*
Difficulty in breathing, inflamed testicles, loss of condition	Parasite	▷*Dipetalonemiasis*
Swollen lymph nodes, dark red mucous membranes in eyes and mouth, weak cough, blood-stained dung	Bacteria	▷*Haemorrhagic septicaemia*
Swollen lymph nodes, bleeding in skin, nose, mouth, anus	Unknown	▷*Swollen glands, khanid*
Dry cough, no stomach movement, enlarged lymph nodes	Bacteria	▷*Haemorrhagic disease*
High fever, dark red blood from mouth, nose and anus, sudden death	Bacteria	▷*Anthrax*
Swellings under skin in shoulder or hind legs. Dark skin on legs, crackling sound when touched. Lameness	Bacteria	▷*Blackquarter*
Stiffness, spasms, trembling	Bacteria	▷*Tetanus*

Major signs	Cause	Disease
Strange behaviour, drooling, excitement	Virus	▷*Rabies*
Weakness, abortions	Virus	▷*Rift Valley fever*

Diseases covered in other chapters

The table above does not include infectious diseases that affect mainly one part of the body. The main ones are listed below.

Major signs	Body parts most affected	Cause	Disease
Pimples, fever, especially in calves	Skin	Virus	▷*Pox, Orf*
Coughing, sneezing, difficulty breathing	Nose, windpipe, lungs	Virus, bacteria	▷*Problems of the nose and lungs*
Diarrhoea	Stomach, intestines	Virus, bacteria	▷*Problems of the stomach and intestines*

Trypanosomiasis

Trypanosomosis, surra
***Louta, ghandi, dukan* (Borana), *atteh, gudho* (Eritrea), *ghandi, dukan* (Gabbra), *surra* (India), *guffar* (Kordofan), *el debab* (Middle East, North Africa, Sudan), *surra* (Pakistan), *lokurucho* (Pokot), *omar* (Rendille), *ltikana, saar* (Samburu), *dhuukaan, dukan* (=*T. evansi*), *korbarar* (= *T. congolense*), *geudhi, ghandi, gindi, suuqiye* (Somali), *lokipi, ltorobwo* (Turkana), *mbori, tahaga* (West Africa)**

Trypanosomiasis is probably the most widespread and economically important disease in camels. It occurs wherever camels are kept, except Australia.

Trypanosomiasis is transmitted from one animal to the other by biting flies (mostly tabanids). It is more frequent in relatively humid areas and rare in extremely dry zones, where there are few flies. The disease occurs seasonally, spreading after the beginning of the rainy season when flies multiply.

Trypanosomiasis can take an acute course, leading to death in 2 weeks to 3 months. Or it can take a chronic course, lasting over several years. The chronic course is more frequent.

Signs

- Reduced appetite and water intake.
- Animal becomes thin, and the hump disappears.

- Intermittent fever.
- Hair dull and rough, lost from tail.
- Swelling (oedema) under the belly or neck, especially visible in the morning.
- Females abort late in pregnancy.
- Newborn calves of infected mothers may die.
- The amount of milk from milking animals drops rapidly.
- The urine may have a characteristic smell.
- The membranes around the eyes are pale (anaemia).
- Watery eyes.
- The animal may become more prone to infection with other diseases, especially ▷*Mange* and pneumonia (▷*Coughs, colds and pneumonia*).
- Sometimes abnormal behaviour, staggering and blindness.
- The animal usually dies in a few months.

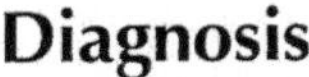

Diagnosis

Trypanosomiasis can be hard to diagnose. Watch for the signs listed above. You can also try the tests described below to confirm that an animal has trypanosomiasis. Various other tests not described here can be done in a specially equipped laboratory.

Traditional tests

- **Sandball test**. Collect a handful of the soil that the camel has urinated on. Shape it into a ball, let it dry for 15 minutes, and then break it open. If the animal has trypanosomiasis, you can smell a typical, sweet smell.
- **Tail-hair test**. Try to pull a hair out from the animal's tail. If it comes out easily and has some tissue sticking to it, this means that the animal has trypanosomiasis.

Modern tests

Trained animal health workers can do special tests to find the trypanosome parasites in the blood of sick animals. ▷*How to collect samples for testing* and *Checking for diseases in the laboratory* for details.

Direct tests look for the trypanosomes themselves in the blood. These tests are not very reliable, as there may not be many trypanosome parasites in the blood, and they can be hard to see (especially if you are inexperienced). So if you do not see any parasites in the blood, you cannot be sure that the animal does *not* have trypanosomiasis.

The trypanosome parasites are present in the blood only at certain times when the animal has a fever. Blood samples should be taken from the ear, and when the animal's body temperature is above normal.

Direct tests include wet blood film, dry blood film and the buffy coat test.

Indirect tests detect changes in the blood rather than the trypanosomes themselves. The same changes can be caused by other diseases, so you cannot be absolutely certain an animal has trypanosomiasis even if the test is positive. Indirect tests include packed cell volume and the mercuric chloride test.

Cause

Trypanosomiasis is caused by small parasites (called 'trypanosomes') that live in the blood. There are several different species of trypanosomes. *Trypanosoma evansi* is the most common in camels. This is carried from one camel to another by biting flies.

In sub-humid parts of Africa, trypanosomiasis caused by *T. congolense* and *T. vivax* can be carried from cattle to camels by tsetse flies. This form of the disease takes a rapid course. It is common in areas with thick vegetation or near rivers.

Trypanosomes are carried by biting flies, especially tabanids. Tsetse flies are less important as carriers in camels than in cattle. It is possible that camel flies (*Hippobosca camelina*, or *takar* in Somali) also transmit the disease, although they are not important carriers.

Prevention

- Avoid fly-infested areas such as thickets and river basins.
- Water animals around noon or at night, when fly activity is low.
- Water animals in small groups so that they do not stay long at wells.
- Repel flies with smoke from cow dung.
- Use pour-on insecticides (synthetic pyrethroids such as permethrin and cypermethrin) to repel flies.
- Inject quinapyramine chloride and quinapyramine methylsulphate mixture (Triquin, Antrycide) at a dose of 5 mg/kg body weight, 3–4 weeks after the start of the rainy season when the danger of infection is greatest. Be very careful to follow the instructions that are supplied with the drug. If too little is used, the parasites can become resistant to the drug.

See ▷*Bites and stings* for more ways of repelling flies.

Treatment

Traditional treatments

Pastoralists have many treatments for trypanosomiasis. Some of these are listed below, but they are not known to be effective.

- The **Pokot** conduct a cleansing rite for fever called *chpkogh*. They also use several herbal remedies:
  - 1 kg of roots of *Clerodendrum* sp. (*chepotet*), crushed and boiled in 5 litres of water. This liquid is cooled and strained, then about 2 litres are drenched.
  - 1 kg of roots and bark of *Acacia reficiens* (*pilil*), crushed and soaked in 5 litres of water overnight. The resulting mixture is strained and 3 litres are used as a drench.
  - 0.5 kg of ash from *Salvadora persica* (*asiokonyon*), mixed with 1 litre of water and then drenched.
  - Dried, pounded fruit and bark of *Zanthoxylum chalybeum* (*songowo*), mixed with water and drenched.

- The **Rendille** bleed sick animals.
- The **Samburu** feed sick animals with sheep's fat or drench them with an extract of *Myrsine africana* (*seketet*). They also:
  - Crush fruits of *Zanthoxylum chalybeum* (*loisuk*), mix them with water, and give as a drink twice a day.
  - Grind 200 g of fresh bark of *Terminalia brownii* (*lbukoi*), boil it in 2 litres of water, and allow it to cool. They then drench the liquid. They may add another 2 litres of water to the bark, boil and drench again the following day.
- The **Turkana** soak 0.5 kg of the crushed roots of *Adenia volkensii* (*loarakimak*) in 2 litres of water for 12 hours. They drench with 2 litres of the liquid.
- In **Mali**, camel herders make sick animals eat pounded millet and billy-goat meat.
- The **Tuareg** in Niger give a sick animal fresh cow's or goat's milk for up to a week. Other remedies include feeding with the meat from a jackal and pouring a mixture of *Boscia senegalensis*, *Cadaba glandulosa* and *Maerua crassifolia* into the nostrils.
- The **Raika** in India treat trypanosomiasis with chilli peppers.

Modern treatments

- Inject quinapyramine chloride and quinapyramine methylsulphate (Triquin, Antrycide) under the skin at a dose of 5 mg/kg body weight. This is effective against both *T. evansi* and *T. congolense*.
- For *T. evansi* only, inject melarsomine (Cymelarsan) into the muscle at a dose of 0.25 mg/kg body weight. This drug comes in ampoules containing 100 mg: enough to treat a 400 kg animal. Dissolve the powder in 20 ml of sterile water before injecting it. This medicine is reported to be safe even in pregnant camels, but is not available in all countries.
- Inject suramin (Naganol) 10% solution (1 sachet of 5 g in 50 ml of sterile water) intravenously at a dose of 10 mg/kg body weight (i.e., 30–50 ml for the average camel weighing 300–500 kg). Do not inject into the muscle, as it is irritating. It is not effective against *T. congolense*.

Isometamidium chloride (Samorin, Trypanidium) is **not recommended** for use in camels. It should not be injected into the muscle as it causes severe irritation. If you do use it, inject it into the vein as a 1% solution (1 g in 100 ml of sterile water) at a rate of 0.25 mg/kg body weight. Make sure that the animal is well rested. Do not use this medicine together with other anti-trypanosomiasis drugs, and do not use too high a dosage. It is effective against both *T. evansii* and *T. congolense*.

Important Do not use diminazene aceturate (Berenil, Trypazen): it is toxic to camels. Homidium chloride (Ethidium) and homidium bromide (Novidium) are not effective, and the animal may get sick again after a few weeks.

References

Bizimana (1994) p. 376–9; Evans et al. (1995) p. 7:1, 7:6, 5:20–1; FAO (1994) p. 184–5; Forse (1999) p. 295–300, 334–6; Higgins (1986) p. 42–9; ITDG and IIRR (1996) p. 126–7; Kaufmann (1998) p. 190–1; Leese (1927) p. 217; Manefield and Tinson (1997) p. 274–6; Projet Cameline (1999) p. 27, 29–30; Rathore (1986) p. 162–7; Schwartz and Dioli (1992) p. 157, 166–7; Sewell and Brocklesby (1990) p. 204–15, 217–21; Wilson (1998) p. 100–2.

Dipetalonemiasis

Dipetalonemiasis is caused by a worm that lives in certain parts of the camel's body. This is a serious problem in Pakistan, affecting many camels there and reducing the camels' condition. It is also found in other areas.

Signs

- Shrunken hump.
- Difficulty in breathing.
- The camel is unable to work.
- The testicles become enlarged.
- The disease lasts a long time.

If you look at a wet blood film through a microscope, you can see the worm larvae ('microfilariae') moving around with snake-like movements. The larvae are 252–292 μm long and 6–7 μm wide (▷*Checking for diseases in the laboratory*).

Dipetalonemiasis can be confused with ▷*Trypanosomiasis*, other internal parasites (▷*Internal parasites [worms]*) and poor nutrition.

Cause

A parasitic worm (*Dipetalonema evansi*) which lives in the spermatic cord, blood vessels in the lung, the heart, the lymph nodes and membranes connecting the internal organs to the body wall (the 'mesentery'). The worm larvae live in the blood.

The disease is carried by *Aedes* mosquitoes. It is not known if it can be carried by other biting insects such as ticks or flies.

Prevention

- Control biting insects (▷*Bites and stings*).

Treatment

- Inject ivermectin (0.2 mg/kg body weight) under the skin. Repeat after 3 weeks.

SCI

References

Higgins (1986) p. 68–9; Manefield and Tinson (1997) p. 74; Sewell and Brocklesby (1990) p. 157.

Haemorrhagic septicaemia

Pasteurellosis

***Khandich, khandicha, quando* (Borana), *khando, qando* (Gabbra), *galtiya, magravala* (India), *ghedda* (N Africa), *khanid* (Rendille), *nalngiarrngarri, ngarngar, nolgoso* (Samburu), *kharar, garir, khud, kurri* (Somali), *aengarre, lorarrurei, longarrue, elukunoit, lobolio, lobolibolio* (Turkana)**

This is an important disease that appears suddenly and can kill animals quickly. It occurs in the rainy season and is sometimes linked to drinking water from puddles. It usually affects only a few animals in a herd, but many (up to 80%) of the sick animals die. It is especially common in areas that get flooded.

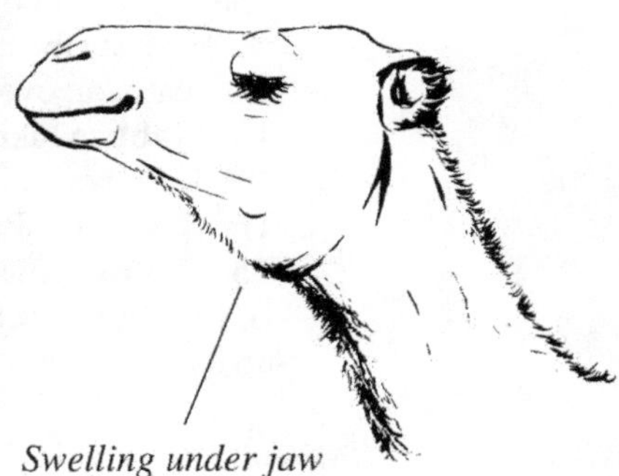
Swelling under jaw

Signs

- ○ Fever over 40°C (this may be the first sign of the disease).
- ○ Swollen, painful lymph nodes, especially in the angle of the jaw and at the bottom of the neck.
- ○ The camel does not chew and may grind its teeth. It does not feed.
- ○ Mucous membranes (in the eyes and mouth) are dark red.
- ○ Frequently belly pain (colic).
- ○ Weak cough, rapid shallow breathing, salivation.
- ○ Rapid pulse.
- ○ Blood-stained or tar-like faeces.
- ○ Coffee- or chocolate-like urine.
- ○ Pregnant females abort.
- ○ Death 2–8 days after the first signs appear.

If the dead animal is cut open, small red or purple spots like flea-bites can be seen on the surface of the internal organs. There may be many haemorrhages (bleeding spots) in the intestines, stomach and lungs. The lungs, liver and spleen can be sent to a laboratory for tests to confirm that the animal has died from the disease. If the laboratory is more than 8 hours' journey away, send a long bone instead (▷*How to collect samples for testing*).

Other diseases with similar signs include ▷*Anthrax*, *Blackquarter* and *Salmonellosis*.

Cause

A bacterium called *Pasteurella multocida*. The disease is carried in the breath of infected animals. It can also be carried in contaminated saliva, discharge from the mouth and nose, and in the faeces.

Prevention

- ○ Separate sick from healthy animals. TRAD
- ○ Avoid contact with sick herds.
- ○ Clean and disinfect camel pens. SCI
- ○ Vaccinate animals against the disease. There are two types of vaccine: one that can be used 1 month before the rainy season, and another that can be used during a disease outbreak. SCI

Treatment

Traditional treatments

It is not known how effective (if at all) the following traditional treatments are.

- ○ The **Samburu** and **Rendille** brand the swollen glands of sick animals.

- The **Turkana** boil 1 kg of crushed leaves of *Salvadora persica* in 2.5 litres of water, allow the mixture to cool, and then drench the animal with it. They repeat the treatment every 4 days until the camel recovers.
- The **Gabbra** take an arm's length piece of root from *Euphorbia heterochroma* (*harken*), boil it in 2 litres of water, then cool it and use the liquid as a drench. The dose for calves is three finger-size roots in 1 litre of water.
- The **Raika** treat sick animals with alcohol and human urine.
- **Indian herders** feed the animal with milk and eggs or *gur* (molasses) to keep up its strength.

Modern treatments

- If the disease is caught in the early stages, treat with antibiotics such as amoxycillin, tetracyclines or sulphonamides (▷*Common medicines*).
- Give 110 mg/kg body weight of sulphadimidine by mouth each day for up to 4 days.

References

Evans et al. (1995) p. 7:29; Forse (1999) p. 283–4; Higgins (1986) p. 103–4; ITDG and IIRR (1996) p. 166; Leese (1927) p. 270; Manefield and Tinson (1997) p. 184; Rathore (1986) p. 171; Schwartz and Dioli (1992) p. 159, 167–9; Sewell and Brocklesby (1990) p. 74–7; Wernery and Kaaden (1995) p. 27–30.

Swollen glands, *khanid*

Kando, kandich, kandicha **(Gabbra),** ***khanid*** **(Rendille),** ***quandich, kud kurri garir*** **(Somali)**

The Rendille term *khanid*, which means 'lymph node', includes virtually all conditions associated with enlarged lymph nodes and bleeding in the skin, nose, mouth or anus ('haemorrhagic conditions'). The disease is short and acute, and if untreated, kills the animal suddenly. Both adults and calves (over 3 months of age) can be affected.

Signs

- Swollen lymph nodes (especially on the head and neck).
- The animal rests more than usual, and at odd hours of the day.
- It stops eating and drinking.
- Watery eyes.
- Fever, shivering.
- Diarrhoea.
- Little or no urine.
- Dullness, rough coat.
- Slight cough, difficulty in breathing.

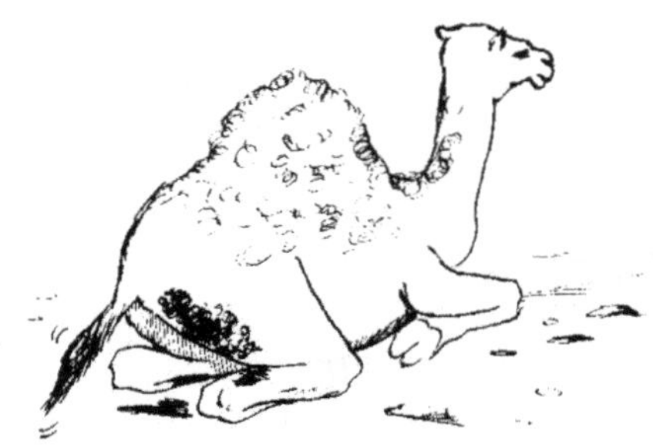

- Sudden death after a short illness.

If you cut the dead animal open, you will see that all the lymph glands are bloody, and there is blood in all the body tissues, especially the intestines. The meat is dark red from blood.

Cause

Not known. May be one of the following diseases: ▷*Anthrax*, *Haemorrhagic disease*, *Haemorrhagic enteritis*, or *Haemorrhagic septicaemia*.

Prevention

- Vaccinate against anthrax. GABBRA, RENDILLE

Treatment

No successful treatment is known. Herders use the following traditional treatments, but with little success.

Traditional treatments

- Feed with sheep-tail fat.
- Soak *gathaha* (a local herb) in water and drench. RENDILLE
- Drench with a mixture made from roots of a tree called *bura*, *burs* or *bursa* (possibly *Acacia elatior* or *Acacia goetzei*). GABBRA
- Boil tobacco in water and drench. GABBRA
- Change the site of the enclosure.
- Brand the lymph nodes.

Modern treatments

- Check the disease signs (see the sections on the diseases listed above under *Cause*) and treat accordingly.
- Inject with penicillin or oxytetracycline antibiotics (▷*Common medicines*).

References

Kaufmann (1998) p. 187–8.

Haemorrhagic disease

Haemorrhagic diathesis, HD, *Bacillus cereus* intoxication

This is a serious disease of camels that affects mainly racing camels in the United Arab Emirates. Up to 50% of the sick animals may die.

Signs

- Fever (up to 41°C).
- Camel stops feeding and ruminating.
- The camel swallows frequently and has a dry cough (▷*Problems of the nose and lungs*).

- The stomach stops moving (press your ear against it to listen for movement).
- Lymph nodes (mostly those on the neck) on one or both sides swell.
- After a few days, the faeces are mixed with blood (either fresh and red or black and tar-like). No diarrhoea.
- After some days, the animal sits down and refuses to get up.
- The animal dies after 3–7 days.
- After the animal has died and is cut open, blood can be seen inside the mouth, nose and windpipe, on the sac around the heart, in the last stomach, on (and inside) the guts, and in the kidneys.

Diseases with similar signs include ▷*Haemorrhagic septicaemia, Haemorrhagic enteritis, Salmonellosis, Colibacillosis* and *Problems of the nose and lungs.*

Cause

A bacterium called *Bacillus cereus.* This may be carried on feed contaminated by cattle dung (for example, alfalfa which has been fertilized with dung). If a camel is fed with grain and other concentrates but not enough roughage, the contents of the rumen (the first stomach) become very acid (▷*Indigestion*). These acidic conditions also help the bacteria multiply quickly and produce harmful toxins.

Prevention

- Provide good-quality, clean feed.
- Do not store freshly cut feed in bundles (as the heat this generates helps the bacteria to multiply). Instead, spread it out on racks in the air.
- Give plenty of roughage in the feed.

Treatment

Treat the animal quickly if you suspect it has haemorrhagic disease. Nevertheless, treatments almost always fail as the disease takes a very rapid course.

- Dissolve 500 g of sodium bicarbonate in water and drench twice a day for at least 2 days. This reduces the acidity in the rumen. SCI
- Inject antibiotics and antipyretics such as Tomanol (a medicine to reduce fever) into the vein (▷*Common medicines*). SCI
- Give a drip with electrolytes, glucose and vitamins. SCI

References

Manefield and Tinson (1997) p. 114, 117; Wernery and Kaaden (1995) p. 19–27.

Anthrax

***Chilmalo* (Gabbra), *mohri, sujhan, sut, garhi* (India), *lokuchum* (Samburu, Turkana), *kud* (Somali)**

Anthrax is a serious disease that can affect camels, other livestock, wild animals and humans. It is highly infectious and leads to death.

Signs

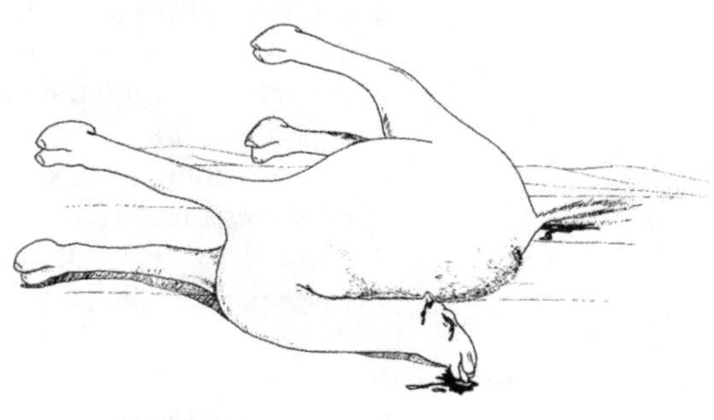

- High fever.
- Rapid death, often without any signs of illness beforehand.
- Often the best animals in the herd are affected.
- Blood coming out of body openings (mouth, nose, anus). This blood is dark red and does not clot.
- Diarrhoea, pain in the abdomen (colic), bloat.
- Fast, irregular pulse and breathing.
- Sometimes painful swellings on the throat and neck.

The Rendille describe a disease called *khanid*, which may be similar to anthrax or haemorrhagic disease (▷*Swollen glands, khanid*).

Watch for the signs above, especially blood coming out of the mouth, nose and anus. The spleen is enlarged 3–5 times its usual size. A trained worker can check the blood of a sick animal for the bacteria (▷*How to take samples for testing* and *Checking for diseases in the laboratory*).

Cause

A bacterium called *Bacillus anthracis*, which remains in the soil for up to 60 years and is extremely resistant to high temperatures and drought. Anthrax is a problem where animals are crowded, for instance at watering holes, salt-licks and livestock markets. The disease is transmitted through grazing close to the ground, and by inhaling dust. Possibly it can also be transmitted through biting flies (tabanids) and nasal bot-flies.

Prevention

Warning! Anthrax is a highly infectious disease that can kill people.

- Avoid grazing where anthrax has previously occurred.
- Be careful when handling animals that are sick with anthrax: avoid touching them or their blood. If you must handle them, wear plastic bags on your hands like gloves.
- Vaccinate camels with Blanthrax vaccine.
- Avoid touching a carcass of an animal that has died of anthrax, and do not open the carcass. *Never* eat the meat of an animal that might have died of anthrax. If you must touch the carcass, wear plastic bags on your hands like gloves.
- Put thorn bushes around and on top of the carcass to prevent predators and vultures from ripping it open and spreading the disease.
- **Important:** To stop the disease from spreading, destroy the carcass by burning rather than burying it. Make sure it burns completely.

Treatment

Traditional treatments

The effectiveness of traditional treatments is not known.

- The **Samburu** take about 6 cm of the root of *Salvadora persica* and an equal weight of leaves. They pound, crush and boil these for 30 minutes in 10 litres of water. They allow the liquid to cool, and then use it as a drench. They repeat the treatment until the animal recovers.

- The **Turkana** brand the swollen parts of the body, and feed boiled goat meat, pounded *Euphorbia triaculeata* mixed with water, or soup made of boiled, unemptied donkey intestines.
- The **Tuareg** mix a red clay called *tamasgeyt* with sheep milk, and pour this into the nostrils of the sick animal. They spread the foam of sheep milk onto the swollen parts of the body.

Modern treatments

- Inject immediately with penicillin (10 000 units/kg body weight) and streptomycin (8 mg/kg body weight) into the muscle twice a day.

References

Bizimana (1994) p. 370–1; Evans et al. (1995) p. 7:26; Forse (1999) p. 141–4; Higgins (1986) p. 98–9; ITDG and IIRR (1996) p. 158–9; Leese (1927) p. 268; Manefield and Tinson (1997) p. 33–4; Projet Cameline (1999) p. 45; Rathore (1986) p. 170–1; Sewell and Brocklesby (1990) p. 33–6; Wernery and Kaaden (1995) p. 18–19.

Blackquarter

Blackleg, gas oedema, clostridiosis
***Lkumur* (Borana, Gabbra), *ngwaat, lokichum* (Pokot), *khadit* (Rendille), *loduseddi* (Samburu), *khut* (Somali)**

This disease affects mostly cattle and sheep, but sometimes camels as well. Young animals aged 8–18 months are susceptible to it.

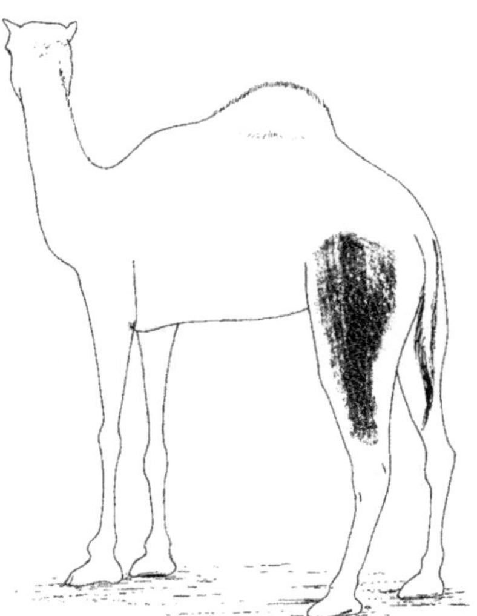

Signs

- Swellings under the skin in the shoulder area or in the hind legs. These swellings are at first hot and painful, but later cold and painless. They make a crackling sound when touched.
- The skin becomes dark.
- Lameness.
- Fever and rapid heart beat.
- The animal stops feeding.
- Death within 2–3 days.

Cause

A bacterium called *Clostridium chauvoei*. This bacterium can survive in the soil for 30 years and withstand temperatures of 100°C. Disease outbreaks are linked to stress, drought, feed with a high fibre content, overcrowding and lack of food.

Prevention

- Vaccinate with Blanthrax vaccine.
- Burn or bury carcasses of animals that have died of blackquarter.

Treatment

- Treat in the same way as for anthrax (▷*Anthrax*). SCI

References

Bizimana (1994) p. 371–2; Evans et al. (1995) p. 7:26; Forse (1999) p. 144–5; Higgins (1986) p. 104; Rathore (1986) p. 172; Sewell and Brocklesby (1990) p. 49–51; Wernery and Kaaden (1995) p. 5–6.

Tetanus

Lockjaw
***Hattal?* (Kordofan), *rekigerri?* (Rendille), *kongoro, nkeeyae lmeut* (Samburu), *tagou?* (Somali)**

Tetanus affects mostly humans and horses; it is rare in camels. The animal's limbs and neck become stiff and unable to move. Even if it is treated, tetanus usually kills infected animals.

Signs

- The animal becomes stiff and stands with its legs splayed (like a sawhorse).
- It startles easily and has spasms.
- A membrane (the 'third eyelid') appears across the eye (▷*Eye problems*).
- The muscles of the hind legs tremble, sometimes very strongly.
- The animal has difficulty in chewing ('lockjaw').
- The tail becomes stiff.
- Later, the animal cannot stand.
- The animal usually starves to death.

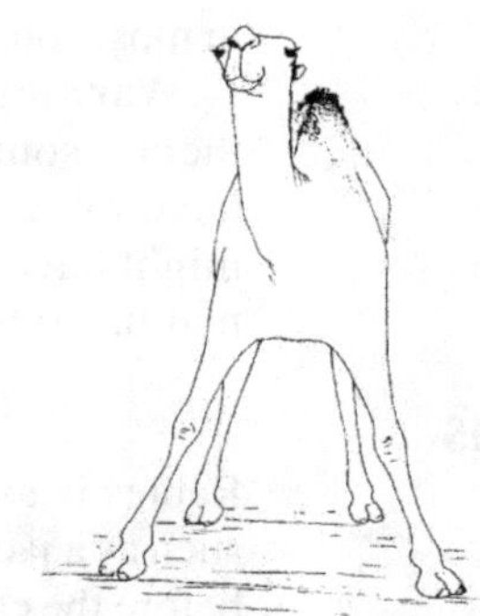

Cause

Deep wounds (caused by sharp objects puncturing the skin, such as dirty surgical instruments or acacia thorns) become infected with a bacterium called *Clostridium tetani*. These bacteria multiply where there is no air – such as in deep wounds. When the symptoms of tetanus appear, the wound has usually already healed.

Prevention

- Clean deep wounds promptly with potassium permanganate or hydrogen peroxide (▷*Wounds and burns*). SCI

Treatment

- Put the animal in a quiet, dark place, or plug its ears and put patches on its eyes.
- Inject 3000 units of tetanus antitoxin under the skin. Inject penicillin for at least 7 days (▷*Common medicines*). Inject propionylpromazine (Combelen) (▷*Sedation and anaesthaesia*). To calm the animal, inject a muscle relaxant such as methocarbamol (Robaxin). SCI
- If the infected wound can be found, open it to expose it to the air, drain out the fluid, and dress it with an antiseptic such as potassium permanganate. SCI
- If the animal cannot eat, feed with milk, oatmeal gruel and linseed gruel by working it into its mouth from the side.

References

Bizimana (1994) p. 74; Evans et al. (1995) p. 7:32; Forse (1999) p. 263–4; ITDG and IIRR (1996) p. 171; Leese (1927) p. 268; Manefield and Tinson (1997) p. 258–9; Rathore (1986) p. 170; Schwartz and Dioli (1992) p. 218–19; Sewell and Brocklesby (1990) p. 58–9; Wernery and Kaaden (1995) p. 71–3.

Rabies

***Siribo* (Borana), *nyanye* (Gabbra), *pagal hona* (India), *sugeri ikaare* (Rendille), *nkwang* (Samburu), *ruqus* (Somali), *ingerep* (Turkana)**

Rabies is a rare but very important disease of camels because it can be transmitted to humans. Rabies *always* kills infected camels, other animals and people. It occurs in most countries in the world.

Warning: Rabies can infect people. If it is not treated immediately, it kills them – sometimes months later. If you are bitten by a camel or dog that may have rabies, consult a doctor straight away. Avoid contact with animals that might have rabies. Inform the veterinary authorities if you suspect that an animal has rabies.

Signs

Rabies is usually transmitted by the bite of an infected predator or other animal, such as a jackal, hyena, dog or mongoose. The bite wounds often heal many weeks before the camel becomes sick.

Rabies can take two forms: 'furious' and 'dumb':

Furious form

- Strange or unusual behaviour.
- The camel may become more aggressive and angry. It may attack other camels.
- The camel may run away from the herd.
- The camel produces a lot of saliva, which runs from its mouth. This saliva is very dangerous because it contains the rabies virus.
- The camel may chew its own body or other objects, or appear to be 'itchy'.
- Male camels may show excessive sexual excitement.
- Near the end of the disease, the camel may yawn continuously.
- The back legs of the camel become weak. The weakness gradually worsens so that the camel cannot stand.
- The animal cannot swallow properly.
- The camel collapses, has difficulty in breathing, and dies.

Dumb form

- This form of the disease is less common in camels than the furious form.
- Dullness, lack of appetite.
- Bellowing.
- Paralysis, inability to get up.
- Drooping of the lower lip.
- Death.

If you suspect that an animal has died of rabies, seek help from a trained veterinary worker. If such a worker cannot be found, bury the carcass (make sure you do not touch the saliva, blood or other body fluids!). The veterinary worker may take the animal's head to a laboratory for tests to find out if the animal did indeed have rabies (▷*How to take samples for testing*).

Other conditions with similar signs include:

- Rut: excitement and aggression in males, a normal part of male behaviour (▷*Rutting*).
- ▷*Trypanosomiasis*.
- Staggering in dehydrated camels (▷*Sunstroke*).
- Cerebral coenuriasis (not covered in this book).
- Listeriosis or other bacterial meningitis (not covered in this book).
- ▷*Nasal bots*.

Cause

Rabies is caused by a virus. An animal suffering from rabies has virus in its saliva. When this rabid animal bites another animal or human, the virus in its saliva infects the bitten animal through the bite wound. Rabid dogs, jackals, hyenas and wolves transmit rabies easily to other animals when they bite them. It can take between 3 weeks and 6 months for the camel to develop rabies after it has been bitten. The further the bite from the animal's brain, the longer it takes for the disease to emerge.

Prevention

- Protect camels from predators like stray dogs, foxes and hyenas.
- In areas where rabies is common, vaccinate against it.
- If a camel is bitten by a mad dog or other predator, clean the wound very carefully with lots of running water and the antiseptic cetrimide (Savlon). Dress the wound with Savlon, which will kill the virus. Separate the camel from the rest

of the herd and watch it very carefully for signs of disease.

- If you suspect that a camel has rabies, inform the local veterinary authorities.
- People who come into contact with a rabid animal (or who are likely to do so) must be vaccinated against the disease.

Treatment

There are no effective treatments for rabies. If rabies is confirmed, the animal must be killed immediately and its carcass burned.

References

Bizimana (1994) p. 100–1; Evans et al. (1995) p. 7:30–2; FAO (1994) p. 229–31; Forse (1999) p. 260–3; Higgins (1986) p. 95–6; ITDG and IIRR (1996) p. 168–70; Leese (1927) p. 264; Manefield and Tinson (1997) p. 199–200; Rathore (1986) p. 169–70; Schwartz and Dioli (1992) p. 217; Sewell and Brocklesby (1990) p. 346–9; Wernery and Kaaden (1995) p. 75–81.

Rift Valley fever

Rift Valley fever is a serious disease that affects animals (especially ruminants) and people and is so far only reported from Africa. Infected camels sometimes have no signs of the disease, but can carry it from one place to another and infect humans and other livestock species. Outbreaks occur only after unusually heavy rainfall.

Signs

- Fever, general weakness and poor appetite.
- Abortions: sometimes all pregnant camels abort.
- Other livestock, especially sheep, are likely to be very sick and die.

Cause

A virus transmitted by mosquitoes.

Prevention

- Vaccination.

Treatment

- None.

References

Evans et al. (1995) p. 7:32; Forse (1999) p. 289; Higgins (1986) p. 97–8; Manefield and Tinson (1997) p. 220; Sewell and Brocklesby (1990) p. 349–52; Wernery and Kaaden (1995) p. 95–6; Wilson (1998) p. 98.

8 Non-infectious diseases

This chapter deals with various non-infectious diseases not covered elsewhere in this book.

Major signs	Cause	See section
Red urine, blood in urine	Kidney problems, plant poisoning	▷*Red urine, Plant poisoning*
Exhaustion, fainting	Convulsions, dizziness, fainting	▷*Sunstroke*
Various: bloat, vomiting, staggering, diarrhoea, paralysis	Eating poisonous plants	▷*Plant poisoning*
Loud, long bellowing; foaming at mouth	Snake bite	▷*Snake bite*
Itchy skin, shivering, difficulty breathing	Allergy to medicine, insect bites, feed, etc.	▷*Allergy*
Eating strange things	Mineral or vitamin deficiency, internal parasites, rabies	▷*Pica, Internal parasites (worms), Rabies*
Animal does not get up	Various causes	▷*Downer*
Animal does not drink; little or no sweat	Unknown: perhaps lack of salt	▷*Dry coat*
Swelling under skin	Various	▷*Oedema*

Red urine

Haematuria
Rut mootra, lahoo mootna (**Punjabi**)

Red urine is caused by blood in the urine. It is not a common problem in camels. It may have several different causes.

Signs

- Urine may range from pinkish to deep red.
- Straining while passing urine; sometimes signs of discomfort in the belly.

Cause

- Infections of the kidneys or other parts of the urinary tract.
- Damage to the kidneys caused by a blow on the back.
- Wounds to the scrotum or penis, possibly caused by bites by other males during the rut season (▷*Rutting*).
- Bladder stones (cause severe pain).
- Parasites in the kidney.
- Plant poisoning.
- Grazing on certain plants: this is not a problem. If this is the cause, it is likely that many animals in the herd will have red urine.

Prevention

- Avoid injuries to the kidney region (the camel's back behind the hump).

Treatment

- **Caused by bladder stones:** Inject with 20–30 ml of Buscopan Compositum or 20–30 ml of Novalgin (a medicine against muscle spasms) into the muscle or vein, and treat as for infections (see next treatment below). SCI
- **Caused by an infection:** Inject an antibiotic such as ampicillin (10 mg/kg body weight into the muscle twice a day for 7–10 days) or norfloxacin (5 mg/kg body weight into the muscle for 7–10 days). Give the camel lots of water to drink (drench with water if it does not drink). SCI
- **Caused by injury:** Press a cold, damp cloth on the wound and then apply an antiseptic dressing (▷*Wounds and burns*). Inject a systemic coagulant such as carbazochrome or vitamin K. Give a urinary antiseptic such as nitrofurantoin (4 g twice a day by mouth) for 10–15 days. Inject an anti-inflammatory drug such as phenylbutazone (10 mg/kg body weight) once a day for 7–10 days. To prevent secondary bacterial infections, inject an antibiotic such as ampicillin (10 mg/kg body weight twice a day into the muscle for 7–10 days) or norfloxacin (5 mg/kg body weight into the muscle for 7–10 days). SCI

References

Evans et al. (1995) p. 7:27; Manefield and Tinson (1997) p. 113–14, 166–8; Rathore (1986) p. 140.

Sunstroke

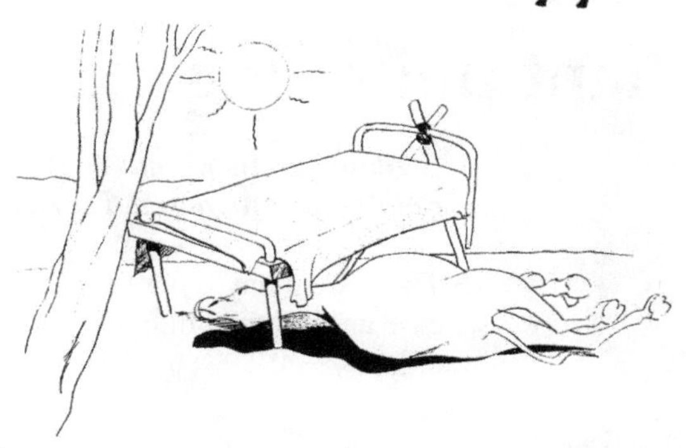

Heat exhaustion
***Red awarng* (Rajasthan)**

In very hot or humid weather, an overworked camel may fall down and lose consciousness. It may die immediately, or remain weak and go off its food and water, possibly dying later. This problem is more common in draught camels and animals that are stall-fed.

Signs

- Convulsions, dizziness, and sudden loss of consciousness.
- The camel does not want to eat or drink.
- It does not respond to movement nearby.
- It seeks shade and hides its head in bushes.

Similar signs can be caused by shock, nervous disorders and ▷*Tetanus*.

Cause

Heat, and deficiency of minerals and vitamins in the feed.

Prevention

- Do not use the animal for draught work in very hot or humid weather.
- Provide mineral and vitamin supplements to stall-fed camels. TRAD+SCI
- Provide a drink made of 1–2 kg of sorghum twice a day. TRAD

Treatment

Traditional treatments

- Put the animal in the shade (or build a shelter over it). TRAD+SCI
- Pour cold water over its head and body. TRAD+SCI
- Throw sand over its body.

Modern treatments

- Give a drip of 7–10 litres of normal saline solution per day for 3 days.
- Give a drip of 3 litres of 20% dextrose saline solution per day for 2 days.
- Drench with 3–4 litres of oral rehydration liquid (9 g salt, 50 g of sugar and 10 g of sodium bicarbonate dissolved in each litre of water) for 7 days.
- Inject the following each day: vitamins AD_3E into the muscle for 3 days, dexamethasone (40 mg into the vein for 3 days), and analgin or paracetamol (e.g., Paracetol 30 ml into the muscle for 2 days). **Caution:** do not give corticosteroids such as dexamathasone to a female camel during the last 4 months of a pregnancy because they can cause an abortion (▷*Abortion*).

References

Bizimana (1994) p. 367–9; Forse (1999) p. 268–70; Projet Cameline (1999) p. 49; Rathore (1986) p. 149.

Plant poisoning

***Goulum* (Arabic), *arda* (Borana), *hada* (Gabbra), *lotil* (Pokot), *loturudei* (Samburu), *gedak* (Somali), *bosoto* (Turkana)**

There are many types of plant poisoning. Some poisonous plants cause severe disease and death, while others cause mild disease such as stomach pain or diarrhoea only.

Signs

Different forms of poisoning result in different signs. Any of the following may result from plant poisoning.

- Bloat, stomach pain (▷*Bloat*).
- Groaning, kicking of the belly.
- Excitement, depression, weakness, loss of co-ordination.
- Stumbling, jumping, running in circles.
- Strange behaviour, such as pressing the head against a post or tree stump.
- Shivering, twitching in the face, head and neck; fits, convulsions; salivation or foaming at the mouth.
- Difficulty in breathing, excessive sweating.
- Uncontrolled urination.
- Diarrhoea, vomiting (▷*Diarrhoea*).
- Stiffness, paralysis, coma and death.

See below for signs that are caused by specific plants.

Cause

Camels usually recognize certain poisonous plants and avoid eating them. However, a camel may eat such plants if it is eating quickly (for example, if it has gone without food for a long time). It is much more likely to eat poisonous plants if it is moved into new grazing areas where it has no experience of the local vegetation.

Prevention

- Know which plants are poisonous and avoid feeding them to camels.
- Avoid grazing in areas with many poisonous plants.

Treatment

Many treatments for poisoning make the animal defecate, so removing the poison from the body. These medicines are called 'purgatives'. They include Epsom salts (magnesium sulphate), castor oil, linseed oil and liquid paraffin.

Drenching with activated charcoal (which comes as tablets) helps prevent the stomach absorbing more poison.

See also the sections below for treatments for poisoning caused by specific plants.

Traditional treatments

- Mix together equal amounts of milk and water. Drench 15 litres a day; repeat as necessary until the animal recovers. SAMBURU, TRAD+SCI
- Make the animal drink as much camel milk as it will take. This will cause diarrhoea, which will help remove the poison from its body. GABBRA, TRAD+SCI

- Mix 4 litres of milk with 6 fresh eggs and 50 g of Omo detergent. Add 100 ml of liquid paraffin oil or castor oil.
- Grind 1 kg of charcoal and mix with 4 litres of water. Drench once a day. Repeat as necessary.

Modern treatments

- Drench with 1 g of activated charcoal for every 20 kg body weight, mixed with water. Repeat once a day for 4–5 days.
- Drench with large amounts of liquids.
- Drench with magnesium salts, linseed oil, castor oil or paraffin oil to make the animal excrete the poison in the faeces.
- Drench with 200 g of kaolin (China clay), mixed with water. Repeat each day for 4–5 days.

Buxus semper virens

***Phappar* (Punjab)**

An abundant plant in Iran and Punjab, Pakistan. Same signs and treatment as *Euphorbia tirucalli* (see below)

Calotropis procera

***Aak* (Hindi)**

Camels do not usually eat this plant, but if they do, they may vomit and have diarrhoea.

Capparis tomentosa

***Gorrahgel* (Borana, Rendille), *gora* (Gabbra), *laturdei* (Samburu), *gamboor*, *gomborlik* (Somali), *ekorokoroite* (Turkana)**

Signs

- The camel's neck becomes twisted into an S-shape (▷*Wry neck*).
- The animal is weak in the legs and staggers.
- The animal convulses and becomes thin.
- Most camels will die within 24 hours after the symptoms start.

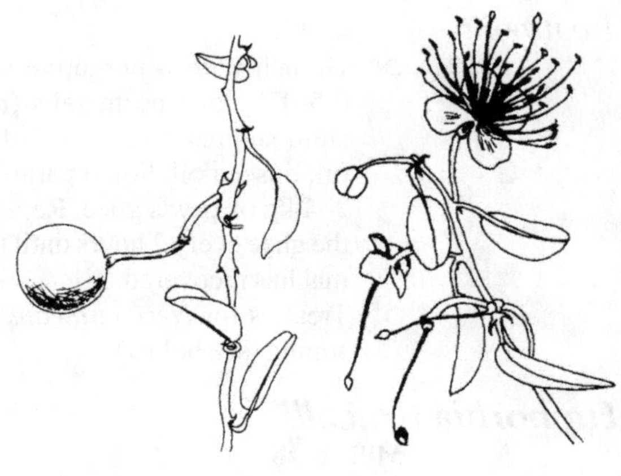

Prevention

- Graze animals away from areas with many *Capparis* shrubs (especially along river banks).

Treatment

- Use one of the treatments for poisoning listed above.

Cassia occidentalis

Senna
***Kesudo* (Hindi)**

Signs

- Diarrhoea.
- The camel will die only if it has eaten a large amount.

Treatment

- Give rice gruel every 3–4 hours.

Daphne oleiodes

Spurge laurel
***Laghunay* (Baluchistan)**

A plant causing similar signs to *Euphorbia tirucalli* (see below). Treat in the same way.

Datura alba/stramonium (?)

Thorn apple
***Dhaturo* (Hindi), *hurna* (Kordofan), *ntuju* (Samburu), *bohamidu* (Somalia), *ebune* (Turkana)**

A bush with large, angular leaves, white, funnel-shaped flowers and prickly fruit. Found on banks of water-courses.

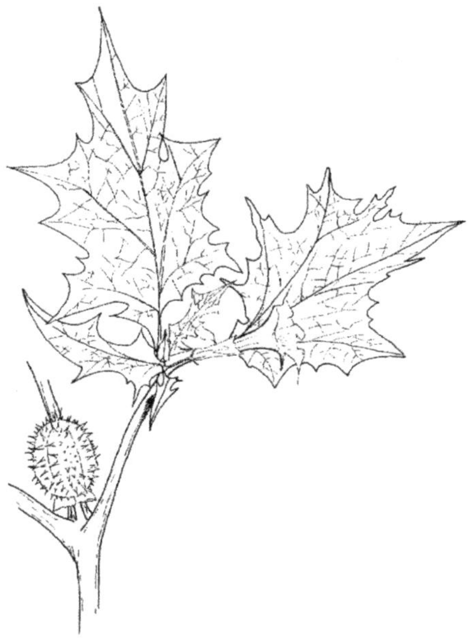

Signs

- The camel becomes very quiet and goes to sleep.
- Bloat.

Treatment

- Drench with a purgative such as 0.5–1 kg of Epsom salts (magnesium sulphate) or 1 litre of castor oil, linseed oil, liquid paraffin, and 2–4 kg of cow's ghee. Repeat with the ghee every 2 hours until the animal has recovered.
- Treat as for *Nerium oleander* poisoning (see below).

Euphorbia tirucalli

Milk-bush
***Irgin* (Somali?)**

A bush with small thorns but no leaves, growing in thickets beside water-courses in Somalia. The milky sap is intensely irritating.

Signs

- Swollen throat, cough.
- Vomiting, pain, straining to defecate, swollen belly.
- Hard, dry dung at first, then becoming soft, then evil-smelling diarrhoea.
- Sometimes severe hiccough.
- The camel may die within 3 days.

Treatment

- Drench with soup made from sheep fat. TRAD+SCI
- Mix 60 ml (12 teaspoons) of turpentine with 1 litre of linseed oil and drench. One hour later, drench with warm ghee and milk. SCI
- Inject 130 mg of arecoline under the skin to make the animal defecate. Then give linseed tea or warm ghee and milk every 4 hours to soothe the inflamed gullet, stomach and intestines. SCI

Lantana indica

Lantana
***Rukri* (Hindi)**

This plant appears to be very poisonous to camels.

Signs

- Diarrhoea.
- Sensitivity to light.
- Quick death.

Treatment

- Drench three times with 250 g of ghee mixed with 250 g of jaggery. TRAD

Nerium oleander

Oleander
***Difli* (Arabic), *kaneer* (Hindi), *kharzarah* (Iran), *nara* (Sindh), *dehr* (Somali)**

Poisoning occurs only in camels not familiar with this plant.

Signs

- 6–8 hours after eating the plant, the camel stops feeding and starts vomiting.
- Dullness, shivering, yawning, staggering.
- Diarrhoea, vomiting, convulsions.
- The camel may die after 1 day.

Treatment

- Drench with 1 kg of Epsom salts (magnesium sulphate).
- Drench with 2–3 litres of linseed oil (*tili ka tel*), or a mixture of 4 litres of milk with 6–10 eggs.
- Inject 130 mg of arecoline under the skin to make the animal defecate. Once a day, mix a little tartaric acid in water and force the animal to drink it. Three minutes later, drench with 3 g of potassium permanganate dissolved in water. SCI
- Inject 0.01–0.1 g of atropine sulphate under the skin. This relaxes the intestines. SCI

Sarcostemma andongenese

Signs

- Paralysis.
- Twisting of the neck, which looks as if it is broken (▻*Wry neck*).

Treatment

- Give a drench of melted sheep fat. TRAD
- Inject with vitamin B.
- Drench with baker's yeast mixed with sugar and water.

Sorghum bicolor

Sorghum
***Jowar* (India)**

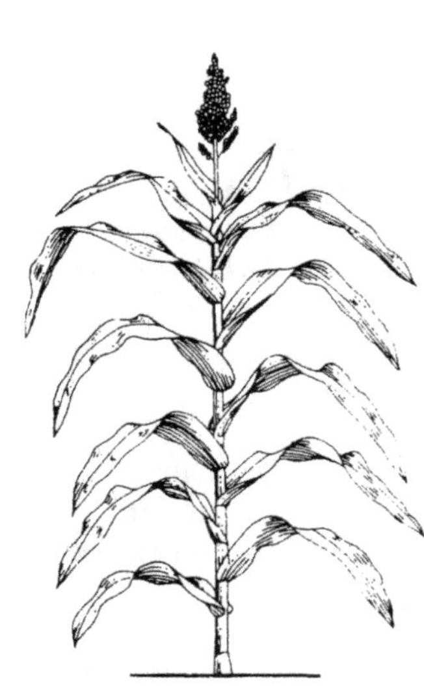

Some farmers abandon sorghum fields during drought because they think the fields are not worth harvesting. Young sorghum or millet plants (before the ears form) are poisonous because they contain cyanide. Cut stunted sorghum and allow it to dry in the sun for 2 full days before feeding to camels: the poison will disappear in this time.

Signs

- Bloat, severe pain in the belly.
- Difficulty in breathing, and death.

Treatment

- Mix up to 25 g of ammonium carbonate with oil and water, and drench.
- Drench with 500–1000 ml of Tympanyl or liquid paraffin. SCI
- Inject 0.01–0.1 g of atropine under the skin. SCI
- As a last resort, puncture the rumen with a trocar and cannula or a sharp knife (▻*Bloat*). SCI

References

Bizimana (1994) p. 381–5; Evans et al. (1995) p. 7:30, 7:37; FAO (1994) p. 225–6, 259; Forse (1999) p. 301–8; ITDG and IIRR (1996) p. 29–36; Manefield and Tinson (1997) p. 189; Rathore (1986) p. 190–4; Schwartz and Dioli (1992) p. 193, 220–1.

Allergy

An allergy is when the body over-reacts to a certain substance. The substance can enter the body if it touches the skin, is injected, or if the camel eats it or breathes it in. The allergy can affect the whole body, or only the part that comes into direct contact with the antigen.

Some animals have allergies to certain substances, while others may not be affected at all.

Signs

- Difficulty in breathing.
- Shivering of the muscles.
- Restlessness.
- Drooling of saliva from the mouth.
- The camel bites or scratches the affected areas.
- Raised skin patches and loss of hair (▷*Skin problems*).

Cause

- Injection of medicines against ▷*Trypanosomiasis*.
- Certain types of vaccines (especially those that are oily).
- Insect bites (such as wasps, bees and ants) (▷*Bites and stings*).
- Sand flies and midges.
- Certain types of feed.

Prevention

- Find out what is causing the allergy and remove it. TRAD+SCI

Treatment

- Inject an antihistamine (▷*Common medicines*). SCI
- Inject corticosteroids such as dexamethasone (▷*Common medicines*). **Caution:** do not give these to a female camel during the last 4 months of a pregnancy because they can cause an abortion (▷*Abortion*). SCI
- For allergies affecting only one part of the body, apply creams containing prednisolone to the affected places. SCI

References

Forse (1999) p. 162; Manefield and Tinson (1997) p. 25–6; Rathore (1986) p. 158.

Pica

***Nandh* (Gabbra), *singate* (Samburu), *megay* (Somali), *ekichoe* (Turkana)**

Pica refers to the licking, chewing and eating of objects, such as stones, bones, pieces of wood, tree bark, soil or faeces. This can lead to blocked guts (⊳*Swallowed objects* and *Blocked intestines*). It can also make the camel infected more easily by diseases such as ⊳*Anthrax*, *Blackquarter* and *Tetanus*.

Signs

- The animal eats peculiar objects, such as bones, metal, faeces, hair, sand or soil.
- The animal becomes thin and weak, and may seek shade.
- Rough, dull hair.
- Reduced milk production.
- Females do not conceive.
- The animal may fall ill easily.

To check for pica, take a blood plasma sample and take it to a laboratory to be tested for mineral concentration. Take a faeces sample to check for intestinal worms (⊳*How to collect samples for testing*).

Cause

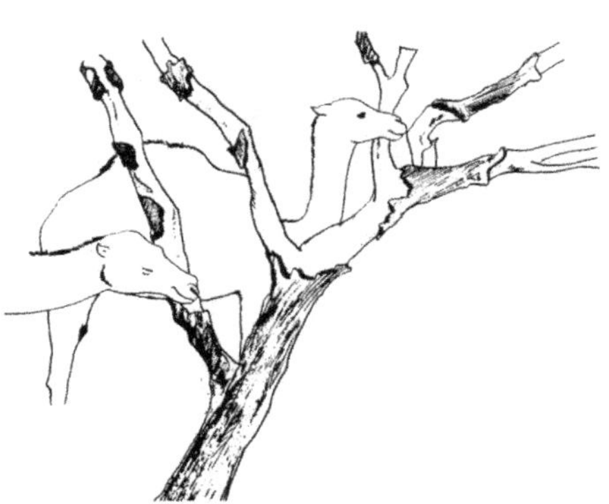

- Lack of salt.
- Lack of certain minerals in the food, such as phosphorus, calcium and iron.
- Vitamin deficiency.
- ⊳*Internal parasites (worms).*
- ⊳*Rabies.*
- Boredom.

Prevention

- Give the camels a mineral supplement.
- Inject with multivitamins and phosphorus.
- In worm-infested areas, deworm the animals regularly.

Treatment

- Take the animals to places with rocks that contain mineral salts so they can lick the rocks or eat the soil. TRAD
- Take the animals to areas with salty grasses. GABBRA
- Take the animals to spring water. GABBRA, TURKANA
- Provide *amakat* (Magadi soda) as a lick. TURKANA
- Provide formulated mineral salts (blocks or powder). SCI

References

Higgins (1986) p. 60, 161; ITDG and IIRR (1996) p. 28; Manefield and Tinson (1997) p. 188; Rathore (1986) p. 160.

Downer

Camels sometimes are not able to get up and walk for a variety of reasons. It can be difficult to determine the cause. Reportedly, camels can be down for weeks, then may suddenly get up and walk away.

Signs

- The camel sits down and refuses to get up for any reason.

Cause

- Weakness: may have many causes. Check for signs of other diseases.
- Muscle injuries.
- Nerve damage.
- Exhaustion, overwork, being tied down for too long, or sedation for surgery (▷*Myopathy*).
- Broken bones in the pelvis, hind legs or back (▷*Broken bones*).
- ▷*Plant poisoning.*
- ▷*Snake bite.*
- Tick paralysis (▷*Ticks*).
- ▷*Rabies.*
- ▷*Haemorrhagic disease.*

Prevention

- Remove ticks regularly.
- Avoid tying animals down for more than 4–5 hours at a time (e.g., for transportation).
- Avoid overworking camels (e.g., forcing them to walk too fast or for too long).

Treatment

- Find out why the camel cannot get up, and treat this problem.
- If the animal is lying on its side, turn it over frequently and encourage it to sit upright.
- Give an anti-inflammatory treatment such as Tomanol or dexamethasone (▷*Common medicines*). **Caution:** do not give dexamethasone or other corticosteroids to a female camel during the last 4 months of a pregnancy because they can cause an abortion (▷*Abortion*). SCI
- Massage and slap the hind limbs to help blood circulation. SCI+TRAD
- Feed with a nourishing diet (maize-meal, oatmeal, dairy meal, bran, molasses, etc). Cut green feed and bring it to the animal. SCI+TRAD
- Inject with vitamin B12 and phosphorus (e.g., Tonophosphan, Catosal) if you suspect nerve or muscle damage. SCI
- Lift the camel up in a sling and let it stand for some time, at least once a day. This helps increase blood circulation and prevents the muscles from getting weak. SCI

References

Manefield and Tinson (1997) p. 75–6.

Dry coat

Anhidrosis, dry coat syndrome, hypohidrosis
***Paseena bund, thakawat, gar'mee* (Punjabi)**

A problem widely recognized by camel herders, although not reported in the veterinary literature. Dry coat syndrome is common in the summer, particularly during rainy days. It usually disappears when the weather becomes cooler.

Signs

- Reduced amount of sweating, or none at all. (A normal draught camel will start sweating within 30 minutes of work during the summer.)
- Unwillingness to drink. This is typical of dry coat syndrome.
- Unwillingness to eat (but the animal continues to chew the cud).
- Rapid loss of condition.
- The animal seeks shade.
- Depression: the animal may sit with its neck resting on the ground.
- Fever (99–103.4°F, 37–40°C) during the morning, possibly higher in the evening. The temperature stays high even when the camel is resting.
- Rapid pulse and breathing, breathlessness.
- The animal becomes tired quickly.

Continuous work in hot, humid conditions can lead to fatigue and similar signs to those above, but has no effect on sweating, and the thirst remains normal. Check also for signs of ▷*Myopathy*.

Cause

The exact cause is not known. Dry coat syndrome may be brought on by:

- Overwork and improper rest.
- Lack of enough salt intake: camels needs 6–8 times more salt than other types of livestock, especially during the summer, when they lose more salt through sweating.

Prevention

- Allow camels to rest properly.
- Reduce the number of working hours during the summer.
- Make sure there is enough salt in the feed and water.
- Provide ghee or molasses (or other feeds rich in fats and carbohydrates) before working the camel for a long time.

Treatment

Traditional treatments

- Force the camel to drink, or drench with water. PUNJAB
- Provide 0.5 kg of salt in the feed or water every 4–8 days. PUNJAB
- Soak 2 kg of chickpeas overnight, and give to the camel to eat in the morning. Repeat for 3–4 days. PUNJAB
- Drench with 250 ml of *Eruca sativa* (*taramira*) oil. This is thought to cool the camel. PUNJAB
- Make a drench of ground garlic, ginger, *Vernonia anthelmintica* (*kalizeeri*),

skimmed milk, jaggery (palm sugar) and common salt. Give 500–700 g of this drench twice a week. PUNJAB

Modern treatments

The following treatments are used in horses, so may be useful for camels.

- Rest for 1 week.
- Make a solution of 120–240 g of commercial oral rehydration salts, plus 0.5 kg of glucose (sugar). Or prepare 3–4 litres of oral rehydration fluid (▷*Calf diarrhoea*). Drench once a day for 1 week.
- Give 5–6 litres of Ringer's lactate–dextrose solution and vitamin B-complex as a drip once a day for 1 week.
- Give 2–3 g of vitamin E in the mouth once a day for 1 week.

References

Forse (1999) p. 166; Sewell and Brocklesby (1990) p. 363–4.

Oedema

An oedema is a swelling caused by the accumulation of fluid in the body tissue. In the camel, these swellings occur mostly under the skin, in the face, under the jaws, under the belly, in the lower limbs and on the udder. It is not a disease in itself, but rather a sign of an underlying disease.

Signs

- Soft, painless swellings on the skin.
- If you press against the swelling with your finger, it leaves a pit that returns to normal only slowly.
- Oedema is particularly visible in the morning.

Cause

Oedema can have various causes:

- Under the belly: ▷*Trypanosomiasis, Internal parasites (worms)*, heart failure, pneumonia (▷*Coughs, colds and pneumonia*) or advanced pregnancy (▷*Pregnancy and birth*). It can also be normal after the camel has drunk a lot of water.
- On the face and under the lower jaw: ▷*Pox, Orf*.
- On the udder before or after birth: ▷*Pregnancy and birth*.
- Around wounds, insect and scorpion bites: ▷*Bites and stings*.
- On the penis sheath: ▷*Trypanosomiasis*.
- On the legs: ▷*Snake bite*, arsenic poisoning, hospitalized camels that need exercise.

Treatment

- Treat the root cause of the swelling (see under *Cause* above, and the relevant section in this book). SCI
- Restrict the amount of water and salt in the diet. SCI

If the swelling is very severe, give a diuretic (a medicine that makes the camel urinate) such as the following. Do not use if the animal is dehydrated and does not urinate. Note: only trained veterinarians should use diuretics.

- Naquasone: 1 bolus in the morning, and one in the evening, or 1 bolus a day for 3 days. (Do not use if the camel is pregnant.)
- Inject 0.5–1 mg/kg body weight of furosemide (e.g., 5 ml of Frusemide) into the muscle or slowly into the vein.

References

Bizimana (1994) p. 365–6; Forse (1999) p. 190; ITDG and IIRR (1996) p. 108; Leese (1927) p. 149; Manefield and Tinson (1997) p. 176–7.

9 Reproduction

This chapter describes reproduction in camels, and various disorders in female and male animals. How to treat calves is covered in the next chapter.

Animal	Problem/topic	See section
Female	Normal pregnancy and birth	▷*Pregnancy and birth*
	Problems during calving	▷*Difficult birth*
	Afterbirth (placenta) does not come out	▷*Retained afterbirth*
	Birth canal hangs out	▷*Prolapse of the vagina or womb*
	Swollen or sore udder, strange-smelling or curdled milk	▷*Mastitis*
	Female does not get pregnant	▷*Female sterility*
	Abortion	▷*Abortion*
Male	Normal breeding behaviour	▷*Rutting*
	Male cannot breed	▷*Breeding-bull problems*
	Castration	▷*Castration*
	Swollen testicles	▷*Dipetalonemiasis*

Pregnancy and birth

Camels are very slow breeders because they breed seasonally, take a long time to sexually mature, and there is a long gap between one calf and the next. Compared with other livestock, female sterility and birth problems are rare, but many calves die.

Female camels become sexually mature when they are about 4 years old, and give birth for the first time at about 5 years of age. The female gives birth 12–13 months after a successful mating.

A mother camel is ready for mating again about 12 months after giving birth (although healthy, well-fed females can be bred again after only about 3 months). On average, females can give birth to a calf every 24–36 months. They can continue to breed until they are 20–30 years old.

Breeding facts

Breeding age in male	At least 6–7 years
Age of female at first calving	4–6 years
Pregnancy length (from mating to birth)	12–13 months (375–390 days)
Calving interval (from birth to birth)	24–36 months
Calf weight at birth	26–51 kg (average of 30–40 kg)
Weaning age	3–18 months, depending on management

Mating

The bull approaches the female, sniffs her genitals, pulls up his upper lip to expose his teeth and sniffs (this is called 'flehmen'), and bites her in the neck and front foot. The female either lies down by herself, or he forces her down by pressing on her neck with his neck. He then sits on top of her.

The bull mounts the female from behind. During mating, the bull gurgles, froths at the mouth, and may blow out his *dulaa* (▷*Rutting*). The breeding act usually takes about 6–10 minutes, although it can last from 3 to 30 minutes.

The bull may mate with the same female several times in the same day. It may be necessary to help a young, inexperienced male by grasping the penis and guiding it into the female camel's vagina.

A female that has conceived will refuse to lie down, and curls up her tail when the bull approaches. If a female does this, you can be sure she is pregnant. This 'tail-up' appears 14–16 days after successful mating – or earlier in females pregnant for the first time. It can also happen if a man (especially a stranger) comes near.

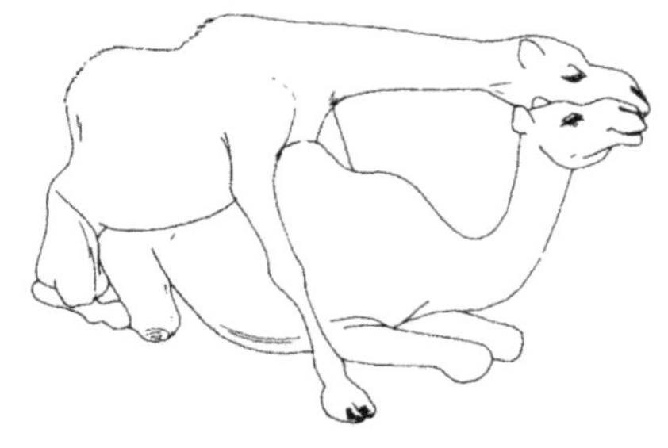

Pregnancy and birth

20 days after successful mating	When a male approaches, the female camel refuses to lie down and curls her tail up. If this continues 2 months later, the female is certainly pregnant.
45–50 days after mating	A skilled person can put his or her hand in the camel's rectum and feel the enlarged left horn of the womb. (Nearly all pregnancies occur in the left horn.)
6 months after mating	The female's belly starts getting bigger.
10–14 days before birth	The muscles above the pelvis between the hips and the tail relax, get softer, and appear to sink.
5–7 days before birth	The female becomes restless, carries the tail in a horizontal position, and tends to wander away from the herd. The udder gets bigger; the vulva swells.
First stage of labour	The female frequently passes urine, lies down and gets up. She moves away from the rest of the herd. This stage lasts 3–24 hours.
Second stage of labour	The water bag becomes visible in the vulva and breaks (it may also break while it is still inside).
30–40 minutes later	The calf is expelled. The mother usually lies down to give birth, but first-time mothers may remain standing. The calf comes out forefeet first, with the head between the forelegs.
Within the next 1–3 hours	The afterbirth (placenta) is expelled.

During pregnancy

- Give the pregnant animal preventive treatment against ▷*Trypanosomiasis*.
- Provide the pregnant animal with enough feed and water, and avoid using it for heavy work.

During and after birth

- It is not normally necessary to help the mother in any way during birth. ▷*Difficult birth* and *Retained afterbirth* for how to deal with problems.
- See ▷*Care of newborn calves* and *Poor mothering and fostering* for how to care for newborn animals.

Controlling pregnancy

Pastoralists who rely on camel milk often try to delay the next pregnancy to lengthen the time the mother will produce milk. They have many ways to do this, including keeping the lactating females separate from males, and reportedly, putting a pebble inside the female's vagina.

References

Evans et al. (1995) p. 6:16–21; FAO (1994) p. 175–8; Forse (1999) p. 48–54; Higgins (1986) p. 113–8; ITDG and IIRR (1996) p. 42–3; Manefield and Tinson (1997) p. 43–5, 177–8, 182–3, 193–6; Rathore (1986) p. 54–6, 100–5; Schwartz and Dioli (1992) p. 63–5, 77–80; Wilson (1998) p. 53–68.

Difficult birth

Dystocia
***Dalmichirir* (Gabbra)**

Most camel births occur without problems because the calf has a streamlined shape, so can come out easily. During a normal birth, it is not necessary to assist the mother in any way. The birth may not be normal because the calf is dead, is in the wrong position inside the womb, or for various other reasons.

Signs

- The calf does not come out after labour begins and the waterbag has burst.

Cause

- The calf is in the wrong position inside the womb. The head may be bent to the side, or the front feet may be bent, preventing the calf from coming out easily.
- The calf is too big to come out.
- The calf is dead.
- The mother is too weak.

Prevention

- Watch the mother closely the last few days before birth.

Treatment

To correct the calf's position

If the camel is from a large breed (such as the Somali), you must be tall and have long arms to correct the calf's position.

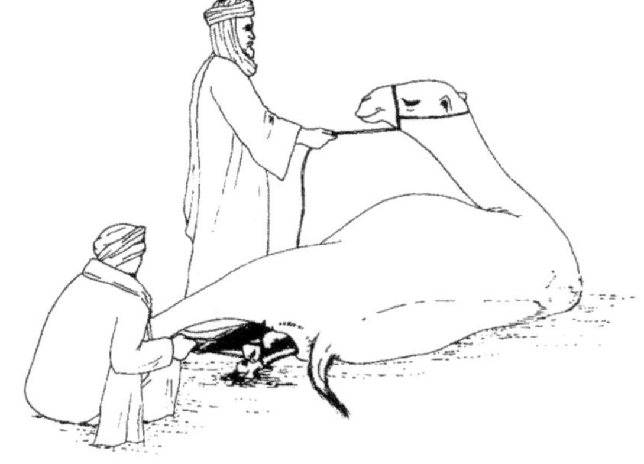

1. Before putting your hand inside the birth canal, remove all your rings and bracelets, cut your nails and wash your hands thoroughly with soap. Mix 1 kg of *amakat* (Magadi soda, sodium bicarbonate) in 5 litres of water, and use this to clean the mother's vulva.
2. Make the mother animal lie on its side and tie it down. If necessary, lubricate your hand with vegetable oil and push it into the birth canal. Push the calf back into the uterus to make space for you to move it. If the calf's neck is bent to one side, reach for the base of the neck and slowly pull the neck until it is straight and the head is between the front legs. Then pull gently on the front legs to bring the calf out. GABBRA, SCI

Caesarean section

***Pet chirana, aaperation karke bachha nikalana* (Hindi)**

A caesarean section is an operation in which you cut open the uterus to pull out the calf (dead or alive). This is a risky operation, and should be done only if other methods have been tried and it is necessary to save the mother's life. It can be done only by a trained veterinarian.

Calf that is dead

If the calf is dead, you will have to cut it up inside the mother and pull it out piece by piece. You will need a small, sharp knife or an obstetric wire and handle, and a blunt metal rod. Make sure that these tools are all sterile. This is a difficult procedure that normally results in the death of the mother if it is done by an untrained person.

1. Sterilize the tools. Tie a strip of the inner layer of *oltepesi* (*Acacia tortilis*) bark around the knife blade to make the exposed sharp edge smaller so it does not cut the mother. To keep the tools clean, do not put them on the ground during the operation.
2. Hold one of the calf's front legs and cut the skin around its wrist joint. Push the metal rod between the skin and the muscles, to separate them up to the shoulder joint. Pull the calf's leg to separate it from its body at the shoulder. Leave the leg skin attached to the body. Repeat for the other front leg.
3. Cut a hole at the base of the calf's neck. Push your hand through it and pull out all the internal organs. Break the ribs by pressing on them. Make sure they do not stick out to harm the mother. Pull the rest of the calf's body out.
4. If the mother survives, watch her carefully: bringing the calf out in this way often results in a prolapsed uterus (▷*Prolapse of the vagina or womb*).

SAMBURU, TURKANA, BEDOUIN, TRAD+SCI

References

Forse (1999) p. 55–9; Gahlot and Chouhan (1992) p. 129–32; Higgins (1986) p. 118–9, 131–2; ITDG and IIRR (1996) p. 45–6; Manefield and Tinson (1997) p. 48–9, 80–1; Rathore (1986) p. 144, 220–1; Wanyama (1997) vol. 2, p. 40–3.

Retained afterbirth

***Dillu itis* (Gabbra), *jerr, jer nahi heerana* (India), *lmodong* (Samburu), *maderr* (Somali), *edungat* (Turkana)**

After the calf is born, the afterbirth (placenta) normally comes out during the next 1–3 hours. It can still come out by itself up to 24 hours later. If it has not come out after 24 hours, you will have to treat the mother. Retained afterbirth is not a common problem in camels.

If the afterbirth does not come out, it will lead to an infection that may kill the mother.

Signs

- The afterbirth does not come out after the calf is born.

Causes

- Unskilled, rough, vigorous pulling on the calf while it is being born (▷*Difficult birth*).
- Premature birth or abortion (▷*Abortion*).
- The womb does not contract.
- Diseases such as brucellosis (not covered in this book).

Prevention

- Do not pull too hard on the calf during a difficult birth. (During a normal birth, it is not necessary to assist the mother in any way.)

Treatment

Traditional treatments

- Pull the placenta out gently. Do not pull it too roughly; instead, put gradual pressure on it over an extended period by rolling it around a stick or tying a stone to it.

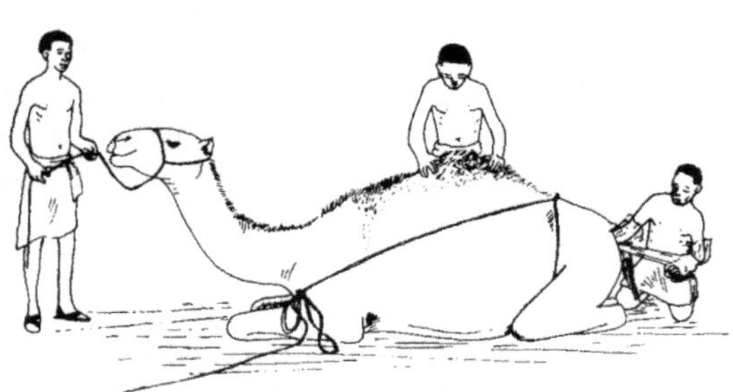

- Drench with 2.5–3 litres of sour camel's milk mixed with salt.
- Encourage the calf to suckle. This stimulates the uterus to contract and helps to expel the placenta.
- Boil roots of *Salvadora persica* (*sokotei* in Samburu, *haech* in Rendille, *adeh* in Gabbra) in water. Allow to cool, then use the liquid to drench the animal. KENYA, TRAD+SCI
- Soak bark of *tilomwa* (*Ziziphus mauritiana*) in water. Boil, then allow to cool before drenching with 3 litres of the liquid. You can also use the bark of *sitot* (*Grewia bicolor*) or *ses* (*Acacia tortilis*). POKOT
- Crush 3–4 shoots of wild sisal (*ewais*) and boil them in 3 litres of water. Allow to cool, then use as a drench. POKOT
- Crush a 200 g piece of bamboo (*bansara, Dendrocalamus strictus*) and mix with water. Pour through a clean cotton cloth to separate out the coarse fibre. Drench the animal with the liquid. After about 2 hours, the afterbirth will come out. RAJASTHAN
- Boil 0.5 kg of *bajra* (pearl millet, *Pennisetum americanum*) in water. Allow to cool, then give to the animal to eat. RAJASTHAN

Modern treatments

- If there is an obvious infection, inject an antibiotic.
- Inject 20–40 international units of oxytocin into the muscle. Carefully remove the placenta by hand. Insert antibiotic boluses into the vagina.

References

Bizimana (1994) p. 349; Evans et al. (1995) p. 7:26; Forse (1999) p. 241–2, 350; ITDG and IIRR (1996) p. 50–1; Manefield and Tinson (1997) p. 184; Rathore (1986) p. 144–5; Wanyama (1997) vol. 2, p. 4–8, 66–71.

Prolapse of the vagina or womb

Aar nikalna **(India)**
Prolapse of the womb: *ormat abui* (Gabbra)
Vaginal prolapse: *arab qab* (Gabbra)

A prolapse is where the vagina or the whole womb pushes through the birth opening (the 'vulva'). It turns inside-out and hangs down outside. Vaginal prolapse is quite common in camels, occurring either in late pregnancy (especially in well-fed animals) or after a difficult birth. If an animal has had one prolapse, it may well have another during its next pregnancy.

Prolapse of the womb (the 'uterus') is very rare in camels.

Signs

- During pregnancy, the vagina may hang out from the vulva. This occurs especially in the evening during the last stages of pregnancy.
- After the birth, the uterus may hang out.

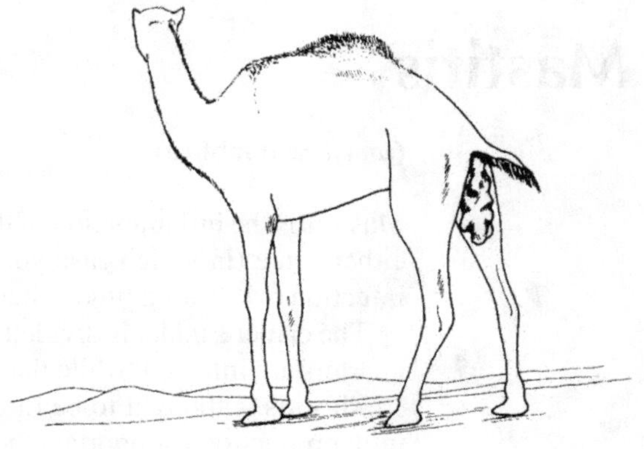

Causes

- After a difficult birth, especially one where the herder has helped but has pulled the calf out too strongly.
- An inherited tendency.

Prevention

- Avoid breeding camels that have suffered from a prolapse.
- Do not use a breeding bull that is much larger than the female.
- Be gentle when assisting the camel during birth.

Treatment

It may not be necessary to treat a prolapsed vagina. To treat a prolapsed vagina or uterus:

1. Calm the camel down (the Gabbra sing to it), or sedate it.
2. Prevent the camel from walking around so that it does not step on the prolapsed tissue.
3. Carefully wash the vagina or womb with soap or an antiseptic, making sure no sand or soil is left on it.
4. Sprinkle all over with a handful of sugar.
5. If possible, inject an epidural anaesthetic between the bones at the top of the base of the tail (▷*Sedation and anaesthesia*).
6. Push the vagina or womb slowly back in through the vulva. This is easier if the back part of the camel is raised up. Lifting the vagina or womb up with a clean piece of cloth (such as a sheet) also makes it easier.
7. Close the vulva with stitches, leaving an opening at the lower end so the animal can urinate. Remove the stitches after 2–5 days. The Gabbra, Somali and Bedouins use a special type of woven basket to close the vulva: this method can be messy and cumbersome. In India, two parallel sticks are used.
8. Inject antibiotics, or apply antibiotics locally, such as putting a bolus into the vagina and putting antibiotic powder on the vulva and stitches (▷*Common medicines*). SCI

References

Bizimana (1994) p. 349–50; Evans et al. (1995) p. 7:30; Forse (1999) p. 76–8, 242–3; ITDG and IIRR (1996) p. 52; Manefield and Tinson (1997) p. 285–7; Projet Cameline (1999) p. 51; Rathore (1986) p. 145; Schwartz and Dioli (1992) p. 81.

Mastitis

***Qamyara* (Gabbra)**

Mastitis is the inflammation of the udder, usually due to bacterial infection. It can be either acute (in which case you may see signs of the disease) or chronic: (a mild infection over a long time, when you may not see signs of the disease).

The camel's udder is divided into four separate quarters. Usually only one or two quarters are infected, while the others are healthy.

Mastitis is thought to be rare in camels, although in Sudan and Somali, where milk production is important, herders think it is an important disease.

A female with an obvious udder problem is difficult to sell. After the lactation is over, the udder shrinks and it is difficult to detect a faulty quarter.

Signs

- The infected quarters of the udder swell and become hard and hot.
- The animal kicks when being suckled or milked.

- The milk seems curdled or coagulated.
- The milk smells strange.
- The milk yield is reduced.
- In acute cases, the milk from infected quarters is clotted and mixed with pus and blood.
- If untreated, treated too late or not treated for long enough, acute mastitis can develop into chronic mastitis.

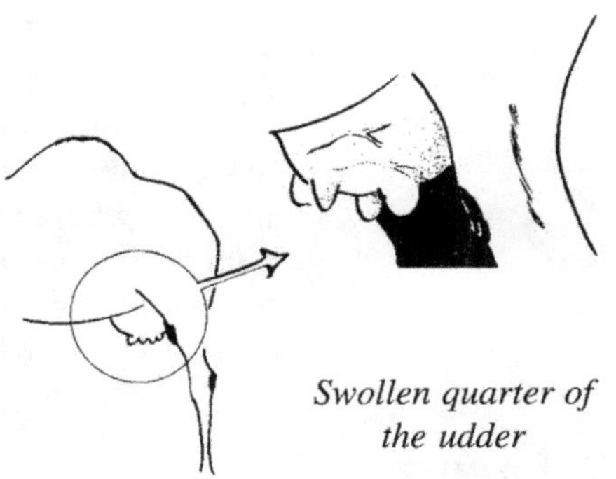

Swollen quarter of the udder

Cause

Mastitis can be caused by a wide variety of bacteria: *Staphylococcus aureus*, *Bacillus*, *Corynebacterium bovis*, *Streptococcus agalactiae*, *Escherichia coli uberis* and *Pasteurella haemolytica*. These bacteria enter the udder through the teat.

Animals may become infected if:

- The animal enclosure is dirty.
- Inexperienced persons are milking (using the wrong milking technique).
- People milk with dirty hands.
- The udder or teats are injured: an obstruction in the teat canal may make milking impossible.
- There are a lot of ticks (especially *Amblyomma* ticks) on the udder (▷*Ticks*).
- The teats are tied with string or with dirty udder covers to prevent the calf from suckling.

Mastitis cannot be transmitted directly from one animal to another. However, it can spread if you milk healthy animals after milking one with mastitis without washing your hands in between.

Prevention

- Wash your hands before milking.
- Clean the udder before milking.
- Milk regularly.
- Regularly remove ticks from the udder.
- Keep the animal enclosure clean and dry.

Treatment

Wash your hands thoroughly after milking or treating an infected animal, to avoid carrying the infection to other animals. TRAD+SCI

Traditional treatments

- It is very important to milk the camel as frequently as possible and to remove all the milk from the udder. Throw this milk away; do not use it or feed it to the calf. Give the calf to another female for fostering, or feed it with milk from another camel (▷*Poor mothering and fostering*). TRAD+SCI
- Rub an ointment such as sheep-wool fat or sheep-tail fat into the affected area.
- Apply an ointment made of *Sesbania sesban* or *Ajuga remota* mixed with butter or a fat made from sheep-tail or goat intestines.
- Burn faeces in a pot and place the pot under the udder so that the udder starts sweating.

Modern treatments

- Apply an antibiotic into the udder through the openings in the teat. You can use the same antibiotics as are used to treat mastitis in cattle. Take care when applying the drug, since each camel teat has two small holes (unlike in cattle where there is only one large hole); you should treat both (▷*Administering medicines*). After applying the antibiotics, massage the udder to distribute the drug.
- If it is too difficult to apply a medicine into the teat, you can inject antibiotics into the vein or muscle instead (▷*Common medicines*).

References

Bizimana (1994) p. 352; FAO (1994) p. 256–7; Forse (1999) p. 244–5, 331; Higgins (1986) p. 105; ITDG and IIRR (1996) p. 53; Manefield and Tinson (1997) p. 152–3; Projet Cameline (1999) p. 41; Rathore (1986) p. 146–7; Wernery and Kaaden (1995) p. 70–1.

Female sterility

Immature reproductive tract: *dabeno* (Gabbra)
Uterine infection: *mala kesa yaa* (Gabbra)

Female camels may fail to become pregnant when they reach maturity or after a previous birth. This is not very common: the percentage of sterile females in Raika breeding herds in India is very low (1%). In Saudi Arabia, too, only 1% of females are sterile. This is also a rare complaint in Kenya.

Sometimes pastoralists try to prevent female camels from becoming pregnant because they want to use them for riding. The Tuareg do this by inserting a pebble into the animal's uterus.

Signs

- The female fails to get pregnant, or becomes pregnant but then aborts early in the pregnancy.
- The female may become very fat and develop a very large hump.

Causes

- Abnormal development of the reproductive tract from birth.
- Infection of the womb (endometritis) due to one of the following bacteria: *Staphylococcus aureus*, *Streptococcus pyogenes*, *Diplococcus*, *Escherichia coli*, *Clostridium*, *Klebsiella*, *Pseudomonas aeruginosa*, *Salmonella*, *Campylobacter fetus* or *Trichomonas fetus*. Many infections that cause sterility may be spread by the breeding bull.
- Injury to the reproductive tract during a previous difficult birth or because of attack by predators such as hyenas.
- Chronic, long-term disease, such as ▷*Trypanosomiasis* or brucellosis.

- Cyst on the ovary (the ovary is the source of the unfertilized eggs in the female).
- The 'corpus luteum' (part of the ovary that produces hormones during part of the heat cycle) produces hormones continuously, preventing the female from coming into heat.
- Malnutrition (▷*Pica*).
- Abnormal tissues in the vagina.

Prevention

- If the animal has a congenital defect (an abnormality from birth), it should not be used for breeding.
- Give young female camels enough good-quality feed to ensure they can conceive and maintain the pregnancy.

Treatment

The appropriate treatment depends on the cause of the problem.

For an infected womb

- Flush the uterus with sour camel's milk mixed with salt. GARI SOMALI
- Sometimes excessive growth (called 'hyperplasia') of the tissue inside the vagina is held responsible for the failure to conceive. Remove this tissue with a knife, and then insert a cloth drenched with turmeric into the vagina. RAIKA

For malnutrition

- Provide additional feed, and inject multivitamins and a stimulant such as 20 ml of Tonophosphan into the muscle or under the skin. SCI

Hormonal imbalance

- The Tuareg know how to remove a persistent corpus luteum by hand. TUAREG

References

Bizimana (1994) p. 346–8; Forse (1999) p. 241, 350–1; Higgins (1986) p. 119–20; ITDG and IIRR (1996) p. 43; Manefield and Tinson (1997) p. 11; Rathore (1986) p. 147; Wernery and Kaaden (1995) p. 56–62.

Abortion

***Iralii* (Borana, Gabbra), *touno* (Pokot), *nkiboroto* (Samburu), *d'ess*, *dhies*, *l'ess* (Somali), *akiyech*, *akiyechum*, *akiecium* (Turkana)**

An abortion is when the mother animal expels the foetus before it is due. This can happen at any time during pregnancy and may be missed in the early stages, since there is little to be seen. The main signs are that the female ceases to lift its tail when the herdsman approaches, and eventually returns to be served by the bull.

Signs

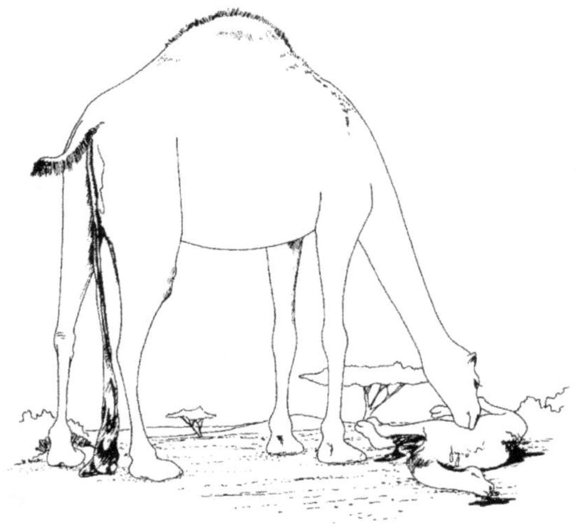

- The animal is restless.
- Blood comes out of the vagina.
- The foetus is expelled.
- The female returns to the bull for mating.

Causes

- ▷*Trypanosomiasis* (causes abortion late in the pregnancy). Herders often think this is the cause.
- Any disease which causes fever can also cause abortion, including ▷*Pox, Salmonellosis, Rift Valley fever*, Q-fever, leptospirosis, brucellosis, trichomoniasis, vibriosis and toxoplasmosis.

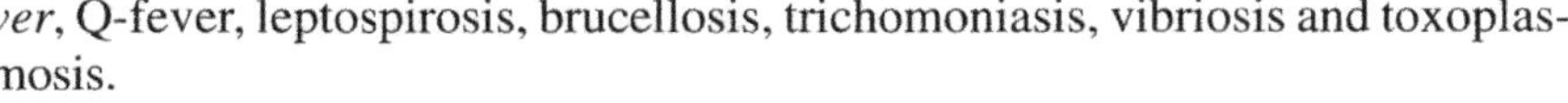

- Nutritional stress, malnutrition.
- Hard work and stress during transport or while travelling during drought.
- Infrequent watering.
- Injection of dexamethasone or other corticosteroids (medicines used against inflammation) during last 4 months of pregnancy (▷*Common medicines, Allergy, Arthritis, Chest sprain, Downer, Foot problems, Myopathy, Sunstroke*).
- Pregnant animals feeding on immature *Acacia nilotica* pods. SAMBURU
- Tradition also holds acacia pods, spiders' webs, caterpillars and the custard-apple tree (*Annona squamosa*, *sitafal* in Hindi) responsible for abortions.

Prevention

- Avoid trypanosomiasis and other infections.
- Feed pregnant females well, give them enough to drink, and do not work them too hard.
- Avoid feeding with immature *Acacia nilotica* pods.
- Do not use corticosteroids (e.g., dexamethasone) or xylazine (Rompun) during the last 4 months of a pregnancy.

Treatment

- Keep the animal quiet in a stress-free environment.
- Keep the female away from bulls.
- Check for trypanosomiasis, and treat if necessary (▷*Trypanosomiasis*).
- If more than one camel in a herd or in an area aborts, try to find out the cause. Take a sample of the foetus, the afterbirth, and the mother's blood. Take these to a laboratory for analysis (▷*How to collect samples for testing*).

References

Bizimana (1994) p. 348–9; Evans et al. (1995) p. 7:26; Forse (1999) p. 238; ITDG and IIRR (1996) p. 44; Manefield and Tinson (1997) p. 19–20; Rathore (1986) p. 146.

Rutting

***Hej* (Arabic), *musth* (India), *waghogh* (Somalia)**

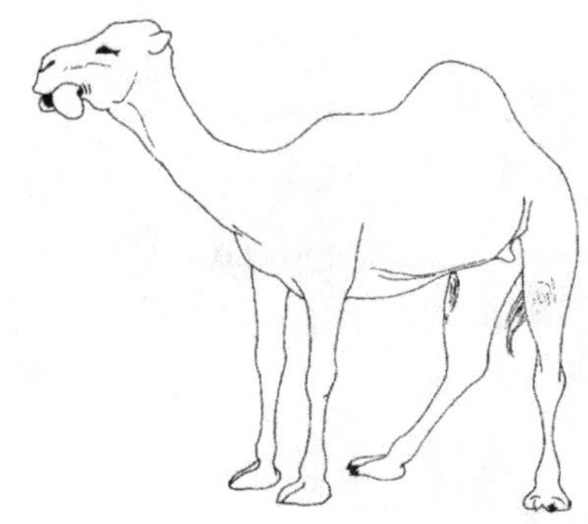

Male camels are sexually mature at 6–7 years of age. They are seasonal breeders; under pastoral conditions, the breeding season, or 'rut', normally occurs for several months a year, usually during the rainy season. In East Africa, there are two rutting seasons.

During this time, male camels become more aggressive and show the signs listed below. Rutting males can be dangerous and have to be handled with care.

The bulls fight each other, and usually the oldest and heaviest bull establishes dominance. He shows fully developed rutting behaviour, while the other males have a subdued version. The dominant bull expends a lot of energy guarding his harem of females from rivals, and has little time for eating, so loses weight during the breeding season. A bull can mate with 50 or more females in the season.

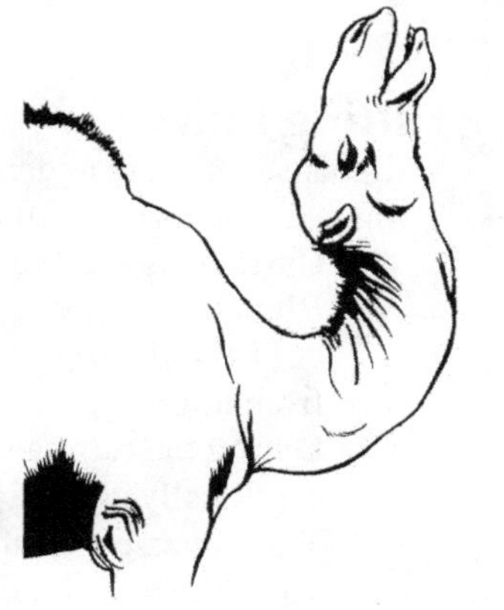

In an all-male herd, the animals do not go through a marked rut.

Signs

- The bull sprays urine and flaps its tail. A urine mark can be seen on the back of the rump of rutting bulls.
- Frothing at the mouth, grinding the teeth.
- Frequent blowing out of the *dulaa* (a part of the soft palate).
- Loud, frequent gurgling.
- The poll glands (on the back of the neck near the head) produce a blackish, foul-smelling liquid.
- The bull rubs his poll glands on objects and his own hump.
- Diarrhoea.
- The bull attacks other male camels and people, often causing injury.

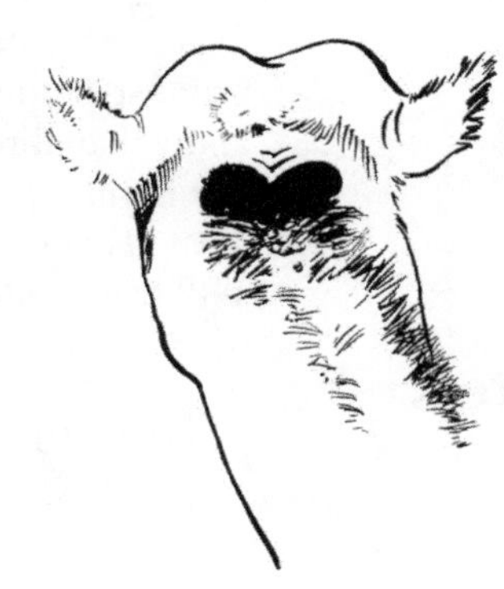

Normal rutting behaviour may be mistaken for ▷*Rabies*.

Rutting seasons

Egypt	March–April
India	November–March
Iran	January–February
Kenya	May, December–January
Kuwait	October–April
Mali	February–March, August–September
Morocco	December–April
Pakistan	December–March
Somalia	June, September–November
Sudan	March–August
Turkestan	January–May

Handling rutting bulls

Because bulls are aggressive during the rutting season, it can be difficult to handle them and to use them for work.

- Castrate the bull to prevent rutting (▷*Castration*). TRAD
- Blunt the large canine teeth by sawing their tips off with a small saw about 0.5 cm from the top. Round off the teeth them with a file. This prevents the bulls from injuring each other during the rut.
- During the rutting season, keep male and female animals separately. Keep exceptionally aggressive bulls away from other males. TRAD
- Tie a muzzle over the bull's mouth to prevent him from biting. TRAD
- Work the bulls hard during the rutting season. TRAD
- Tie the tail of the bull to one side to prevent it from spraying urine and dung around. TRAD

Managing breeding males

- It is often necessary to manage the bull's activities, for example, to prevent him from spending too much time with any one female. Do not let him mate with more than three females a day, and prevent him from mating with females that are immature or too small (▷*Difficult birth*).
- Provide sufficient, high-quality feed during the rutting season to prevent the bull from getting too thin.

References

Evans et al. (1995) p. 6:15–16; FAO (1994) p. 176; Forse (1999) p. 51; Higgins (1986) p. 22–3, 114; Leese (1927) p. 90–1; Manefield and Tinson (1997) p. 43–5; Rathore (1986) p. 100–1; Schwartz and Dioli (1992) p. 62–3, 75–6; Wilson (1998) p. 49–51.

Breeding bull problems

In rare cases, male camels selected for breeding are not able to do so.

Signs

- The bull does not go into rut and shows no interest in mounting female camels (▷*Rutting*).
- He is not able to mount a female.
- He is not able to insert his penis into the female's vagina.
- The female camels do not become pregnant (▷*Pregnancy and birth*).

Causes

- Abscess on the chest (▷*Chest-pad abscess*).
- Exhaustion.
- Bull is young (4–5 years).
- Inflammation of testicles, penis or sheath.
- The opening of the penis sheath is too tight.
- Injuries on the scrotum or testicle by bites of other camels, jackals or hyenas.
- Arthritis in the hind legs, or spine problems (▷*Arthritis*).
- Lack of libido.
- Low numbers of sperm in the semen.

Prevention

- Keep male camels apart to prevent fights.
- Limit the number of females each male serves.
- Give strengthening tonics (such as ghee and jaggery) to breeding males before, during and after the breeding season.

Treatment

- Treat an injury or inflammation of the penis, sheath or scrotum with an antiseptic dressing. Inject a systemic antibiotic such as long-acting Terramycin into the muscle (▷*Wounds and burns* and *Common medicines*).

References

Forse (1999) p. 237; Gahlot and Chouhan (1992) p. 135–45; Manefield and Tinson (1997) p. 184–6, 232; Rathore (1986) p. 141–3.

Castration

***Kolansiti* (Gabbra), *ngelemata* (Samburu), *dhufan* (Somali Kenya), *aleldougi* (Turkana)**

Camel breeders castrate male camels for several reasons:

- To control breeding.

- To make the animals easier to handle, especially those meant for work (but not for carrying a pack, as castrated males develop a large hump which interferes with the pack).
- To reduce the animals' aggressiveness and urge to fight, so reducing the risk of injuries (▷*Rutting*).
- To fatten the male.
- In case of bite wounds or injuries to the testicles.

Camels should be castrated after they reach the age of 4–5 years. If an older animal has to be castrated, do not do it during the rutting season, as at this time there is more blood in the sex organs, and profuse bleeding may kill the animal.

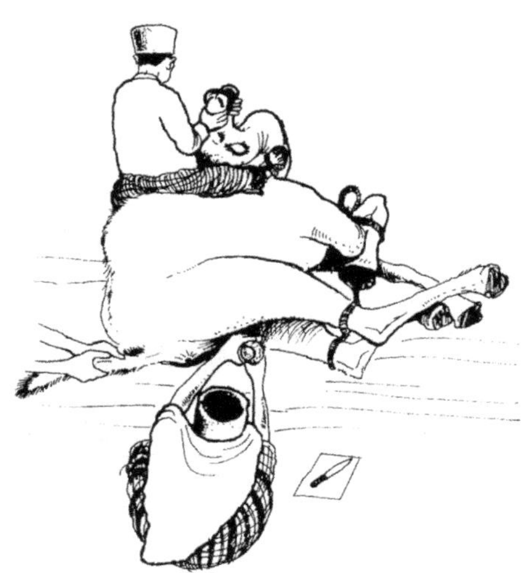

Treatment

It is best to use surgery to castrate camels. This involves cutting open the scrotum, cutting the spermatic cord (the cord that joins the testes to the body), and removing the testes.

Non-surgical methods common in cattle and other livestock (where sticks or a hammer are used to crush the spermatic cord without cutting open the skin) are difficult in camels because the scrotum is tight and the skin on the scrotum is thick.

Traditional treatments

- Tie the bull down on its chest or on its side. Make a cut into the scrotum. Pull out the testicle, cut the spermatic cord with a red-hot knife, and remove the testicle. Repeat with the other testicle. Fill the wound with salt, and sew the lips of the wound together. Brand the animal three or four times on the top of the thighs and bring the animal to good pasture so it can regain its strength. TUAREG AJJER
- After castrating the animal, wash the wound with lukewarm water and apply a powder made of dried *eteteleit* (*Acalypha fruticosa*) leaves. Repeat every 4 days until the wound heals. TURKANA
- After castrating the animal, cut an aloe (*Aloe secundiflora*) leaf and collect the juice. Apply 1 teaspoonful of the juice onto the wound and then dust the wound with ash. SAMBURU

Modern treatments

1. Restrain the bull and inject a sedative (▷*Sedation and anaesthesia*).
2. Tie the hind legs together and pull them forward to expose the testes. Inject a local anaesthetic into each of the testes and the spermatic cord: 10 ml into each spermatic cord and 10 ml into each testis.
3. Wait 2–5 minutes for the anaesthetic to take effect.
4. Wash the scrotum thoroughly with soap and water, and paint antiseptic on it.

5. Hold the testis in your hand and squeeze it at the base to force the testis out.
6. Use a sharp, disinfected knife or scalpel to make a cut, 5–10 cm long, vertically along the inner side of the scrotum. The testis pops out as you squeeze the scrotum.
7. Push back the fats and membrane covering the testicle while pulling the testis out.
8. Tie off the cord with catgut. Crush and cut the spermatic cord with an emasculator, or cut it with scissors below where it is tied. Or wind the cord around a clean piece of wood or your finger, and pull it until it snaps.
9. Remove the testicle.
10. Repeat the same procedure for the other testicle, if necessary making a second cut in the scrotum.
11. Leave the cut open to allow fluid to drain out.
12. Spray the wound with antibiotic aerosol spray.
13. Inject the animal with a broad-spectrum, long-acting antibiotic (▷*Common medicines*).
14. Untie the camel, beginning with the hind legs. Roll the animal into a sitting position so it can stand up.

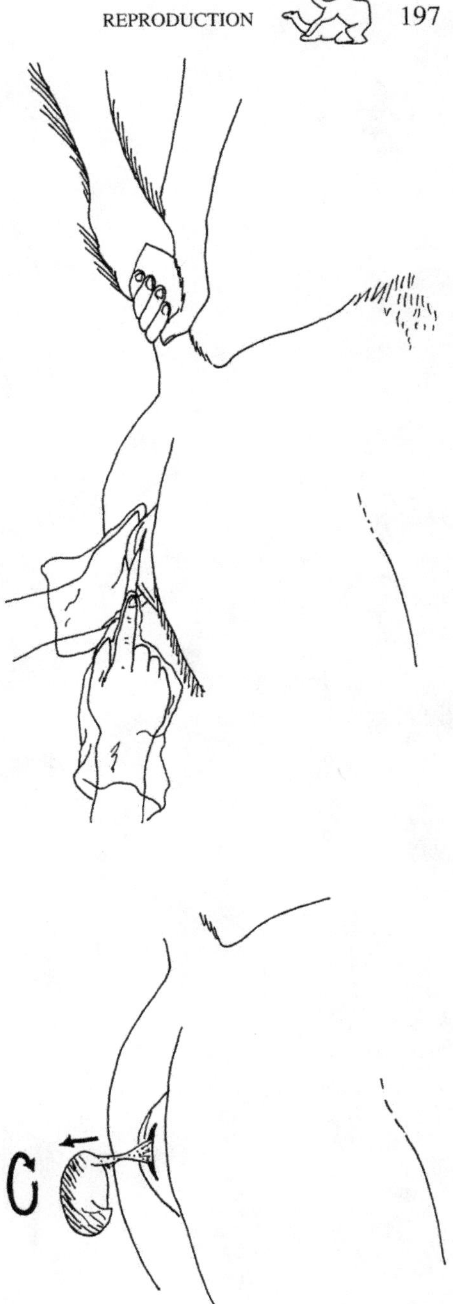

References

Bizimana (1994) p. 348; Evans et al. (1995) p. 7:21–2; Forse (1999) p. 79–82; Higgins (1986) p. 133; ITDG and IIRR (1996) p. 63–5; Leese (1927) p. 94; Manefield and Tinson (1997) p. 57–8; Projet Cameline (1999) p. 55; Rathore (1986) p. 219–20; Schwartz and Dioli (1992) p. 129–30, 141; Wilson (1998) p. 76–8.

10 Calves

This chapter covers the care of newborn calves and major problems unique to calves. See other chapters for problems that affect both calves and adult camels.

Signs	**See section**
Care of calves immediately after birth	⊳*Care of newborn calves*
Mother ignores calf; mother dead	⊳*Poor mothering and fostering*
Swollen navel	⊳*Navel ill*
Calf has diarrhoea	⊳*Calf diarrhoea, Colibacillosis, Diarrhoea, Salmonellosis*
Watery, sunken eyes, pus in eye	⊳*Saam*

Care of newborn calves

Birth is usually easy in camels. The mother likes to separate herself from the rest of the herd. ⊳*Pregnancy and birth* for information on normal birth, and ⊳*Difficult birth* for what to do if there are problems.

When it is born, the calf is covered by a whitish membrane. The mother guards her calf, but she does not lick it, nor does she eat the afterbirth. The umbilical cord breaks when the mother gets up.

A normal newborn calf weighs 26–51 kg (average of 30–40 kg).

Helping the calf breathe

The calf starts breathing after the umbilical cord has broken. Sometimes you have to help a calf to start breathing.

- Clear the mucus from the nostrils with your fingers. TRAD+SCI

- Pour cold water over the calf. TRAD+SCI
- Hold the calf upside-down. TRAD+SCI
- Tickle the calf's nostrils with a straw to make it sneeze mucus out of its nose. TRAD+SCI
- Use a commercial respiratory stimulant (e.g., Respirot). SCI
- Dissolve 9 g of salt, 50 g of glucose and 10 g of sodium bicarbonate in 1 litre of sterile water and give as a drip. SCI

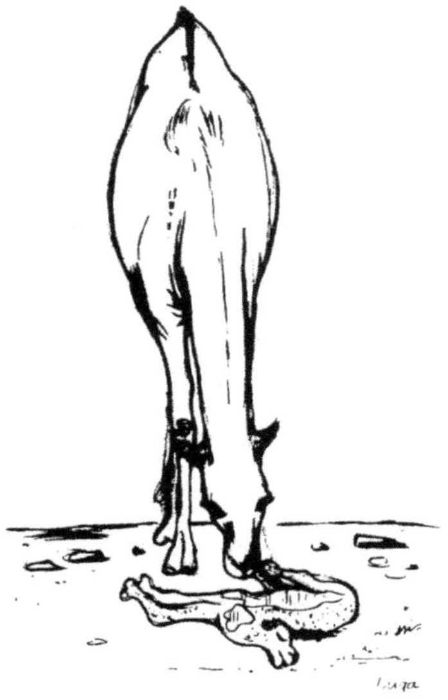
The newborn calf is covered with a white membrane.

Umbilical cord

The umbilical cord breaks about 10 cm from the calf's body.

- After the umbilical cord breaks, dip the end in iodine solution to prevent infection. SCI

Suckling

Calves normally try to stand up soon after birth and will be standing and suckling within 2 hours. They should suckle as soon as possible and be given some help. The calf suckles until it is 3–18 months old, depending on the management system.

It is important that the newborn calf drinks enough colostrum (the mother's first milk) within the first 6 hours after birth. Colostrum contains antibodies that protect the calf from diseases. It also helps the calf to pass its first faeces. See ▷*Poor mothering and fostering* if the mother will not let the calf suckle.

Note, however, that too much colostrum can cause diarrhoea (▷*Calf diarrhoea*). Good milking mothers that have already delivered two or three times produce a large amount of colostrum: more than the calf needs. Make sure the calf does not drink too much.

Many camel pastoralists believe that too much colostrum is not good for the calf and restrict or even prevent the calf from drinking it. This practice causes many calves to die.

Calves that have been born too soon (low body weight, lack of pigmentation and short, silky hair) or are too weak to stand, need to be fed by bottle.

- If the mother has no milk, massage the udder to encourage milk let-down.
- Inject 20–40 international units of oxytocin into the vein to increase the milk flow. After the calf has suckled, milk the udder out

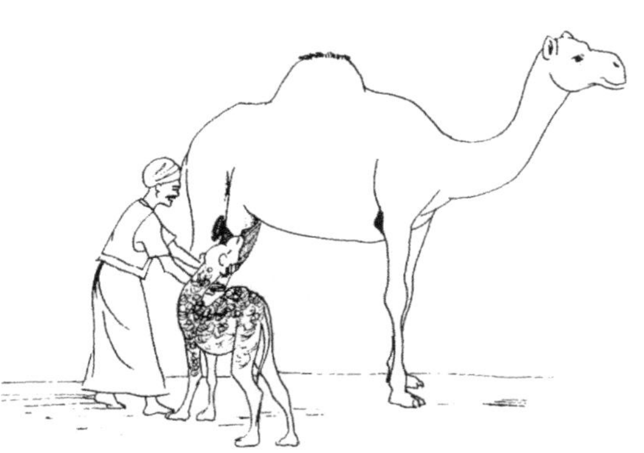

completely to prevent mastitis. SCI

- Milk the mother and feed the colostrum to the calf. SCI
- If no colostrum is available, take 1–2 litres of blood from the mother and drench the calf with it within 6 hours after birth. SCI
- If you have a freezer, collect colostrum from a mother whose calf has died and keep it frozen. If a mother dies or has no milk, you can thaw the colostrum and give it to the newborn calf. SCI

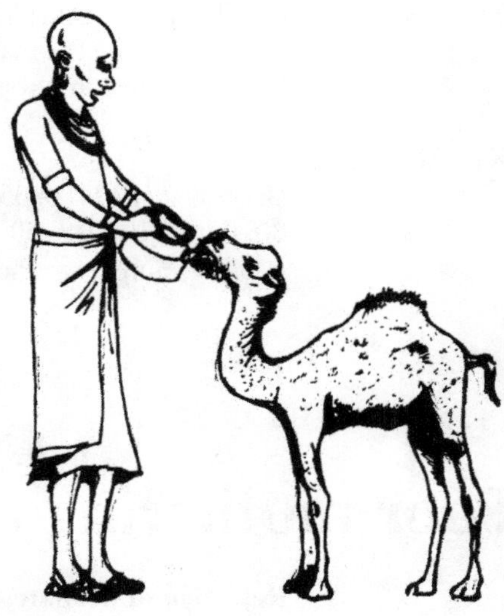

Faeces

A calf's first faeces (dung) are dark and pasty. They should come out within 24 hours after birth. If this does not occur, do one of the following.

- Spoon-feed the calf with some cooking oil (but *not* castor oil).
- Mix oil or liquid paraffin with an equal amount of warm water. Put it into a syringe (without a needle!) and squirt this liquid into the calf's rectum.
- Put your finger into the calf's rectum and massage carefully. Take care not to injure the rectum.

Calf health

Camel calves are delicate creatures. A large proportion of calves die during their first year: around 30% in East African pastoral systems. Many die because they do not get enough milk, since the herders also live off camel milk. In India, where people rely less on camel milk, only about 10% of calves die before weaning.

Calves are prone to ▷*Diarrhoea*, *Constipation*, *Navel ill* and vomiting. See also ▷*Calf diarrhoea* and *Colibacillosis*.

Weaning

The calf begins to feed on grass when it is 2–3 months old, and can be weaned at 4 months. Many pastoralists leave the calf with its mother until it is at least 1 year old.

If the calf is weaned early, introduce it slowly to solid feed to avoid diarrhoea.

To wean a calf, do one of the following:

- Tie a cloth or basket over the mother's udder.
- Tie a muzzle over the calf's mouth. Remove the muzzle to allow the calf to graze.

Pastoralists have many other techniques for weaning calves, or for restricting the amount of milk it drinks (so making more available for people to drink). These include the following (Schwarz and Dioli (1992) have pictures of these):

- They push two acacia thorns through the calf's upper lips from inside, fixing them in place with acacia resin. If the calf tries to suckle, it pricks the mother's udder, and the mother will kick it away. The thorns are removed after 7–10 days.
- They cut a thin flap of skin from the calf's nostrils, forming two dangling skin flaps.
- They cut a thin flap of skin from the top of the calf's nose, and tie bark around this so it stands upright.

- They cut a thin strip, about 10 cm long, in the back of the calf's tongue, separating it from the rest of the tongue with a layer of camel hair.
- They tie a thin rope in a figure of 8 around the two parts of the calf's upper lip.

References

Bizimana (1994) p. 350; Evans et al. (1995) p. 7:24–5, 30, 33; FAO (1994) p. 179–80; Forse (1999) p. 59–64; Manefield and Tinson (1997) p. 50–2, 68; Rathore (1986) p. 56–7; Schwartz and Dioli (1992) p. 64, 119–22.

Poor mothering and fostering

Rejection of neonate, maternal failure
***Nkibata e lashe* (Samburu), *ilmadid* (Somali)**

Some camel mothers refuse to allow their calves to suckle. If a mother dies, it is necessary to persuade another female to accept the calf as her own. Pastoralists use various methods to persuade the mother (or foster-mother) to accept the calf.

Signs

- The female kicks or tries to bite the calf when it tries to suckle.
- The female does not pay attention to the calf.
- The female has no milk.

Cause

- The mother has gone through a difficult or painful birth.
- The problem runs in some family lines.
- The mother is inexperienced.
- The udder is painful (▷*Mastitis*).

Prevention

- Help promptly if the birth is a difficult one (▷*Difficult birth*).
- Select for breeding good females from a good mother.

Treatment

Traditional treatments

Many other traditional treatments are used, apart from those described here.

- Allow the new mother to smell her calf all over. Do not disturb her.
- Lift the calf and help it suckle.

POKOT

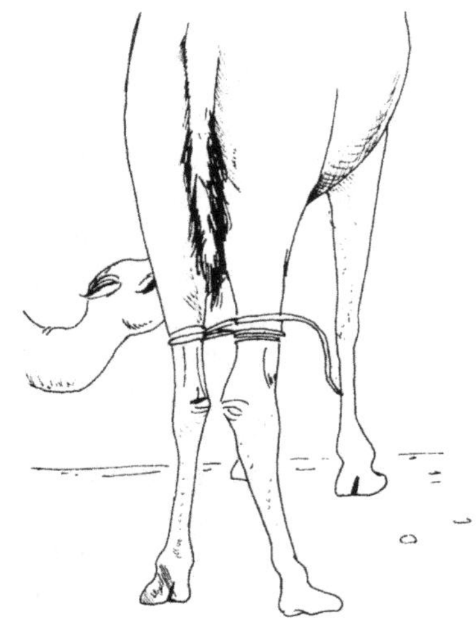

Hobble on hind legs

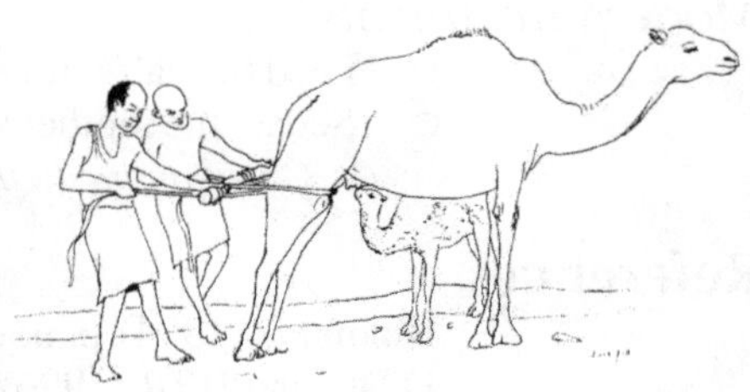

Pulling the mother's legs back to allow the calf to suckle

- Pull the mother's hind legs back with ropes to prevent her from kicking the calf away. KENYA
- Hobble the mother by tying a loop of rope around her back legs. KENYA
- Blindfold the mother while the calf is suckling. POKOT

The main purpose of the treatments below is to make the mother uncomfortable, so giving the calf a chance to suckle.

- Herders in **East Africa** bend one of the mother's front legs up and tie the fetlock to the forearm so the animal is forced to stand on three legs. She will not be able to kick the calf when it tries to suckle (⊳*Restraining*).
- They may pass a thin rope through the mother's nose, then tie it to a tree so that the head is pulled upwards. After a few hours, the mother will 'forget' the calf and concentrate on minimizing the discomfort, allowing the calf to suckle.
- If other remedies fail, East African herders close the mother's anus with two wooden sticks tied together with thin rope. At the same time, they tie soft bark-fibres around the nostrils so the camel is forced to breathe through her mouth. They leave the mother tied this way for up to 8–10 hours. They then bring the calf and persuade it to suckle. (This method causes the mother a lot of pain.)
- The **Gabbra, Samburu and Somali** tie the mother's upper lip with a thin rope, then twist and pull it.
- The **Samburu** take the mother and calf to an isolated place and tie the mother on the ground. They bring a dog very close to the calf to scare it. The mother will try to protect the calf from the dog, so forming a mother–calf bond.
- The **Raika** put a ball of straw and twigs into the vulva, then close the anus and vulva with two horizontal sticks tied together. Leave the calf with the mother and persuade it to suckle.

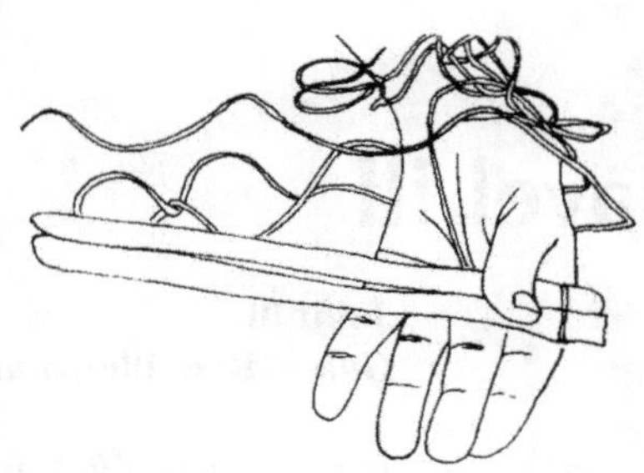

Sticks used to close the mother's anus (above); closing the anus (below and bottom)

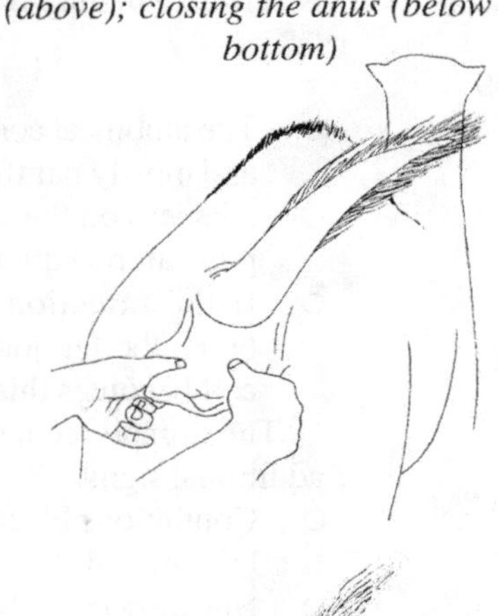

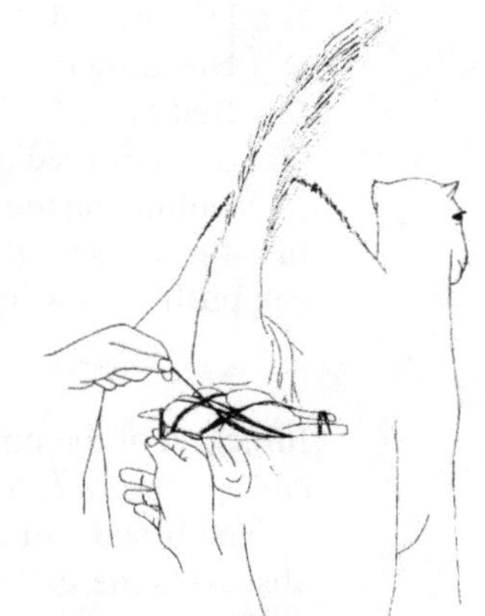

Modern treatments

- Feed the calf with milk using a bucket or teapot.
- Sedate the mother with a small dose of a tranquillizer (e.g., xylazine, Rompun, ▻*Common medicines*). Then allow the calf to suckle.

References

Bizimana (1994) p. 350–1; Evans et al. (1995) p. 5:14, 5:20; Forse (1999) p. 63; ITDG and IIRR (1996) p. 47; Manefield and Tinson (1997) p. 106; Schwartz and Dioli (1992) p. 113–18, 139; Wanyama (1997) vol. 2, p. 14–21; Wilson (1998) p. 60.

Navel ill

Joint ill
***Gulor* (Rendille), *andurgiigi* (Somali)**

In newborn calves up to 2 weeks of age, the umbilical cord can become infected. This infection can spread into the body and kill the calf. The Rendille believe that it is heritable mainly from the bull.

Signs

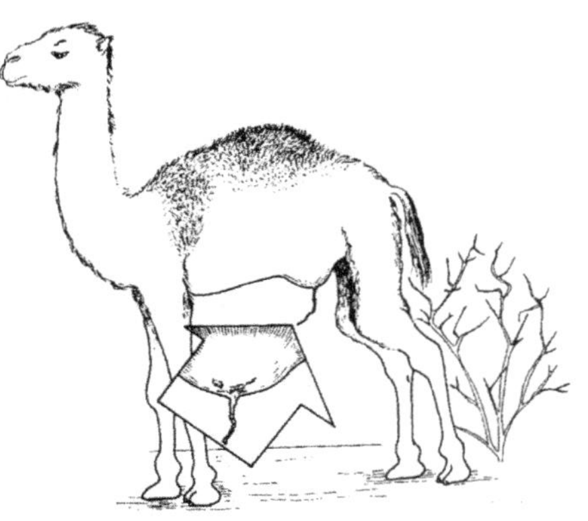

- The umbilical cord is swollen, moist and mostly painful.
- Abscess on the navel, from which pus can be squeezed.
- If the infection spreads into the body, the leg joints swell, and the calf becomes thin and dies.

The Somali recognize the following additional signs:

- Continuous bleeding from the umbilical cord.
- Bleeding from the nose.
- Red eyes.
- Sometimes diarrhoea.

Swelling on the navel can also be caused by an umbilical hernia (where a loop of intestines pushes through the muscle wall). Press on the swelling: if it is soft and you can push it back into the body, it is probably a hernia.

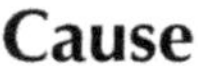

Cause

Infection of the umbilical cord by the bacteria *Actinomyces pyogenes*, *Streptococcus* sp. or *Staphylococcus* sp.

The blood can carry the bacteria into the liver, lungs, spleen or joints, causing abscesses there.

The infection can occur if:

- Conditions during birth are unhygienic (dirty).
- The umbilical cord is damaged during birth.
- The cord breaks off too short, or hangs down too far.

Prevention

- Ensure that the female gives birth in a clean place.
- Help at birth only if the mother has obvious problems delivering the calf (▷*Difficult birth*).
- If possible, wash your hands carefully before touching the mother or calf during birth.
- Do not pull or cut the umbilical cord: it will break by itself. If the cord dangles down a long way, tie a knot in it, but do not cut it: the end will break off by itself when it has dried.
- Keep the umbilical cord clean. It should dry quickly.
- Disinfect the navel directly after birth with iodine solution. SCI
- If the navel bleeds, soak a piece of clean string in iodine (or other antiseptic) and tie it around the navel. Or disinfect the navel with iodine and tie a knot in it to stop the bleeding. SCI
- Treat calves with antibiotics (an injection or as a cream) if other calves in the herd are already infected. SCI
- The Rendille do not breed from a bull thought to transmit this condition. RENDILLE

Treatment

Important Before cutting open a swelling on the navel, make sure it is an abscess, not an umbilical hernia (see *Signs* above).

Traditional treatments

- Wash the wound with boiled, salty water. GABBRA
- Wash the infected area with warm, salty water and apply butter on it. SOMALI
- Apply juice of *Aloe secundiflora* to keep flies off. SAMBURU
- Wash the navel with lukewarm water. Pound dry *eteteleit* (*Acalypha fruticosa*) leaves. Apply 1 tablespoon of the leaf powder to the navel every 4 days. The plant has a strong smell and drives flies away. TURKANA
- If the swelling is an abscess with pus, disinfect a sharp knife by holding it in the fire, and carefully make a cut to drain the pus. Treat the cut with fresh *hagar* gum (from *Commiphora erythraea*) to aid healing and to repel flies. SOMALI

Modern treatments

- Treat with broad-spectrum antibiotics as soon as the first sign of navel ill appears (▷*Common medicines*).
- If only the navel is affected, open the navel abscess when it ripens, clean it and disinfect it. You can speed up the ripening of the abscess by washing or dipping it in warm, salty water. You can also use warm, salty water to wash the abscess wound once it is open. Apply antibiotics (in an injection or as a cream) if available (▷*Common medicines*).

References

Forse (1999) p. 251–2; ITDG and IIRR (1996) p. 48–9; Kaufmann (1998) p. 189–90.

Calf diarrhoea

Milk scours, dietetic diarrhoea
Khurag **(Arabic, Sudan),** ***albahti, lbartey, albata*** **(Borana, Gabbra),** ***loleo, colera, lolei'a, ekuruton*** **(Pokot),** ***ngiriata, nkorotit, kepi-ngocheki*** **(Samburu),** ***dab, adeya*** **(Somali)**

Diarrhoea is common in calves, and many die from it. This is one reason that camel herds grow in size only slowly.

Signs

- The faeces are white and liquid, like milk: 'milk scour'.
- The diarrhoea is yellowish and watery (in calves up to 4 weeks old): rotavirus or coronavirus infection.
- The calf weakens and loses condition.
- The animal may stop suckling.
- The animal may have fever.
- The stomach may swell.

▷*Problems of the stomach and intestine*.

Causes

- Drinking too much milk (milk scour) (▷*Care of newborn calves*).
- Virus infection (rotavirus or coronavirus).

Make sure that the diarrhoea is not caused by another problem. Watch the calf carefully, as milk scour or virus infections can easily develop into a bacterial diarrhoea (▷*Colibacillosis*).

Prevention

- Ensure that the newborn calf drinks colostrum (the mother's first, thick milk).
- Avoid over-feeding.

Colostrum

Colostrum is the first milk produced by the mother after giving birth. This milk is a rich food. It also helps protect the calf from disease (like a vaccine).

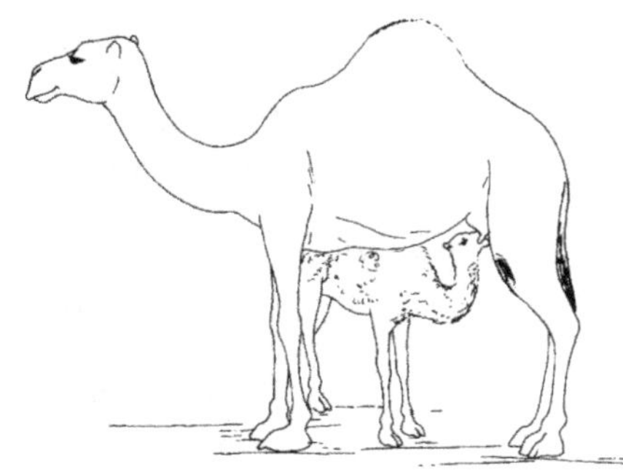

Make sure the calf drinks colostrum as soon after birth as possible. If necessary, help it suckle from the mother's udder. Help it drink small amounts at regular, 1-hour intervals (▷*Care of newborn calves*). Do not let it drink too much, as this may cause diarrhoea.

Treatment

Restricting the amount of milk the calf drinks and providing it with oral rehydration solution (see below under *Modern treatments*) will cure the calf within 1–2 days. If diarrhoea continues, you should suspect other causes and use the appropriate treatment (▷*Colibacillosis* and *Diarrhoea*).

Traditional treatments

- Soak *Capparis cartilaginea* (*chepkogh*) in 0.5 litre of water, then give the liquid as a drench to a calf with scours. POKOT
- Chop up the bark of *Maerua crassifolia* tree (*umacho* or *dumasho* in Gabbra, *ldumei* in Samburu, *dume* in Rendille and Somali, *ereng* in Turkana) and boil it in water. Allow the liquid to cool, strain it, and drench the calf 2–3 times per day. GABBRA, TRAD+SCI

Modern treatment

- Stop feeding milk for 24 hours. Instead, feed with oral rehydration liquid. You can buy this from shops (follow the instructions on the packet carefully). You can also make your own rehydration fluid (see directions below).

How to make oral rehydration liquid

1. In each litre of clean, boiled water, dissolve 9 g of salt, 50 g of sugar and 10 g of sodium bicarbonate. Or mix 5 tablespoons of sugar and 1 tablespoon of salt with 2 litres of water.
2. Keep the liquid in a clean, sealed bottle.
3. For newborn calves give 0.5 litres by mouth, four times during the first day. Be careful! Weak calves may not suckle properly. Make sure that you give the liquid slowly and that it does not go into the calf's lungs. If the calf is weak, gently use a syringe (without a needle) to feed the calf.
4. On the second day, mix the rehydration fluid with an equal amount of milk.

References

Evans et al. (1995) p. 7:32; FAO (1994) p. 259; Forse (1999) p. 345–6; Manefield and Tinson (1997) p. 73–4; Projet Cameline (1999) p. 37–8; Rathore (1986) p. 122–3; Sewell and Brocklesby (1990) p. 352–4.

Colibacillosis

Colibacillosis is diarrhoea caused by infection with *Escherichia coli* bacteria. It usually occurs as a secondary infection following milk scour, rotavirus or coronavirus infections (▷*Calf diarrhoea*). At first only one calf may be ill, but the disease can spread easily to others. If untreated, they may die within a few days.

Signs

- The calf is weak, frequently lying, resting or sleeping.
- It has no appetite (the mother's udder is full).
- It has watery, yellowish diarrhoea.
- It has a high body temperature (above 40°C).
- The animal becomes dehydrated: lift a fold of skin between your fingers and thumb, then release it. It the skin fold returns to its normal position only slowly, the calf is dehydrated. Another sign of dehydration is sunken eyes.
- Animals usually die after 2–3 days if they are not treated.

- The infection can develop into a generalized septicaemia (blood poisoning), resulting in high fever and perhaps death.

See also the sections on ▷*Calf diarrhoea* and *Diarrhoea*.

Cause

Escherichia coli bacteria. Calves are usually infected from 3 weeks of age onwards, when they start playing around and licking and eating all sorts of objects. Since the *E. coli* bacteria are everywhere, calves will inevitably eat some. At the same time they have lost much of the disease immunity given to them by the mother's first milk (the 'colostrum'). Dirty enclosures increase the danger of infection.

Prevention

- Keep enclosures clean.
- Make sure the calf receives the mother's first milk (▷*Care of newborn calves*).
- Treat other animals early to stop the disease from spreading.
- Separate sick animals from healthy ones.

Treatment

Treat quickly to stop the disease early and to avoid it spreading to other animals.

- Pound 300 g of the roots of *egis* (*Cissus quadrangularis*) and mix with 0.5 litre of water. Allow to stand for 12 hours. Drench the animal with the mixture. Repeat every morning and evening. The calf should not be allowed to suckle for 12 hours before the treatment starts. SAMBURU, TURKANA
- Inject (or give in the mouth) antibiotics such as ampicillin or enrofloxacin. Since many *E. coli* strains have developed resistance to specific antibiotics, you should submit faecal samples to the veterinarian to determine the best type of antibiotic to use (▷*How to collect samples for testing*). However, as the tests may take too long, do not wait for the results, but start giving broad-spectrum antibiotics immediately (▷*Common medicines*). In severe cases, inject these into the vein. SCI
- Use oral rehydration liquid (▷*Calf diarrhoea* for instructions). SCI

References

ITDG and IIRR (1996) p. 151; Manefield and Tinson (1997) p. 64–5; Wernery and Kaaden (1995) p. 40–2.

Salmonellosis

Salmonellosis is a serious bacterial infection that affects calves over 2 weeks of age. It starts as a gastro-enteritis with diarrhoea, but especially in younger calves it can develop into a form where bacteria enter the blood (known as blood poisoning or 'septicaemia'). It often kills the calf. Animals that recover often have the bacteria in their faeces for a long time, so may infect other animals.

The disease can infect other animal species and people. It is especially dangerous for small children, old people and people with poor immunity (such as AIDS sufferers). Be careful when handling infected animals.

In many countries, you must inform the government health or veterinary officer immediately if you suspect an animal has salmonellosis. It is the most important disease of suckling calves, killing up to 20% of them.

Signs

- Yellowish or greenish-grey, foul-smelling diarrhoea.
- Faeces often contain blood.
- Often fever.
- Dehydration: sunken eyeballs, dry mucous membranes.
- In very acute cases, animals die 24–48 hours after the disease signs appear. More usually, the animal dies after 1–2 weeks.

If the disease develops into the septicaemic form:

- The body temperature rises rapidly.
- The animal becomes dull and does not react.
- The animal rests and does not get up.
- It has difficulty breathing.
- It has unco-ordinated movements.
- Other parts of the body (lungs and joints) may become inflamed.

Some camels may carry salmonella without appearing to be ill. However, they may infect other camels and people.

Salmonellosis can be diagnosed for certain only by culturing the bacteria in a laboratory. Take several samples of faeces at different times because the bacteria may not be present in all of the samples.

Many other diseases can also cause diarrhoea (▷*Problems of the stomach and intestines* and *Diarrhoea*).

Cause

Bacteria of the genus *Salmonella*. The disease is passed on by an animal eating feed or drinking water contaminated with faeces from infected animals.

Prevention

- Make sure that calves get as much colostrum (the thick, yellowish first milk) as possible, as early as possible (▷*Care of newborn calves*).
- Vaccinate breeding females before or during pregnancy (the antibodies will be transferred to the newborn calves).
- Immediately separate sick animals from healthy ones. Move the healthy animals' enclosure away.
- People treating sick calves should not handle healthy calves at the same time.
- Keep new animals coming into the herd separate at first. Watch them carefully, especially if they have diarrhoea.
- Use drinking troughs rather than ponds to water animals. Keep the drinking water clean and free of contamination by faeces.

Treatment

If you suspect an animal has salmonellosis, treat it immediately. If it is not treated within 24–48 hours, the animal is likely to die. Once the septicaemic form has developed, treatment is usually not successful – especially if the infection has moved into the lungs.

- Give oxytetracycline antibiotic by mouth as well as through injection (▷*Common medicines*). SCI

- Inject with enrofloxacin 5 mg/kg body weight (e.g., Baytril, ▷*Common medicines*). SCI
- Treat with oral rehydration fluid (▷*Calf diarrhoea* for instructions). SCI
- Give a drip of 5 litres or more of lactated Ringer's solution mixed with sodium bicarbonate (▷*Administering medicines*). SCI

References

Forse (1999) p. 235–6; Higgins (1986) p. 102–3; ITDG and IIRR (1996) p. 155–6; Manefield and Tinson (1997) p. 229; Rathore (1986) p. 175; Sewell and Brocklesby (1990) p. 90–7; Wernery and Kaaden (1995) p. 37–40.

Saam

***Saam* (Rendille, Gabbra), *ilgoff* (Somali)**

Saam and *ilgoff* affect only suckling calves – mainly between 6 and 12 months of age, although the Somali say that some die during the first month of life.

The Rendille and Gabbra cannot relate the disease to any particular cause. They believe that *saam* is caused by mothers of the infected calves being milked by women, or by men who have sexual intercourse. The Somali relate *ilgoff* to the smell of perfume of women or men. Some herders believe the problem is related to bad teeth.

Most infected animals die.

Signs

- Watery eyes.
- Sunken eyes (the eye sockets are enlarged).
- Oozing pus in the eye, may lead to blindness.
- Anaemia.
- Dullness and loss of condition (starting from the tail – hence the name of the disease in Somali).
- Sometimes a big stomach (pot belly).
- Sometimes fever and joint pains.
- The animal becomes very thin and dies.

Cause

Possibly caused by parasites, or by dirty hands of the person milking, and hence dirty teats which might infect the calf when suckling. *Saam* may be a bacterial enteritis or joint ill (▷*Navel ill*), or a mixture of several diseases.

Prevention

Herders often try to prevent the disease by sending animals at risk to the mobile herds, where they are herded by young warriors only, or keep them at home and have the mothers milked only by young boys or very old men.

- Apply Nilzan (a medicine against intestinal worms). SOMALI
- Inject with Samorin (a medicine against trypanosomiasis).

Treatment

There is no effective treatment known. Injecting tetracycline antibiotics apparently has no effect.

Traditional treatments

- Treatment using a plant called *darken* (?) is sometimes successful. SOMALI
- Drench with the urine of an unmated heifer or lamb, or with soup made from sheep fat or the head of a sheep or goat. SOMALI
- Remove two upper and two lower teeth, then brand on the cheeks. SOMALI

References

Kaufmann (1998) p. 190.

Appendices

Disease names in local languages

Uncertain names are marked with '?'.

Afar (Ethiopia)

Coughs, colds and pneumonia *kharoo*

Algeria

Coughs, colds and pneumonia (autumn pneumonia) *rnaze*

Arabic

Calf diarrhoea *khurag*
Coughs, colds and pneumonia *nahaz*
Myopathy *makiola*
Nasal bots *al-naghaf*
Plant poisoning *goulum*
Rutting *hej*

Borana (Kenya)

Abortion *iralii*
Blackquarter *lkumur*
Calf diarrhoea *albahti, lbartey, albata*
Contagious skin necrosis *dulla*
Coughs, colds and pneumonia (respiratory diseases in general) *dougouda, ene kouffa*
Diarrhoea *albati*
Haemorrhagic septicaemia *khandich, khandicha, quando*
Mange *chitto*
Orf *humbururu, mburur*
Plant poisoning *arda*
Rabies *siribo*
Ringworm *robbi, ropi*
Ticks *shelem, shini*
Trypanosomiasis *louta, ghandi, dukan*

Eritrea

Trypanosomiasis *atteh, gudho*

Gabbra (Kenya)

Abortion *iralii*
Anthrax *chilmalo*
Blackquarter *lkumur*
Broken bones *chachaba*
Burns *gubatu*
Calf diarrhoea *albahti, lbartey, albata*
Castration *kolansiti*
Constipation *udao dabab*
Contagious skin necrosis *dula, kharfat, garfat, hilaliit*
Coughs, colds and pneumonia (general) *kufa', qufa*
Coughs, colds and pneumonia (cold, influenza) *furri*
Diarrhoea *albati*
Difficult birth *dalmichirir*
Eye problems *dhaasi*
Female sterility (immature reproductive tract) *dabeno*
Female sterility (uterine infection) *mala kesa yaa*
Fleas *tuffi njiraa*
Haemorrhagic septicaemia *khando, qando*
Lice *injirre*
Mange *chitto*
Mastitis *qamyara*
Mosquitoes *binni*
Nasal bots *rhamu*
Orf *humbururu, mburur*
Pica *nandh*
Plant poisoning *hada*
Pox *abdarra, aftara, baga?, irgo*
Prolapse of the vagina *arab qab*

Prolapse of the womb *ormat abui*
Rabies *nyanye*
Retained afterbirth *dillu itis*
Ringworm *robbi, ropi*
Skin abscesses *mala, malah*
Swollen glands, *khanid* *kando, kandich, kandicha*
Ticks *chilim, shilmi, yagar, yakhal*
Trypanosomiasis *ghandi, dukan*
Tsetse flies *dug, duga*
Wounds *madaa*
Wry neck *simpiro, chachabsa*

India (see also *Punjabi* and *Rajasthan*)

Chest-pad abscess *adder, adder badhana, adder ki chot*
Anthrax *mohri, sujhan, sut, garhi*
Arthritis *ras bharna*
Broken jaw *jabadi tutana, jadi tutana*
Chest sprain *maachijana, maachhijgaya*
Constipation *pet band hona*
Contagious skin necrosis *jooling*
Coughs, colds and pneumonia *khassi*
Dermoid *foda, maid*
Diarrhoea *dast*
Difficult birth (caesarean section) *pet chirana, aaperation karke bachha nikalana*
Dislocated kneecap *chitki, chatkan, saran*
Ear infection *kaan bahana*
Eye problems (corneal opacity) *fula*
Haemorrhagic septicaemia *galtiya, magravala*
Injured *dulaa* *gulla phansa, ghayal hona*
Lice *jehun, khosa*
Lungworms *khurak*
Mange *khaj, khujli, paam, paanv, pom*
Myopathy *kumri*
Nasal bots *magaz ki kera*
Orf *moomri*
Pox *chechak, mata*
Prolapse of the vagina and womb *aar nikalna*
Rabies *pagal hona*
Retained afterbirth *jerr, jer nahi heerana*
Ringworm *daad, taat*
Rutting *musth*
Saddle sores *chandi, palan ka ghaw*
Tail gangrene *leathery, poonchh sookna, ponchh mein, keeda lagna*
Teeth problems *dant bhadhana, daadh badhana, ubad-khabad dhadh*
Torn nostrils *naas phatna*
Trypanosomiasis *surra*
Wry neck *wadi*

Kazakhstan

Orf *auzdik*

Kordofan (see also *Sudan*)

Coughs, colds and pneumonia *ghudda, al fahada, habub*
Mange *gerrab*
Tetanus *hattal?*
Ticks *gudad*
Trypanosomiasis *guffar*
Wry neck *kasara*

Moorish

Coughs, colds and pneumonia *n'haz*

North Africa

Haemorrhagic septicaemia *ghedda*
Trypanosomiasis *el debab*
Foot problems (cracked or worn pads) *talhas*

Pakistan

Trypanosomiasis *surra*

Pokot (Kenya)

Abortion *touno*
Blackquarter *ngwaat, lokichum*
Calf diarrhoea *loleo, colera, lolei'a, ekuruton*
Coughs, colds and pneumonia *psosoi, songoghowio, erukum, arrkum*
Orf *ngirimen*
Plant poisoning *lotil*
Pox *mokoyon*
Trypanosomiasis *lokurucho*

Punjabi (see also *India*)

Red urine *rut mootra, lahoo mootna*
Dry coat *paseena bund, thakawat, gar'mee*

Rajasthan (see also *India*)

Bloat *afra, pet jam hona, pet rukana*
Blisters in the mouth *mooh upadana, mooh ke chhale*
Blocked intestines *aant ka anta, ant ruk jana, ant ka but*

Broken foot *pag tutana, pagtali kanne tutfut*
Broken leg *nali ka tutuna, far ka tutuna, larle kulhe ki haddi ka tutana*
Contagious skin necrosis *phoda*
Indigestion *apach, badi*
Sunstroke *red awarng*

Rendille (Kenya)

Blackquarter *khadit*
Contagious skin necrosis *garfat, kharfat*
Coughs, colds and pneumonia *yaharr, dahassi*
Diarrhoea *harr, diggheharr*
Haemorrhagic septicaemia *khanid*
Mange *haddo*
Nasal bots, *senghelel*
Navel ill *gulor*
Pox *afturro, afturu*
Rabies *sugeri ikaare*
Saam *saam*
Skin abscesses *mala, malah*
Swollen glands *khanid*
Tetanus *rekigerri?*
Ticks *shilim, chillim, turdach*
Trypanosomiasis *omar*
Wry neck *dahasi*

Samburu (Kenya)

Abortion *nkiboroto*
Anthrax *lokuchum*
Biting flies *lajuigani*
Blackquarter *loduseddi*
Broken bones *ngilata e loito*
Calf diarrhoea *ngiriata, nkorotit, kepi-ngocheki*
Castration *ngelemata*
Contagious skin necrosis *lomgoi, ngamanyeni*
Coughs, colds and pneumonia *nkorroget, loroget, lchama, lbus bus*
Diarrhoea *ngorotit*
Eye problems *moyian yoonkouyek*
Fleas *losusu*
Haemorrhagic septicaemia *nalngiarngarri, ngarngar, nolgoso*
Intestinal parasites *kinyoot, ltuma, ltumai, ndumai*
Leeches *lmolog*
Lice *lache*
Mange *ilbebedo, lpepedo*
Mosquitoes *nkajing'ani*
Nasal bots *marsomwa*
Orf *non-kutukie, lopedo*
Pica *singate*
Plant poisoning *loturudei*
Poor mothering and fostering *nkibata e lashe*
Pox *afturro, abituro*
Rabies *nkwang*
Retained afterbirth *lmodong*
Ringworm *ngamunyeni, nkamunyani*
Skin abscesses *ngemek, ntubui*
Snake bite *onyoto la surai*
Tetanus *kongoro, nkeeyae lmeut*
Ticks *ilmangeri, lmanjeri, lmansher, ltunturi*
Trypanosomiasis *ltikana, saar*
Tsetse flies (and panganids) *lpupoi*
Wounds *ngoldonyot*

Somali (Kenya, Somalia)

Abortion *d'ess, dhies, l'ess*
Anthrax *kud*
Blackquarter *khut*
Broken bones *jab* (Somali Ethiopia)
Burns *gubush*
Calf diarrhoea *dab, adeya*
Camel flies (*Hippobosca camelina*) *takar*
Castration *dhufan* (Somali Kenya)
Contagious skin necrosis *dalleham, dhaleeco, dulla, garfat, ma'ah, maha*
Coughs, colds and pneumonia *ah, dhugato, dugub, erghib, kharid dugub, oof, laxawgal*
Diarrhoea *har, hardik*
Eye problems *itwaren*
Fleas *injit*
Foot problems (infected toes) *suul*
Foot problems (punctured foot) *ragat*
Haemorrhagic septicaemia *kharar, garir, khud, kurri*
Intestinal parasites *bahala*
Leeches *calacuul*
Lice *injir*
Mange *addha, addo, chitto*
Mosquitoes *kanea*
Nasal bots *sangaale*
Orf *ambarrur, mburur*
Pica *megay*
Navel ill *andurgiigi*
Plant poisoning *gedak*
Poor mothering and fostering *ilmadid*
Pox *afrur, furuk*
Rabies *ruqus*
Retained afterbirth *maderr*
Ringworm *ambarr, robi*
Rutting *waghogh*
Saam *ilgoff*
Skin abscesses *mal, mala, malah bahtin, waglal*
Swollen glands *khanid quandich, kud kurri garir*

Tetanus *tagou?*
Ticks *shilin, yakhal*
Trypanosomiasis *dhuukaan, dukan (= T. evansi), korbarar (= T. congolense), geudhi, ghandi, gindi, suuqiye*
Tsetse flies *gendi*
Wounds *boog*
Wry neck *shimper, gudanki, simpiro, gusam*

Sudan

Abscess of the neck lymph nodes *habis*
Calf diarrhoea *khurag*
Contagious skin necrosis *al ni'aita, na'eita*
Stomach worm (*Haemonchus longistipes*) *dud, hulaa, humar*
Mange *gerab*
Orf *kulait, abu shalamboo*
Pox *jedari*
Ringworm *gara'a, goub*
Ticks *gurad*
Trypanosomiasis *el debab*
Wry neck *haboub*

Tuareg (West Africa)

Coughs, colds and pneumonia *abunzhur, torza*
Foot problems (ulcerative dermatitis) *makales*

Turkana

Abortion *akiyech, akiyechum, akiecium*
Anthrax *lokuchum*
Biting flies *ng'ichuchu*
Broken bones *abila*
Burns *nganoman*
Castration *aleldougi*
Contagious skin necrosis *lelebunai*
Coughs, colds and pneumonia *loukoi, lotai*
Diarrhoea *colera, loleo*
Eye problems *edeke ankonyen*
Fleas *ng'ikorobotio*
Haemorrhagic septicaemia *aengarre, lorarrurei, longarrue, elukunoit, lobolio, lobolibolio*
Intestinal parasites *ngirtan, nyiritan*
Leeches *ngidike*
Lice *elachit, ng'ilach*
Mange *ametina, ekoikoi, emitina*
Mosquitoes *ng'isuru*
Nasal bots *ekurrut*
Orf *ngiborwok, mburuwok*
Pica *ekichoe*
Plant poisoning *bosoto*
Pox *ettune, ngiborwok*
Rabies *ingerep*
Retained afterbirth *edungat*
Ringworm *akiserit, akisorit, epara, ekithariit*
Skin abscesses *adjumei, abus, ngubuthien, lobus*
Snake bite *akanyyat*
Ticks *emadang, ngimadang*
Trypanosomiasis *lokipi, ltorobwo*
Tsetse flies *lopodokong'or*
Wounds *ngajemei*

West Africa

Foot problems (cracked or worn pads) *talhas*
Trypanosomiasis *mbori, tahaga*

Yaa Galba (Kenya)

Coughs, colds and pneumonia *qufaa*

Medicinal and poisonous plants

Uncertain names are marked with '?'. Poisonous plants are marked with ☠. Note that some poisonous plants are also used in medicines.

abach (Turkana)
NASAL BOTS

Acacia bussei
galool (Somali)
COUGHS, COLDS AND PNEUMONIA; WOUNDS AND BURNS

Acacia laeta
MANGE

Acacia mellifera
iti (Samburu), *kitir* (Sudan)
EYE PROBLEMS; INTERNAL PARASITES (WORMS); MANGE

Acacia nilotica
garrad (Arabic)
DIARRHOEA; INTERNAL PARASITES (WORMS); SADDLE SORES; WOUNDS AND BURNS

Acacia nubica
DIARRHOEA

Acacia reficiens
pilil (Pokot)
TRYPANOSOMIASIS

Acacia senegal
cadad (Somali)
WOUNDS AND BURNS

***Acacia* spp.**
CARE OF NEWBORN CALVES

Acacia tortilis
ses (Pokot)
DIFFICULT BIRTH; RETAINED PLACENTA

Acalypha fruticosa
eteteleit (Turkana)
CASTRATION; NAVEL ILL; TICKS; WOUNDS AND BURNS

Adansonia digitata
SADDLE SORES; WOUNDS AND BURNS

Adenia volkensii
loarakimak (Turkana)
COUGHS, COLDS AND PNEUMONIA; TRYPANOSOMIASIS

Adenium aculeatum
dhalaandax (Somali)
COUGHS, COLDS AND PNEUMONIA

***Adenium obesum*, desert rose**
MANGE

***Aerva* spp.**
hamboy (Somali)
WOUNDS AND BURNS

Aerva tomentosa
CONSTIPATION

Ajuga remota
MASTITIS

Albizia anthelmintica
kamakiten (Pokot), *ekapakiteng* (Turkana)
INTERNAL PARASITES (WORMS); LUNGWORMS

***Allium sativum*, garlic**
DRY COAT

Aloe broomii
TICKS

Aloe secundiflora
CASTRATION; NAVEL ILL

***Aloe* spp.**
WOUNDS AND BURNS

Aloe vera
WOUNDS AND BURNS

anthatha (Gabbra)
BITES AND STINGS

apetet (Turkana)
LUNGWORMS

Avicennia africana
MANGE

***Azadirachta indica*, neem**
BITES AND STINGS; MANGE

Balanites aegyptiaca
aborak (Tuareg)
MANGE; WOUNDS AND BURNS

Balanites rotundifolia
ebei (Turkana)
EYE PROBLEMS

Boscia coriacea
edung (Turkana)
BITES AND STINGS; EYE PROBLEMS

Boscia senegalensis
CONSTIPATION; FOOT PROBLEMS; TRYPANOSOMIASIS

Boswellia hildebrandtii
sungululwa (Pokot)
DIARRHOEA

***Brassica* sp., mustard**
EAR INFECTION

bura, burs* or *bursa (Gabbra)
possibly *Acacia elatior or Acacia goetzei*
SWOLLEN GLANDS, *KHANID*

Cadaba glandulosa
TRYPANOSOMIASIS

Cadaba rotundifolia
epuu (Turkana)
BITES AND STINGS

Calligonum comosum
MANGE

Calotropis procera ☠
aak (hindi, Rajasthan), *etesuro* (Turkana)
BITES AND STINGS; COUGHS, COLDS AND PNEUMONIA; MANGE; PLANT POISONING; WOUNDS AND BURNS

Capparis cartilaginea
chepkogh (Pokot)
CALF DIARRHOEA

Capparis spinosa
MANGE

Capparis tomentosa ☠
gorrahgel (Borana, Rendille), *gora* (Gabbra), *laturdei* (Samburu), *gamboor, gomborlik* (Somali), *ekorokoroite* (Turkana)
PLANT POISONING

***Capsicum annuum*, chilli pepper**
LEECHES; TRYPANOSOMIASIS

Caralluma socotrana
gowracata (Somali)
CONTAGIOUS SKIN NECROSIS

***Caralluma* sp.**
lokurusio (Turkana)
WOUNDS AND BURNS

***Cassia occidentalis*, senna** ☠
kesudo (Hindi)
PLANT POISONING

Cassia senna
INTERNAL PARASITES (WORMS)

Cissampelos pareira
malutyan (Pokot)
COUGHS, COLDS AND PNEUMONIA

Cissus producta
BITES AND STINGS

Cissus quadrangularis
egis (Turkana)
COLIBACILLOSIS

***Citrullus colocynthis*, bitter apple**
handal (Lahawiyin, Rashaida, Shukriya)
CONSTIPATION; INTERNAL PARASITES (WORMS); MANGE; ORF; POX

***Clerodendrum* sp.**
chepotet (Pokot)
TRYPANOSOMIASIS

Commiphora africana
MANGE

Commiphora erythraea
hagar (Somali)
BITES AND STINGS; NAVEL ILL; SKIN ABSCESSES; TICKS; WOUNDS AND BURNS

Commiphora incisa
damaji (Somali)
TICKS

Commiphora myrrha
malmal (Somali)
WOUNDS AND BURNS

***Commiphora* sp.**
habagar (Gari Somali)
MANGE

***Commiphora* sp.**
saar (Somali)
CONSTIPATION

Cordia sinensis
marer (Somali)
EYE PROBLEMS

Cucumis aculeatus
qalfoon (Somali)
COUGHS, COLDS AND PNEUMONIA

Cucumis colocynthis
MANGE

***Cucumis* sp.**
qaro (Somali)
COUGHS, COLDS AND PNEUMONIA

Cucurbita maxima
MANGE

***Curcuma longa*, turmeric**
CHEST-PAD ABSCESS; CHEST SPRAIN; EYE PROBLEMS; FEMALE STERILITY

***Cymbopogon nerrvalus* (?)**
nal (Sudan)
TICKS

Cymbopogon schoenanthus
MANGE

Cyperus alternifolius
sokwon (Pokot)
COUGHS, COLDS AND PNEUMONIA

Daphne oleioides ☠
laghunay (Baluchistan)
PLANT POISONING

***darken* (Somali)**
SAAM

***Datura alba, D. stramonium* (?), thorn apple** ☠
dhaturo (Hindi), *hurna* (Kordofan), *ntuju* (Samburu), *bohamidu* (Somalia), *ebune* (Turkana)
PLANT POISONING

***Dendrocalamus strictus*, bamboo**
bansara (Rajasthan)
RETAINED PLACENTA

Derris indica
MANGE

Diospyros scabra
eelim (Turkana)
LUNGWORMS

Entada leptostachya
gacmo-dheere (Somali)
COUGHS, COLDS AND PNEUMONIA

Eruca sativa
taramira (Punjab)
DRY COAT, MANGE

***Eucalyptus* sp.**
bahra-saf (Somali)
BITES AND STINGS

***Eucalyptus* sp.**
NASAL BOTS

Euphorbia balsamifera
BITES AND STINGS; MANGE

Euphorbia gossypina
cinjir (Somali)
MANGE

Euphorbia heterochroma
harken (Gabbra)
HAEMORRHAGIC SEPTICAEMIA

Euphorbia robecchii
dharkeyn (Somali)
COUGHS, COLDS AND PNEUMONIA; EYE PROBLEMS; MANGE

Euphorbia somalensis
falanfalho (Somali)
MANGE

***Euphorbia tirucalli*, milk-bush** ☠
irgin (Somali?)
PLANT POISONING

***Euphorbia* sp.**
lparaa (Samburu)
CONTAGIOUS SKIN NECROSIS; MANGE; WOUNDS AND BURNS

Euphorbia triaculeata
ANTHRAX; BLACKQUARTER

***Ferula* spp., asafoetida**
hing (Raika)
CONSTIPATION

Ficus populifolia
balan baal (Somali Ethiopia)
WOUNDS AND BURNS

gathaha (Rendille)
SWOLLEN GLANDS, *KHANID*

Grewia bicolor
sitot (Pokot)
RETAINED PLACENTA

Gutenbergia somalensis
nagaadh (Somali)
COUGHS, COLDS AND PNEUMONIA

Jatropha curcas
habat almuluk (Shukriya, Lahawiyin, Rashaida)
INTERNAL PARASITES (WORMS)

Juniperus phoenicea
MANGE

Khaya senegalensis
SADDLE SORES

***Lantana indica*, lantana** ☠
rukri (Hindi)
PLANT POISONING

***Lawsonia inermis*, henna**
RINGWORM

***Linum usitatissimum*, linseed**
PLANT POISONING

Maerua crassifolia
umacho or *dumasho* (Gabbra), *dume* (Rendille), *ldumei* (Samburu), *dume* (Somali), *ereng* (Turkana)
CALF DIARRHOEA; FOOT PROBLEMS; TRYPANOSOMIASIS

millet
TRYPANOSOMIASIS

Myrsine africana
seketet (Samburu)
TRYPANOSOMIASIS; WOUNDS AND BURNS

***Nerium oleander*, oleander** ☠
difli (Arabic), *kaneer* (Hindi), *kharzarah* (Iran), *nara* (Sindh), *dehr* (Somali)
PLANT POISONING

***Nicotiana tabacum*, tobacco**
kif (pipe tobacco, Tuareg)
EYE PROBLEMS; FOOT PROBLEMS; LEECHES; NASAL BOTS; SWOLLEN GLANDS, *KHANID;* TICKS

odha (Gabbra)
WRY NECK

***Pennisetum americanum*, pearl millet**
bajra (Rajasthan)
RETAINED PLACENTA

***Phoenix dactylifera*, date**
FOOT PROBLEMS

***Piper nigrum*, pepper**
COUGHS, COLDS AND PNEUMONIA

qorsa worana (Gabbra)
SKIN ABSCESSES; WOUNDS AND BURNS

***Ricinus communis*, castor oil plant**
BLOCKED INTESTINES; MANGE; PLANT POISONING; WOUNDS AND BURNS

Salvadora persica
adeh (Gabbra), *asiokonyon* (Pokot), *haech* (Rendille), *sokotei* (Samburu), *esokon*, (Turkana)
ANTHRAX; BITES AND STINGS; BLACKQUARTER; HAEMORRHAGIC SEPTICAEMIA; RETAINED AFTERBIRTH; TRYPANOSOMIASIS; WRY NECK

Sarcostemma andongenese ☠
PLANT POISONING

***Sesamum indicum*, sesame**
INTERNAL PARASITES (WORMS); MANGE

Sesbania sesban
BITES AND STINGS; MASTITIS

sisal (wild)
ewais (Pokot)
RETAINED PLACENTA

Solenostemma argel
WOUNDS AND BURNS

***Sorghum vulgare*, sorghum** ☠ (young plants)
jowar (India)
CONTAGIOUS SKIN NECROSIS; PLANT POISONING

Tamarix aphylla
MANGE

tambo (Gabbra: a local tobacco plant)
CONSTIPATION

Terminalia brownii
lbukoi (Samburu)
TRYPANOSOMIASIS

Thuja articulata
MANGE

Trichilia emetica
ekuyen (Turkana)
LUNGWORMS

Vernonia anthelmintica
kalizeeri (Punjab)
DRY COAT

Withania somnifera
EYE PROBLEMS

Ximenia americana
ORF

Zanthoxylum chalybeum
songowo (Pokot), *loisuk* (Rendille, Samburu), *eusugu* (Turkana)
COUGHS, COLDS AND PNEUMONIA; DIARRHOEA; TRYPANOSOMIASIS

***Zingiber officinale*, ginger**
BLISTERS IN THE MOUTH; DRY COAT

Ziziphus mauritiana
tilomwa (Pokot)
DIARRHOEA; RETAINED PLACENTA

Common medicines

The list below contains the names and dosages for most of the medicines mentioned in this book.

The active ingredient or generic name is given in **bold** type (e.g., **Phenylbutazone**). Note that some medicines have more than one generic name.

This is followed, where available, by the dosage (in g or mg) of the active ingredient per kg of the animal's body weight. For example, if the dosage is 10 mg/kg, and the animal weighs 429 kg, you should give 10 × 429 = 4290 mg = about 4.3 g of the active ingredient. ▷*Estimating a camel's weight and age* and *Using the right amount of medicine* for how to calculate dosages.

Experts sometimes disagree about the best dosage to give, and dosages may vary with the type and severity of the disease. Check the relevant section in the book and use the dosage printed there, if it is different from the one in this list.

If no body weight is given, the dosages given are for an adult camel weighing 400–500 kg. Use less medicine for smaller animals and calves.

Some names of common commercial remedies containing this active ingredient are also given. These are printed in normal type (e.g., Algesin). Because each firm producing a medicine gives it a different name, it is impossible to list all of them here.

Commercial medicines come in various forms (pills, powders, liquids, etc.) and concentrations. They may also contain water, substances to make the medicine stick together, and other ingredients. The list contains dosages of the most common preparations, where these are known. However, you should always check the instructions that come with the medicine to make sure.

*Active ingredient or generic name (**bold**)* — *Dosage of active ingredient (per kg of camel's body weight)* — *Common commercial medicine(s) with this ingredient*

Phenylbutazone (8–10 mg/kg): Algesin (3–12 ml), inject into the muscle

Dosage of commercial medicine — *How to use*

How to read an entry in this list of medicines

Important: If one of the medicines in the list is not available, do not assume that you can use another one in the same part of the list. First check the relevant chapter in the book. **Always check the instructions on the packet or label before using the medicine.**

▷*Equipment and medicines* contains a list of the most commonly used medicines and supplies.

Analgesics and anaesthetics

To treat pain

▷*Constipation, Difficult birth, Sunstroke* (see also *Sedatives and anaesthetics* below)

Analgin: Analgin (15–30 ml): inject into the muscle or vein

Metamizole: Novalgin (20–40 ml), inject into the muscle or vein

Paracetamol: Paracetol (10–50 ml), inject into the muscle

Antibiotics

To prevent and treat diseases caused by bacteria

▷*Abscesses on the lymph nodes, Anthrax, Blisters in the mouth, Broken jaw, Contagious skin necrosis, Coughs, colds and pneumonia, Dermatophilosis, Difficult birth, Eye problems, Haemorrhagic septicaemia, Khanid, Lungworms, Red urine, Salmonellosis, Surgery, Swallowed objects, Tetanus, Torn nostrils, Wounds and burns*

Antibiotics prevent the growth of bacteria, or kill bacteria.

- **Narrow-spectrum** antibiotics, such as penicillin and streptomycin, have an effect on only a few types of bacteria.
- **Broad-spectrum** antibiotics are effective against a wide variety of bacteria. They include oxytetracycline, ampicillin, enrofloxacin, and combinations of penicillin and streptomycin.

Bacteria are becoming resistent against oxytetracycline, making this medicine less effective. A promising new antibiotic is marbofloxacin.

Antibiotics have to be given repeatedly until 48 hours after the disease signs have disappeared. If you stop treatment too soon or give too low a dosage, the bacteria may become resistant and the medicine will be ineffective.

Ampicillin, penicillin, streptomycin and enrofloxacin should be administered every 12 hours.

Oxytetracycline is effective for 24 hours, but also comes in a 'long-acting' form that lasts for 3–5 days.

If the animal's condition does not improve after 2–3 days, consider using a different antibiotic, rechecking the diagnosis (▷*Diagnosing and treating diseases*), or consulting a skilled veterinarian.

Do not eat or drink the meat, blood or milk of an animal for several days after treating it with antibiotics. The number of days depends on the type of antibiotic. Check the instructions that come with the medicine.

Amoxycillin (2–7 mg/kg): Moxel, Clamoxyl, inject into the muscle (broad spectrum)
Ampicillin (10 mg/kg): Vetampin, inject into the muscle (broad spectrum)
Enrofloxacin (5 mg/kg): Baytril, inject into the muscle, or by mouth (broad spectrum)
Nitrofurantoin (4 g): Furadantin, by mouth (broad spectrum)
Norfloxacin (5 mg/kg): Norbactin, inject into the muscle, or by mouth (broad spectrum)
Penicillin (10 000–22 000 units/kg): Penicillin G, inject into the muscle
Streptomycin and penicillin: Penstrep (2–3 ml/50 kg), inject into the muscle (broad spectrum)
Sulphadimidine (5–10 g/50 kg): Sulphadimidine, by mouth (sulphonamide)
Sulphanilamide: powder to treat wounds
Tetracycline: spray to treat wounds
Tetracycline/oxytetracycline (5 mg/kg): Terramycin, Alamycin, inject into the muscle or vein (broad spectrum)
Long-acting tetracycline (20 mg/kg): Terramycin LA (1 ml/10 kg), inject into the muscle (broad spectrum)

Antihistamines

To reduce irritation

▷*Allergy, Bites and stings, Pox, Snake bite*
Pheniramine maleate: Avil (5–10 ml), inject into the muscle

Anti-indigestion

To treat indigestion

▷*Indigestion, Red urine*
Hyoscine: Buscopan Compositum (20–30 ml), inject into the muscle or vein
Ruminodigest, Bykodigest Antacid (320 g), drench

Anti-inflammatory

To treat inflammation

▷*Allergy, Arthritis, Chest sprain, Downer, Foot problems, Myopathy, Red urine, Sunstroke*
Dexamethasone* (10–30 mg): Dexone-5, Voren, inject into the muscle or vein
Dimethylsulphoxide: DMSO, on the skin
Methylprednisolone* (200 mg): Depo Medrol, inject into the muscle
Dexa-Tomanol* (5 ml/100 kg), inject into the muscle or vein, or under the skin
Phenylbutazone (8–10 mg/kg): Algesin (3–12 ml), inject into the muscle
Prednisolone* (200 mg), inject into the muscle, apply as cream on skin
Tomanol (5 ml/100 kg): inject into the muscle or vein, or under the skin
*Contains corticosteroids. Should not be given to camels in the last 4 months of pregnancy.

Antiseptics

To clean wounds and skin before and after surgery

▷*Broken jaw, Care of newborn calves, Castration, Injured dulaa, Navel ill, Prolapse of the vagina or womb, Skin problems, Teeth problems.* See also *Disinfectants* below.
Alcohol (70% solution)
Gentian violet
Hydrogen peroxide (0.2–3% solution)
Potassium permanganate (1 g/litre water)
Povidine iodine: Betadine
Tincture of iodine (2–5% solution in alcohol)
Tincture of iodine/glycerine mixture (1 part iodine solution, 30 parts glycerine)
Lorexane ointment
Metacresolsuphonic acid formaldehyde: Lotagen (0.2% solution)
Acriflavine (0.1% solution)
Dermaclens, Otoderm

Ayurvedic drugs

Ayurvedic drugs are popular in India. The following preparations have been found helpful to treat camels.
Caflon, Catcough, for coughing
Charmil, for skin problems, mange, wounds
Diaroak, Neblon, for diarrhoea
Ectosep, for skin problems
Himax, for wounds
Maggacite, against maggots

Dewormers (anthelmintics)

To treat internal parasites (worms)

▷*Internal parasites (worms), Lungworms*

Albendazole (7.5 mg/kg): Valbazen, by mouth
Fenbendazole (5–7.5 mg/kg): Panacur, by mouth
Oxfendazole (4.5–5 mg/kg): Systamex, by mouth
Thiabendazole (90 mg/kg): Thibenzole, by mouth
Diethylcarbamazine citrate (22 mg/kg): Franocide 40% (2.5 ml/50 kg), inject into the muscle (against lungworms)

Disinfectants and sterilization

To keep surgical instruments sterile

See also *Antiseptics* above
Alcohol (70% solution)
Clorox
Dettol
TCP
Savlon

Diuretics

To make the animal urinate

▷*Oedema*

Furosemide (0.5–1 mg/kg): Frusemide, Lasix, inject into the muscle, or by mouth (follow instructions)
Trichlormethiazide/dexamethasone*: Naquasone (1–2 boluses), by mouth

*Contains corticosteroids. Should not be given to camels in the last 4 months of pregnancy.

Fungicides

To treat fungal infections

▷*Ringworm*

Enilconazole (0.2%): Imaverol (1ml in 50 ml water), wash/spray
Nystatin (100 000 units/g ointment): Mycostatin, on the skin

Hormones

To help in birthing problems

▷*Care of newborn calves, Retained afterbirth*

Oxytocin (20–40 international units): inject into the muscle

Insecticides and acaricides

To combat insects and mites, repel flies

▷*Bites and stings, Dipetalonemiasis, Ear infection, Internal parasites (worms), Lice and fleas, Lungworms, Nasal bots, Ticks, Trypanosomiasis*

Amitraz (250 mg/litre): Taktic, Triatix, Amitak (2 ml/litre water), wash/spray
Benzene hexachloride (0.025–0.05%): Gammatox, BHC, wash/spray
Deltamethrin (1%): Butox (2–4 ml/litre water), wash/spray
Diazinon (0.05–0.1% solution = 0.5–1 g/litre): Neocidal, Bremer dip, Coopers dip (0.05–0.1% solution), wash/spray
Ivermectin (0.2 mg/kg = 200μg/kg): Ivomec (1 ml/50 kg), inject under the skin
Trichlorfon (2.5 g/50 kg): Neguvon, by mouth
Quintiophos (0.02%): Bacdip (10 ml in 18 litres water), wash/spray
Cypermethrin (1 mg/kg): Ectomin, pour on animal's back (fly repellent)
Permethrin: Stomoxin MO, pour on animal's back (fly repellent)

Laxatives, purgatives

To make the animal defecate

▷*Bloat, Constipation, Indigestion, Plant poisoning*

Arecoline (130 mg), inject under the skin
Epsom salts (magnesium sulphate) (250 g dissolved in large amount of water): drench
Neostigmine sulphate (1 mg/50 kg): Neostigmine, inject under the skin
Camelax, drench
Furlax paste, by mouth
Tympanyl (350 ml), drench

Lubricants

To make instruments slippery

(e.g., for putting into the mouth, anus or vagina)

Paraffin jelly: Vaseline
Cooking oil
Ghee

Muscle relaxants

To relax the muscles

▷*Tetanus*

Methocarbamol: Robaxin, follow instructions, inject into the vein

Rehydration

To restore liquid to a dehydrated animal

▷*Bloat, Blocked intestines, Calf diarrhoea, Colibacillosis, Diarrhoea, Dry coat, Salmonellosis, Sunstroke*

Lactated Ringer's solution: give as drip

Sodium bicarbonate (3.5% solution in water): give as drip

Oral rehydration liquid (9 g salt, 50 g sugar and 10 g sodium bicarbonate per litre of water), drench

Hydrate, drench

Lectade, drench

Sedatives

To calm the animal (e.g., for surgery)

▷*Sedation and anaesthesia*; see also *Analgesics and anaesthetics* above

Diazepam (200–300 mg): Valium, inject into the vein

Propionylpromazine (0.2–0.5 mg/kg): Combelen, inject into the muscle

Xylazine (0.25–0.5 mg/kg [minor surgery], 1–2 mg/kg [complete immobilization]): Rompun, inject into the muscle or vein

Xylazine and ketamine (0.4 mg/kg xylazine and 5.0 mg/kg ketamine into the muscle, or 0.25 mg/kg xylazine and 3–5 mg/kg ketamine into the vein): Ketanest, Vetalar, inject

Yohimbine HCl: Antagonil, inject into the vein (reverses the effect of xylazine)

Lignocaine hydrochloride (2%): Lignocaine, Lidocaine, inject (for local anaesthesia)

Stimulants

To stimulate the muscles

▷*Downer*

Catosal, inject into the muscle

Tonophosphan (20 ml), inject into the muscle or vein, or under the skin

Trypanocides

To treat trypanosomiasis

▷*Trypanosomiasis*

Melarsomine (0.25 mg/kg): Cymelarsan, inject into the muscle

Quinapyramine sulphate and quinapyramine chloride (5 mg/kg): Triquin, Antrycide, Tribexin (0.25 ml/10 kg), inject under the skin

Suramin (10 mg/kg): Naganol, Antrypol, inject into the vein

Vaccines

To protect animals against infectious diseases

Vaccines (some traditional) are available for ▷*Anthrax, Blackquarter, Haemorrhagic enteritis, Haemorrhagic septicaemia, Orf, Pox, Rabies, Rift Valley fever, Ringworm, Salmonellosis* and *Tetanus*

Do not use these medicines on camels

Certain cattle medicines are (or are thought to be) poisonous for camels. They include:

- **Diminazene aceturate** (Berenil, Trypazen), **homidium** (Ethidium, Novidium), **isometamidium chloride** (Samorin, Trypanidium), used against ▷*Trypanosomiasis* in cattle.
- **Tetramisole** (Levamisole), used against ▷*Intestinal parasites (worms)* in cattle.
- **Griseofulvin**, used against ▷*Ringworm* in cattle.

Do not use these medicines on pregnant female camels

Corticosteroids can cause abortion if used in the last 4 months of pregnancy. They include:

- **Dexamethasone** (Dexone-5, Voren)
- Dexa-Tomanol
- **Methylprednisolone** (Depo Medrol)
- **Prednisolone**
- **Trichlormethiazide/dexamethasone** (Naquasone)

References

FAO (1994) p. 252–9; Forse (1999) p. 324–53; Manefield and Tinson (1997) p. 323–50; Projet Cameline (1999) p. 58–9; Quesenberry (1990) p. 242–60.

Units of measurement

Keep a set of containers, such as spoons, cups and bottles, to measure medicines in. Write on each container the number of millilitres of liquid it can contain. If you know the volume of one container (such as a bottle with the volume marked on it), you can easily work out how much the others hold. For example, count how many bottles of water you need to fill a bucket. To get the volume of the bucket, multiply the volume of the bottle by the number of bottles used.

- Syringes and droppers have volume markings to show you how much they hold.
- Keep separate containers to measure medicines and poisons (such as acaricides).
- Clean containers carefully after using them, and do not use them for anything else – especially not to prepare food.

Liquid

- 1 litre of water weighs 1 kilogram (1 kg).
- 1 millititre (1 ml) of water weighs 1 gram (1 g).
- 1 ml = 1 cubic centimetre (1 cm³, 1 cc).
- 1/1000 ml of water weighs 1 milligram (1 mg).

Spoons

- 1 teaspoon = 5 ml
- 3 teaspoons = 1 tablespoon = 15 ml

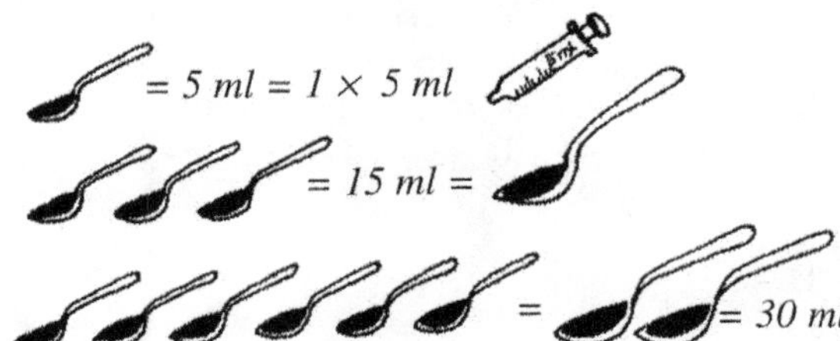

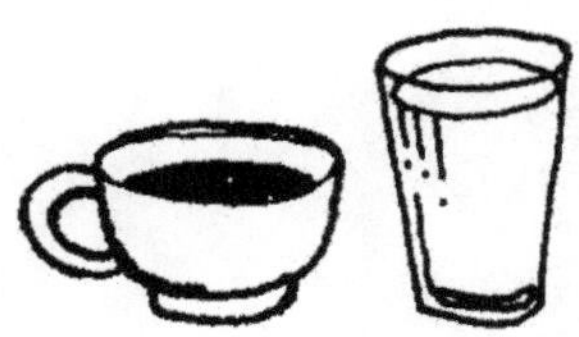

Cups and glasses

The size of cups and drinking glasses varies from country to country and even within a country. Work out how much a cup or glass contains by filling a bottle of known volume with cupfuls of water.

Dropper

- 60 drops = 5 ml = 1 teaspoon = 5 grams

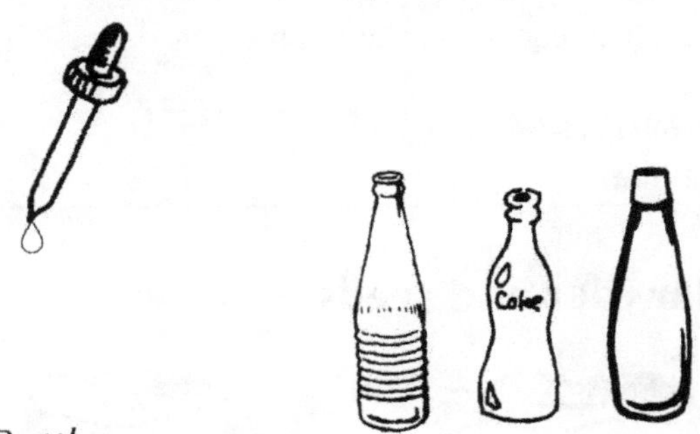

Bottles

Bottles are often marked with their volume. Common sizes are 120 ml, 200 ml, 320 ml, 375 ml, 750 ml, and 1 litre.

- Screw bottle-cap = 7.5 ml = 1.5 teaspoons
- Small Coke bottle = 237 ml
- Small, 'export' beer bottle (Kenya) = 300 ml
- Beer bottle (Kenya) = 500 ml
- Treetop bottle (Kenya) = 700 ml
- Spirit or wine bottle = 700 or 750 ml

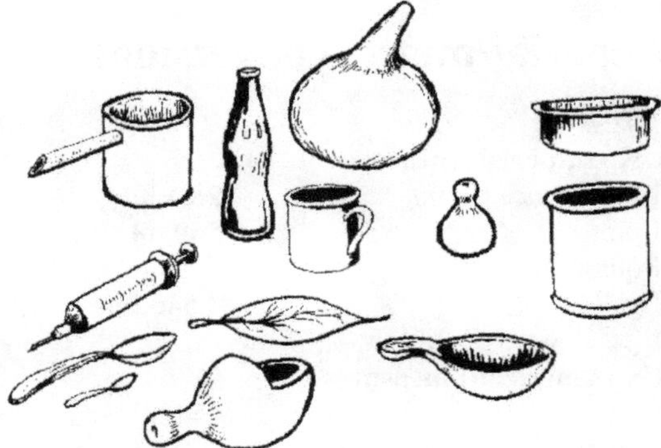

Other containers

Other containers include buckets, jerry cans, gourds, tin cans, cooking pots and water skins. Find out how much each container holds and mark this on it.

- Buckets come in various sizes. A common one is 2 gallons (7.5 litres).
- Do not use containers that have held pesticides for preparing or storing medicines!

See the table on the next page to estimate the weight of ingredients. If the ingredient you want to measure is not in the table, choose the one that is most like it.

A tin that contains this amount of water…	…contains this many grams of:				
	water	flour	sugar	butter	nuts
50 ml	50	26	42	48	24
100 ml	100	53	84	96	48
200 ml	200	105	169	192	95
237 ml (e.g., small Coke bottle)	237	125	200	227	113
250 ml	250	132	211	239	119
568 ml (1 Imperial pint)	568	299	479	544	271
1 litre	1000	527	844	958	477

Powder and seeds

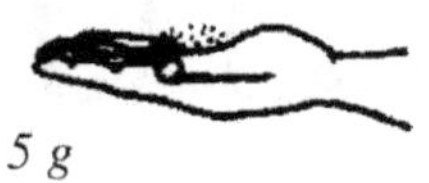

5 g

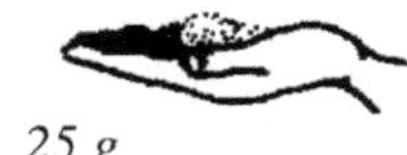

25 g

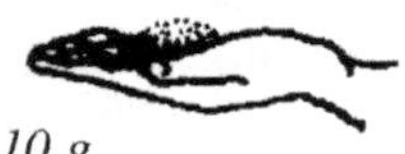

10 g

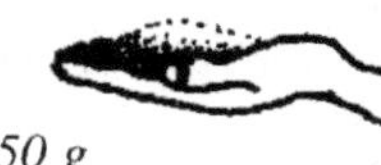

50 g

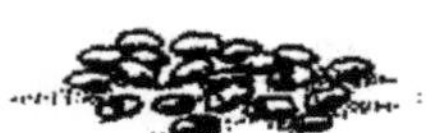

20 peanuts = 10 g

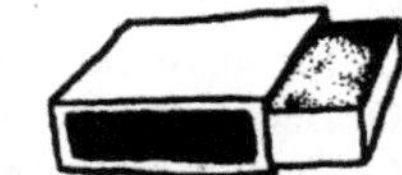

small matchboxful of powder = 50 g

Imperial/metric conversions

Volume

UK (Imperial) measures

1 fluid ounce (fl oz)	=	28.4 ml
1 pint	=	568 ml
1 quart	=	1136 ml
1 gallon	=	4.546 litres

US (American) measures

1 pint	=	454 ml
1 quart	=	909 ml
1 gallon	=	3.785 litres
1 ml	=	0.035 fl oz
1 litre	=	1.76 pints (UK)
	=	2.2 pints (US)

Length

1 inch	=	25.4 mm
1 foot	=	30.48 cm
1 cm	=	0.39 inch
1 m	=	39.37 inches

Weight

1 ounce (oz)	=	28.3 g
1 pound (lb)	=	0.454 kg
1 g	=	0.035 oz
1 kg	=	2.205 lb

Temperature

1 degree Centigrade (°C) = 1.8° Fahrenheit (°F)
1 degree Fahrenheit (°F) = 0.56° Centigrade (°C)

Freezing point of water	= 0°C	= 32°F
Boiling point of water	= 100°C	= 212°F

Normal body temperatures

Camels	= 37.5°C	= 99.5°F
Humans	= about 37°C	= 98.6°F

Temperature conversions

To convert from Fahrenheit to Centigrade:

°C = (°F–32) × 5 ÷ 9

To convert from Centigrade to Fahrenheit:

°F = (°C × 9 ÷ 5) + 32

°C		°F
35	=	95
36	=	96.8
37	=	98.6
38	=	100.4
39	=	102.2
40	=	104
41	=	105.8
42	=	107.6
43	=	109.4

References

IIRR (1994); IIRR (1996); ITDG and IIRR (1996).

Contributors' profiles

The contributors' specializations are given in **bold**.

Hamid Agab

Researcher/supervisor, Al Rajhi Co. for Agriculture, Camel Project, PO Box 2373, Al Qaseem, Buraidah, Saudi Arabia; tel/fax +966-6-323 9388; fax +966-6-392 0183; email: watpp@shabakah.com

Skin diseases

A Sudanese citizen, Hamid Agab holds BVSc and MVSc degrees, and a certificate of specialization from CIRAD-EMVT, France. He was formerly director of the Al-Showak Camel Research Centre, Sudan, and assistant professor with the Animal Health and Research Corporation of Sudan.

Mohamed Fadl Ahmed

Dept of Parasitology, Faculty of Veterinary Science, Khartoum North 13314, Sudan; tel +249-11-313 654 or +249-11-466 938; fax +249-11-312 638 or +249-11-774 732; email: fadlm@hotmail.com

Internal parasites

Mohamed Fadl holds BVSc, MVSc and PhD degrees. He has worked with camels since 1984, specializing in helminthology. He is an assistant professor at the University of Khartoum's Faculty of Veterinary Science. He is a Sudanese national.

Darlington Akabwai

Veterinarian, PARC-VAC of OAU/IBAR/PARC, Box 30786 Nairobi, Kenya; tel +254-2-226 447; fax +254-2-583 358

John Akkara

Consultant, 39 Narang Colony, Janakpuri, New Delhi 110058, India; tel +91-11-5510441

Veterinary extension

John Akkara, an Indian citizen, holds BVSc, MSc and PhD degrees. Formerly principal specialist/coordinator with Action for Food Production, he has worked with camels in Gujarat, and on community-based projects in Phalodi district in Rajasthan. He has conducted veterinary, paraveterinary, training and NGO programmes throughout India.

Stephen Ashdown

Livestock consultant, Downlands, East Dean, Chichester, W Sussex PO18 0JA, UK; tel +44-1243-811 357; fax +44-1243-811 270; email: AshdownSF@aol.com

Camel production

Stephen Ashdown holds a degree in veterinary medicine, an MSc in tropical animal production, and an MA in rural development. He has worked on projects to decentralize livestock services, vaccinate stock against rinderpest, and conduct research on paraveterinary programmes. He is a British citizen.

Muhammad Athar

Lecturer, Department of Clinical Medicine & Surgery, Faculty of Veterinary Science, University of Agriculture, Faisalabad 38040, Pakistan; tel +92-41-302 81 to 89, ext 436; fax +92-41-636 369, 647 846; email: sannalab@khawaja.net.pk

Veterinary preventive medicine, camel medicine

Muhammad Athar is a Pakistani veterinarian who lectures at the University of Agriculture, Faisalabad. He holds DVM and MSc degrees.

Nyotomba (Bonnie) Bonaventure

Artist, PO Box 68308, Nairobi, Kenya; tel +254-2-338 389, tel/fax +254-2-212 176

Art

Bonnie Nyotumba has worked as a designer/painter for Bellerive Foundation, Care–Kenya, *Rainbow* magazine, Jacaranda Designs, Don Bosco, and the International Institute of Rural Reconstruction.

Set Bornstein

Laboratory veterinarian, National Veterinary Institute, PO Box 7073, Uppsala 75007, Sweden; tel +46-18-674 155, +46-1-592 5408; fax +46-18-309 162; email: set.bornstein@sva.se

Skin parasites

A Swedish citizen, Set Bornstein earned his DVM and DTVM degrees in 1968, an MSc in 1975, and a PhD in 1995. He has a wide range of experience with camels, including as a veterinary adviser to the Somali Camel Research Project in the 1980s.

Andy Catley

Veterinarian, PO Box 30786, Nairobi, Kenya; tel +254-2-226447; fax +254-2-667 8299; email: catley@bigfoot.com; internet: http://www.vetwork.org

Community-based animal health services in dryland areas

Andy Catley holds BVetMed and MSc degrees. He has worked with animal health programmes in the Horn of Africa and currently works for both the International Institute for Environment and Development (IIED) and Vetwork UK. He has published on ethnoveterinary medicine, camel management and health practices, and participatory methods in veterinary medicine. He is a British national.

Maurizio Dioli

Herlandsvn 111, 5264 Garnes, Norway; tel.+47-55-240 965; email: berte@online.no

Diseases, health care and management of camels

Maurizio Dioli is an Italan veterinarian, based in East Africa. He has extensive experience providing health services to pastoral nomads and teaching in Ethiopia, Kenya and Somalia/Somaliland. He co-authored *The one-humped camel in Eastern Africa*. He has also worked in Cambodia, Italy, Namibia and Uganda.

Christopher Rashid Field

Consultant in arid lands and wildlife, PO Box 485, Nanyuki, Kenya; tel +254-176-22637, 32352; fax +254-176-32883

Trypanosomiasis, haemorrhagic septicaemia, bronchopneumonia, abortions

Chris Field is an independent consultant and camel raiser in Kenya. A British citizen, he holds a BA in natural sciences and a PhD in zoology. He has conducted research and done consultancies in Kenya, Tanzania, Uganda and Tunisia on both wildlife and camels. Until 1996 he was leader of FARM Africa's Camel Improvement and Pastoralists Development Project. He is interim chairman of the Kenya Camel Association and owns a herd of over 100 camels.

Tarun Kumar Gahlot

Editor, Journal of Camel Practice and Research, *Dept of Veterinary Surgery and Radiology, Veterinary College, 67 Gandhi Nagar West, near Lalgarh Palace, Bikaner 334001, India; tel +91-151-527 029, 521 282; fax +91-151-540 274, email: tkedjcpr@jp1.dot.net.in*

Surgery

T. K. Gahlot holds BVSc&AH and MSc degrees, and a PhD in veterinary surgery and radiology. He has published over 100 scientific papers, including some 50 on camels. He is editor of the *Journal of Camel Practice and Research*, and has written and edited several books on camel veterinary medicine. He is an Indian citizen.

Andrea Gervelmeyer

A2221 Animal Production and Health Section, Joint FAO/IAEA Division of Nuclear Techniques in Food and Agriculture, International Atomic Energy Agency, PO Box 100, 1400 Vienna, Austria; tel +43-1-2600 21606; fax +43-1-2600 7; email: A.Gervelmeyer@iaea.org; internet: http://www.iaea.or.at/programmes/rifa/d3/

Laboratory techniques

Andrea Gervelmeyer is a German veterinarian who holds postgraduate diploma and PhD degrees from the Free University of Berlin. In 1997, she helped establish a field laboratory for the diagnosis of trypanosomiasis, intestinal and skin parasites of camels in Sadri, Rajasthan. She now works at the International Atomic Energy Agency, where she is responsible for livestock disease-control projects in Africa.

Christian Hülsebusch

Centre for Agriculture in the Tropics and Subtropics, Institute for Animal Production, University of Hohenheim (480), 70593 Stuttgart, Germany; tel +49-711-459 3173, 459 3170; fax +49-711-459 3290; email: huelse@uni-hohenheim.de

Dryland animal husbandry, pastoralism

Christian Hülsebusch holds a degree in agriculture from the University of Bonn and the German equivalent of an MSc in animal production from the University of Hohenheim. He has conducted research on camels and other livestock in Kenya for the University of Hohenheim. From 1994 to 1996 he studied the relationship between colostrum and health of newborn camels in Kenya. He is a German national.

Vitthal Kamble

Artist, Badhir Mook Shikshan Kendra Pune, SMRUTI, 805 Bhandarkar Road, Pune 4, India; tel +91-212-373 296, 523 477

Art

An Indian national, Vitthal Kamble holds a diploma in fine art. Since leaving college, he has worked as a comic illustrator and designer for Raj Pocket Books and Manoj Pocket Books, Delhi.

Brigitte Angelika Kaufmann

Centre for Agriculture in the Tropics and Subtropics, Institute for Animal Production, Univeristy of Hohenheim (480), 70593 Stuttgart, Germany; tel +49-711-459 3173, 459 3170; fax +49-711-459 3290; email: bkaufman@uni-hohenheim.de

Pastoral camel husbandry

Brigitte Kaufmann studied agriculture at the universities of Bonn and Hohenheim. She has conducted several field studies on camel production in Kenya, and on goat production in Burundi. She has recently published an analysis of pastoral camel husbandry in northern Kenya. She is a German citizen.

Ilse Köhler-Rollefson

Consultant, Pragelatostrasse 20, 64372 Ober-Ramstadt, Germany; tel +49-6154-53642, 52309; fax +49-6154-53642; email: gorikr@t-online.de

Pastoralism, camels, livestock genetic resources

A German veterinarian, Ilse Köhler-Rollefson is founder of the League for Pastoral Peoples. She has worked with camel pastoralists in Jordan, Sudan and India, focusing on their traditional knowledge. She collaborates with Lokhit Pashu-Palak Sansthan, an NGO working with camel pastoralists in Rajasthan. She recently completed her 'habilitation' degree in the history of veterinary medicine at the University of Munich. She is currently promoting the conservation and development of indigenous livestock breeds.

B J Linquist

PO Box 259, Marsabit, Kenya; tel/fax +254-183 2095; email: bdavid@maf.org

Reproduction, general

BJ Linquist is a American veterinarian who has worked on ethnoveterinary medicine with Gabbra nomads in Kenya since 1988. She has a DVM and a masters of preventive veterinary medicine and epidemiology from the University of California–Davis. Much of her clinical experience has been with camel problems and diseases. She has also worked on decentralized animal health programmes and relief-and-development efforts. She owns a small herd of camels.

Evelyn Mathias

Independent consultant, Weizenfeld 4, 51467 Bergisch Gladbach, Germany; tel +49-2202-932 921; fax +49-2202-932 922; email: evelynmathias@netcologne.de

Ethnoveterinary medicine, indigenous knowledge

Evelyn Mathias holds a Dr med vet degree from the University of Giessen, and an MS in international development studies from Iowa State University. She co-ordinated the production of a set of manuals on ethnoveterinary medicine in Asia (IIRR 1994) and co-organized the first international conference on ethnoveterinary medicine in Pune, India, in 1997. She currently moderates an email discussion group on ethnoveterinary medicine. She is a German citizen.

Ghulam Muhammad

Associate Professor and Chairman, Department of Clinical Medicine & Surgery, Faculty of Veterinary Science, University of Agriculture, Faisalabad 38040, Pakistan; tel +92-41-30281 to 89, ext 436; fax +92-41-647 846, 636 369; email: sannalab@khawaja.net.pk

Veterinary preventive medicine, camel medicine

Ghulam Muhammad is associate professor and chair of the Department of Clinical Medicine and Surgery, University of Agriculture, Faisalabad. He holds DVM, MSc and PhD degrees.

Paul Mundy

Development communication specialist, Weizenfeld 4, 51467 Bergisch Gladbach, Germany; tel +49-2202-932 921; fax +49-2202-932 922; email: paulmundy@netcologne.de; internet: http://www.netcologne.de/~nc-mundypa

Development communication

Paul Mundy is a British development communication specialist based in Germany. He has a PhD in communication from the University of Wisconsin-Madison. He has co-ordinated over 20 workshops to produce easy-to-understand information materials, including those on ethnoveterinary medicine in Asia (IIRR 1994) and Kenya (ITDG and IIRR 1996).

Babiker Elhag Musa

Camel Affairs, Diwan of Royal Court, Muscat 111, Oman; tel +968-539 623, fax +968-893 802

Reproduction

Babiker Musa is a professor at the University of Khartoum. A Sudanese citizen, he holds BVSc, MVSc, MS and PhD degrees, and has worked with camels for more than 25 years. He established the Camel Research Unit in Khartoum and Showak. He is editor of a newsletter on camels and referee on camels for the International Foundation for Science. He currently manages the camels of the Royal Court in Muscat.

Augustine Namanda

Veterinarian, PO Box 795, Nanyuki, Kenya; tel +254-176-32352, 32882; fax +254-176-32883

Camel health

Augustine Namanda holds a bachelor's degree in veterinary medicine. He has worked closely with camels for 3 years, with experience in health care, data collection and analysis. He has been participating in an on-going attempt to characterize Kenya's camel breeds. He is a Kenyan citizen.

Atmaram Pund

Artist, Badhir Mook Shikshan Kendra Pune, SMRUTI, 805 Bhandarkar Road, Pune 4, India; tel +91-212-373 296

Art

Atmaram Pund holds a diploma in fine art. Since leaving college, he has worked as a comic designer and illustrator for Raj Pocket Books and Manoj Pocket Books, Delhi. He is an Indian citizen.

Hanwant Singh Rathore

Director, Lokhit Pashu-Palak Sansthan, c/o Vyas Travels, Bus Stand, Sadri 306702, District Pali, Rajasthan, India; tel +91-2934-85086, 85045; fax +91-2934-85582

Raika pastoralists, India

Hanwant Singh Rathore is founder member and director of LPPS, an NGO working with Raika camel pastoralists in Rajasthan. He has been working and interacting with the Raika since 1991. LPPS aims to develop animal health services that suit the needs of rural livestock owners and integrate traditional and modern approaches.

Shravan Singh Rathore

Consultant veterinarian, Lokhit Pashu-Palak Sansthan, Bhagwan Mahaveer Colony, Sadri District, Pali, Rajasthan, India; tel +91-2934-3686, +91-291-46591

Skin diseases

Shravan Singh Rathore holds a BVSc&AH degree. He has worked for 2 years with Raika and Bisnai herders for LPPS (an Indian NGO) at Sadri, Rajasthan. He has also worked as a veterinarian for the government of Rajasthan.

Jacob Wanyama

Project Manager, Intermediate Technology Development Group, PO Box 39493, Nairobi, Kenya; fax +254-2-710 083; email: wanyama@itdg.or.ke

Camel diseases and husbandry

A Kenyan citizen, Jacob Wanyama holds a BVM degree, and has studied camel diseases and husbandry at Ben-Gurion University of the Negev. For 6 years until 1992, he was responsible for examining and selecting breeding camels and monitoring newly purchased camels for the GTZ Camel Promotion Programme in Samburu, Kenya.

Richard Iriga Wanyiri

Artist, PO Box 52477, Nairobi, Kenya; tel +254-2-811 506, 226 348

Art

Richard Wanyiri has a diploma from the Buru Buru Institute of Fine Art. He has worked with NGOs engaged in the fields of shelter, health, human rights and gender issues.

Fran White

Horseshoes, Sibsey Northlands, Boston, Lincolnshire, PE22 OUA, UK; email: fnwhite@aol.com

Animal health in Samburu communities

At the time this book was drafted, Fran White was studying for a degree in agriculture (animal production science) at the University of Newcastle-upon-Tyne. She spent 1 year in northern Kenya collecting data on animal health for Samburu Aid. She is a British citizen.

Glossary of technical terms

This manual avoids using technical terms if at all possible. Sometimes, however, using a technical word cannot be avoided. This glossary contains such words and other terms found in books on veterinary medicine and animal husbandry.

▷*Italics* refer to sections in this manual; SMALL CAPS refer to other entries in the glossary.

Abdomen. The belly.
Abomasum. Fourth STOMACH of a RUMINANT.
Abortifacient. Substance that causes abortion or miscarriage.
Abortion. Miscarriage: when the FOETUS is expelled before it is due (▷*Abortion*).
Abscess. A collection of PUS in the tissue.
Acaricide. Chemical used to control TICKS (external PARASITES).
Actinomyces. A type of disease-causing BACTERIA.
Active ingredient, active principle, a.i. Ingredient or chemical component of a drug which has a healing effect.
Acute. Critical, sudden and of short duration.
Aetiology, etiology. The cause of a disease.
Afterbirth. PLACENTA and other membranes that come out after birth (▷*Pregnancy and birth*, *Retained afterbirth*).
a.i. ACTIVE INGREDIENT.
AI. ARTIFICIAL INSEMINATION.
Alimentary. Pertaining to, or caused by, food.
Alimentary canal. The DIGESTIVE TRACT.
Allergen. Substance that may cause an allergic response.
Allergy. Hypersensitivity of the body cells to specific substances, such as an ANTIGEN OR ALLERGEN, resulting in rashes or other reactions (▷*Allergy*).
Amakat (Turkana). Natural salt rocks.
Anaemia. Below-normal number of red blood cells and quantity of HAEMOGLOBIN in blood.
Anaesthetic. A medicine that stops all feeling. It makes the animal (or the part of the body it is applied to) numb (▷*Sedation and anaesthesia*).
Analgesic. A medicine that reduces pain but does not cause numbness.
Anhidrosis. Absence of sweating (▷*Dry coat*).
Anthelmintic. Substance that removes intestinal worms from the host animal (▷*Internal parasites [worms]*).
Anthrax. Disease cause by a bacterium called *Bacillus anthracis* (▷*Anthrax*).
Antibiotic. A chemical substance produced by a micro-organism that kills (or inhibits the growth of) other MICRO-ORGANISMS.
Antibody. A protein in the blood that is produced in response to an ANTIGEN.
Anticoagulant. Substance that prevents or slows down blood clotting.
Antidote. A treatment which counteracts or destroys the effect of POISONS or other medicines.
Antiemetic. Substance that relieves vomiting.
Antigen. Substance that may induce an IMMUNE RESPONSE (e.g., BACTERIA, toxins).
Antihistamine. Substance used to treat ALLERGY and colds.
Anti-inflammatory. Counteracting INFLAMMATION.
Antipyretic. Substance that lowers body temperature to the normal level; used against fever.
Antiseptic. Substance that destroys or inhibits disease-causing BACTERIA.
Antispasmodic. Substance that prevents or relieves muscular spasms or cramps.
Antivenin. Substance that counteracts the POISON from an animal, such as a ▷*Snakebite*.
Anus. The opening at the end of the INTESTINES where the dung comes out.
Artery. A vessel that carries the blood away from the heart to other parts of the body.
Arthritis. INFLAMMATION of JOINTS (▷*Arthritis*).
Artificial insemination, AI. Breeding by putting semen into the vagina or uterus without sexual contact.
Ascariasis. Infestation by an intestinal PARASITE called *Ascaris* (▷*Internal parasites [worms]*).
Ascarid. A roundworm NEMATODE (a type of PARASITE) found in the INTESTINES.
Astringent. Substance that shrinks tissues and prevents secretion of fluids from wounds.

***Bacillus cereus* intoxication.** HAEMORRHAGIC DISEASE (▷*Haemorrhagic disease*).
Bacterium, bacteria. Tiny MICRO-ORGANISMS, some of which cause disease.
Balling gun. Tool to apply pills, capsules and BOLUSES (▷*Administering medicines*).
Balm. A soothing or healing medicine.
Blackleg. BLACKQUARTER.
Blackquarter. Disease caused by a bacterium called *Clostridium chauvoei* (▷*Blackquarter*).
Bladder. The organ that holds the urine.
Blister. A VESICLE, a skin lesion.

Bloat. The build-up of gases in the STOMACH or INTESTINES (▷*Bloat*).

Boil. Infected, painful, hard swelling of the skin.

Bolus. A ball or tablet of medicine (▷*Administering medicines, Traditional medicines*).

Branding. Marking the skin with a hot iron (▷*Branding*).

Broad-spectrum medicine. A medicine effective against several disease-causing MICRO-ORGANISMS.

Bronchus, bronchi. The pair of air passages at the end of the TRACHEA, leading to the lungs.

Bronchitis. Inflammation of the BRONCHI.

Buffy coat. Reddish-grey layer in a centrifuged tube, consisting of white blood cells between the red blood cells and the SERUM (▷*Checking for diseases in the laboratory*).

Caesarean section. Operation to cut the uterus open and pull the calf out (▷*Difficult birth*).

Calf diarrhoea. DIARRHOEA in calves caused by too much milk or by a virus (▷*Calf diarrhoea*).

Cancer. A malignant, cellular TUMOUR.

Canines. The pointed teeth beside the INCISORS; they can grow very large in male camels (▷*Estimating a camel's weight and age*).

Cannula. Tube attached to a TROCAR.

Capillary tube. Thin tube with a very small inside diameter.

Carcass. Dead body of an animal.

Castration. Removal of TESTICLES (▷*Castration*).

Catarrh. INFLAMMATION of nose and mucous membranes.

Catgut. An absorbable, sterile thread made from the small intestine of sheep; used as a SUTURE material.

Cauterization. The burning of flesh with a hot iron or a chemical.

Centrifuge. Piece of laboratory equipment that spins very fast. Used to separate parts of a liquid from one another, such as components of a blood sample (▷*Checking for diseases in the laboratory*).

Cervix. The narrow, front part of the UTERUS.

Cestodes. Tapeworms (▷*Internal parasites*).

Chronic. Persisting for a long time.

Closed fracture. Broken bone where the skin remains intact.

Clostridiosis. BLACKQUARTER (▷*Blackquarter*).

***Clostridium*.** A type of disease-causing BACTERIA.

Cold struck. WRY NECK (▷*Wry neck*).

Colibacillosis. Disease caused by a bacterium called *Escherichia coli* (▷*Colibacillosis*).

Colic. Pain caused by gas in the STOMACH or intestines.

Colostrum. Thick yellow milk, rich in ANTIBODIES, protein and micro-nutrients, produced by mothers after giving birth.

Compress. A dry, often warm, substance applied firmly to a part of the body (see also FOMENTATION) (▷*Administering medicines*).

Concentrate. A carefully formulated mixture of nutrients.

Concoction. A preparation from crude materials, made by combining different ingredients.

Congenital. Present at and existing from the time of birth.

Congested. Closely packed.

Congestion. Abnormal accumulation of blood in part of the body.

Conjunctiva. The membranes around the eyeball.

Conjunctivitis. Inflammation of the CONJUNCTIVA.

Constipation. Infrequent or difficult bowel movement with hard dung (▷*Constipation*).

Contagious. Diseases which are readily passed on to others.

Contagious skin necrosis. A skin disease (▷*Contagious skin necrosis*).

Contamination. Introduction of MICRO-ORGANISMS, for example when using surgical instruments that are not STERILE.

Contusion. Bruise, injury where the skin is not broken.

Convulsion. A violent, involuntary contraction of the muscles.

Cornea. The transparent part of the eyeball.

Corneal opacity. Whitish film on the eyeball.

Corneal ulcer. Injury of the CORNEA.

Corpus luteum. Part of the OVARY that forms after OVULATION and produces HORMONES during part of the HEAT cycle.

Corticosteroids. Type of HORMONES; their synthetic equivalents are used as drugs. Corticosteroid drugs are used to treat certain diseases and decrease inflammation and itching.

***Corynebacterium pyogenes*.** A type of disease-causing BACTERIA.

Cud. The ball of food that RUMINANTS chew and then swallow again.

Cyst. A closed sac or capsule containing a liquid or semisolid substance.

Decoction. Medicine made by boiling ingredients in water (▷*Traditional medicines*).

Decongestant. Substance that reduces CONGESTION or swelling.

Defecate. Passing of faeces.

Deficiency. A lack or shortage.

Dehydration. Lack of water in the body.

Dermatitis. Inflammation of the skin.

Dermatomycosis. RINGWORM (▷*Ringworm*).

Dermatophilosis. A skin disease caused by FUNGUS (▷*Dermatophilosis*).

Dermatophytosis. RINGWORM.

Dermoid. Egg-shaped growths on the skin (▷*Dermoids*).

Detergent. Cleansing substance.

Diagnosis. The determination of a disease. It includes the name of the disease, its cause, and the PROGNOSIS.

Diarrhoea. Frequent passing of thin, watery faeces (▷*Diarrhoea*).

Digestive tract. The tube through which food passes: the mouth, OESOPHAGUS, STOMACH, INTESTINES and ANUS.

Dipetalonemiasis. Disease caused by a parasitic worm called *Dipetalonema evansi* (▷*Dipetalonemiasis*).

Discharge. Substance excreted by the body, such as PUS.

Disinfectant. A chemical that kills MICRO-ORGANISMS.

Dislocation. Bone displaced from a joint.

Diuretic. A drug or preparation that causes urination.

Dosage. The determination and regulation of the amount, frequency and number of DOSES.

Dose. The quantity of a medicine to be administered at one time.

Downer. Disease where a camel refuses to get up; can have various causes (▷*Downer*).

Drench. Forcing the animal to drink a liquid medicine (▷*Administering medicines*).

Dressing. Material used to cover and protect a wound.

Drip. Slow, drop-by-drop injection of a liquid into a vein (▷*Administering medicines*).

Dry coat syndrome. ANHIDROSIS, absence of sweating (▷*Dry coat*).

Dulaa. Soft palate of camels.

Dysentery. INFLAMMATION of the large INTESTINES, with liquid and bloody DIARRHOEA and painful straining.

Dystocia. Difficult birth (▷*Difficult birth*).

Echinococcosis. Disease caused by small tapeworms (▷*Hydatid disease*).

Ecthyma. Infection of the skin with large pustular VESICLES.

Ectoparasite. EXTERNAL PARASITE.

Eczema. Inflammatory skin disease characterized by redness, itching and formation of scales and crusts.

Edema. OEDEMA.

EDTA. A substance (ethylenediaminetetraacetic acid) that stops blood from clotting.

Electuary. A medicinal preparation consisting of a powdered drug made into a paste with honey or syrup.

Embryo. A new calf in the earliest stage of development. Becomes a FOETUS.

Emetic. Substance that causes vomiting.

Encephalitis. INFLAMMATION of the brain.

Endoparasite. PARASITE that lives inside the body (in the intestines, lungs, etc.) (▷*Internal parasites [worms]*).

Enema. Liquid preparation introduced into the RECTUM (▷*Administering medicines*).

Enteritis. INFLAMMATION of the INTESTINES.

Enterotoxaemia. HAEMORRHAGIC ENTERITIS (▷*Haemorrhagic enteritis*).

Eosinophil. Type of white blood cell (▷*Checking for diseases in the laboratory*).

Epidemic, epizootic. A sudden outbreak of disease in a relatively small area (see also PANDEMIC).

Epidural anaesthesia. Injecting an ANAESTHETIC into the canal of the backbone (▷*Sedation and anaesthesia*).

Epsom salts. Magnesium sulphate.

Estrus, oestrus. HEAT.

Etiology, aetiology. The cause of a disease.

Expectorant. Substance to remove fluid from the LUNGS and TRACHEA.

Expiration. Breathing out.

External parasite. PARASITE that lives on the surface of the body (on the skin, in the skin, in the ears, etc.).

Faeces, feces. Dung.

Fetus. FOETUS.

Fever. Increase in the body temperature; an abnormally high body temperature.

Firing. Application of a red-hot iron to the skin (▷*Branding*).

Flatulence. Excessive gas formation in the DIGESTIVE TRACT.

Foetus, fetus. The developing young calf in the UTERUS.

Fomentation. Application of a warm, moist substance such as a wet cloth to ease pain and INFLAMMATION (see also COMPRESS) (▷*Administering medicines*).

Foreign body. Any object not normally found in the body.

Fracture. Breaking of a bone.

Fungus, fungi. A group of MICRO-ORGANISMS, some of which cause diseases.

Galactagogue. Substance that promotes milk flow.

Gangrene. Death of body tissue.

Gas oedema. BLACKQUARTER.

Gastro-enteritis. INFLAMMATION of the STOMACH and INTESTINES characterized by pain, NAUSEA and disease micro-organisms.

General anaesthesia. Giving an ANAESTHETIC to make the animal lose consciousness and not feel pain anywhere in the body (▷*Sedation and anaesthesia*).

Gestation. Period of pregnancy, term of life of EMBRYO/FOETUS within the UTERUS (▷*Pregnancy and birth*).
Ghee. Clarified, semi-fluid butter made from milk (common in India).
Giemsa. A dye to stain blood samples used to check for blood PARASITES.
Gland. An aggregation of cells that secrete or excrete materials.
Glucose. Table sugar.
Goitre. Enlargement of the thyroid gland caused by IODINE DEFICIENCY (▷*Goitre*).
Gram-positive. Types of BACTERIA that are coloured deep purple in Gram's method (a laboratory test to determine the type of bacteria).
Gur (India). Molasses.

Haematocrit. The volume percentage of red blood cells in the whole blood (▷*Checking for diseases in the laboratory*).
Haematoma. A swelling filled with blood.
Haematuria. Blood in the urine (▷*Red urine*).
Haemoglobin. Protein found in red blood cells.
Haemorrhage. Bleeding.
Haemorrhagic disease. Disease caused by *Bacillus cereus* bacteria (▷*Haemorrhagic disease*).
Haemorrhagic enteritis. Disease caused by *Clostridium* bacteria (▷*Haemorrhagic enteritis*).
Haemorrhagic septicaemia. Disease caused by *Pasteurella multocida* bacteria (▷*Haemorrhagic septicaemia*).
Heart. Organ in the chest that pumps blood around the body.
Heat. The time when the female accepts the male for mating and can become pregnant.
Helminthiasis. Disease caused by worms (▷*Internal parasites [worms]*).
Heparin. A substance that stops blood from clotting.
Hereditary. Characteristics passed from parents to offspring.
Hernia. The abnormal protrusion of the INTESTINES through the PERITONEUM, or part of another organ through the membrane or muscle that contains it.
Hormones. Chemicals formed by GLANDS in the body; they control the activity of organs.
Hydatid cyst. Fluid-filled sac with young tapeworms in it (▷*Hydatid disease*).
Hygiene. The science of health and its preservation.
Hyperplasia. Excessive growth of tissue or an organ.
Hypnotic. Induces sleep.

Ilgoff. Somali name for a calf disease of unknown cause (▷*Saam*).
i.m. INTRAMUSCULAR.
Immersion oil. Oil used to examine objects under a microscope using a special lens.
Immune. Resistant to a disease due to the formation of ANTIBODIES.
Immune response. Reaction of the body to an ANTIGEN: production of ANTIBODIES that fight a disease-causing organism.
Immunity. Body's defence against disease; can be passed to offspring through COLOSTRUM or through exposure, VACCINATION or INOCULATION.
Incision. Cutting the skin or tissue.
Incisors. Flat teeth at the front of the mouth (▷*Estimating a camel's weight and age*).
Infection. Disease caused by MICRO-ORGANISMS.
Infectious. Caused by infection, able to cause infection.
Infertile. Not able to reproduce.
Infested. Over-run by large numbers.
Inflammation. The reaction of living tissues to injury, INFECTION or irritation; characterized by pain, swelling, redness and heat.
Infusion. Herbal medicine made by adding water to plant ingredients in a pot, covering, and allowing to stand, usually for about 15 minutes. An infusion can be either hot or cold (▷*Traditional medicines*).
Injection. The forcing of liquid into a part of the body (e.g., under the skin, into the vein or muscle) (▷*Administering medicines*).
Inoculation. Introduction of disease-causing MICRO-ORGANISMS or other material to stimulate IMMUNITY.
Insecticide. Chemical that kills insects.
Internal parasites. PARASITES that live inside the body (▷*Internal parasites [worms]*).
Intestines. Part of the DIGESTIVE TRACT between the STOMACH and ANUS.
Intramammary. Into the udder.
Intramuscular, i.m. Into the muscle (▷*Administering medicines*).
Intravenous, i.v. Into the vein (vessel that carries blood towards the heart) (▷*Administering medicines*).
Iodine deficiency. Shortage of iodine in the body.
Iris. The coloured part of the eye.
i.v. INTRAVENOUS.

Jaggery. A palm sugar made in India.
Joint. The point where bones meet (e.g., the knee).
Joint ill. NAVEL ILL.
Jugular vein. Large blood vessel in the side of the neck.

Keratitis. INFLAMMATION of the CORNEA.
Khanid. Rendille name for a disease of unknown cause, affecting the LYMPH NODES (▷*Swollen glands, khanid*).

Kidney. Pair of internal organs that filter wastes from the blood and produce urine.

Kumri. Camel disease in Rajasthan, causing shivering of the back legs (▷*Myopathy*).

Larva, larvae. Immature stage in the life cycle of an insect; maggot, caterpillar.

Larynx. Voicebox.

Lateral recumbency. Lying on the side.

Laxative. Substance that encourages DEFECATION.

Leeches. Segmented worms, some of which suck blood (▷*Leeches*).

Lesion. Alteration of skin or other body parts due to disease or injury.

Liniment. A medicated liquid, usually containing alcohol, camphor and an oil, applied to the skin to relieve pain or stiffness.

Liver. Large, reddish-brown organ that secretes bile and is important in digestion.

Local anaesthesia. Applying an ANAESTHETIC only to a part of the body to stop pain in this part; the animal remains conscious (▷*Sedation and anaesthesia*).

Lockjaw. TETANUS (▷*Tetanus*).

Lower respiratory tract. The LUNGS and PLEURA (the membrane that lines the chest cavity).

Lung. Pair of organs in the chest that take in air, used for breathing.

Luxation. DISLOCATION (▷*Dislocated kneecap*).

Lymph node. Solid lump on lymph vessels which helps to protect the body against disease (▷*Abscesses on the lymph nodes*).

Lymphadenitis. INFLAMMATION of lymph nodes (▷*Abscesses on the lymph nodes*).

Lymphocyte. Type of white blood cell (▷*Checking for diseases in the laboratory*).

Magadi soda. Rock salt from Magadi, in Kenya.

Maggot. The LARVA stage of a fly.

Malnutrition. Poor nutrition caused by an inadequate or unbalanced diet.

Mandible. The bone of the lower jaw (▷*Broken jaw*).

Mange. Skin disease caused by MITES (▷*Mange*).

Mastitis. INFLAMMATION of the udder (▷*Mastitis*).

Membrane. A thin layer of tissue that covers a surface or lines a cavity.

Micro-organism. Very small organism, microbe, that can be seen only using a microscope. Micro-organisms include BACTERIA, FUNGI, VIRUSES and PROTOZOA. Micro-organisms that cause diseases are called PATHOGENS or germs.

Milk scours. CALF DIARRHOEA (▷*Calf diarrhoea*).

Milk teeth. Temporary teeth (▷*Estimating a camel's weight and age*).

Mites. Small PARASITES found in the skin, coat and ears.

Molars. Cheek teeth (▷*Estimating a camel's weight and age*).

Monocyte. Type of white blood cell (▷*Checking for diseases in the laboratory*).

Mucous membrane, mucosa. Membrane lining the RESPIRATORY and DIGESTIVE TRACTS and other parts of the body. It secretes MUCUS.

Mucus. Slimy material formed to protect parts of the body.

Mycosis. Disease caused by FUNGUS.

Mycotic. Caused by FUNGUS.

Myiasis. Invasion of the body by fly LARVAE (▷*Nasal bots*).

Myopathy. A disease affecting the muscles (▷*Myopathy*).

Narcotic. A drug, which, in moderate doses, alleviates pain, reduces sensibility, produces sleep; in large amounts, induces stupor, coma or convulsions.

Nasal bots. Fly MAGGOTS living in the back of an animal's nose (▷*Nasal bots*).

Nausea. Upset STOMACH, tending to vomit.

Navel. Umbilicus, belly button, where the UMBILICAL CORD is attached during GESTATION.

Navel ill. Infection of the navel cord in newborn animals (▷*Navel ill*).

Necrosis. Death of tissue.

Nematodes. Roundworms (▷*Internal parasites [worms]*).

Nerves. Fibres that carry messages between the brain and other parts of the body.

Neutrophil. Type of white blood cell (▷*Checking for diseases in the laboratory*).

Nictitating membrane. The THIRD EYELID.

Nutrient. Nourishing substance.

Nymph. Stage in the life of an insect, after the LARVA stage.

Oedema, edema. Abnormal accumulation of fluids in the tissues (▷*Oedema*).

Oesophagus. The tube that goes from the mouth to the STOMACH.

Oestrus, estrus. HEAT.

Omasum. Third STOMACH of a RUMINANT.

Open fracture. Broken bone that damages the muscles and tissue around it and pierces through the skin.

Oral. Belonging to, or taken through, the mouth.

Orf. A disease caused by a VIRUS (▷*Orf*).

Otitis. Ear infection (▷*Ear problems*).

Ovary. The organ of a female animal that produces the egg or ova.

Ovulation. The discharge of eggs from the OVARY.

Packed cell volume. HAEMATOCRIT (▷*Checking for diseases in the laboratory*).
Pancreas. Internal organ that secretes fluids into the intestine and blood, and is important in digestion.
Pandemic. An outbreak of disease occurring over a very wide area, affecting a large percentage of the population (see also EPIDEMIC).
Paralysis. Inability to move a muscle or group of muscles, often coupled with loss of sensation in the affected area.
Parapox. ORF (▷*Orf*)
Parasites. Organisms which have a harmful effect or cause a disease; usually refers to worms, TICKS, fleas, mites, lice, LEECHES, etc.
Parenteral administration. A method of giving medication that is not through the DIGESTIVE TRACT (e.g., by injection).
Parturient. Giving birth or pertaining to birth.
Parturition. The act of giving birth; calving.
Pasteurellosis. HAEMORRHAGIC SEPTICAEMIA (▷*Haemorrhagic septicaemia*).
Patella. Kneecap (▷*Dislocated kneecap*).
Pathogen. Something that causes a disease, especially a MICRO-ORGANISM.
PCV. PACKED CELL VOLUME.
Pedestal. A camel's chest-pad (▷*Chest-pad abscess*).
Pelvic. The area around the ANUS and the hips.
Penis. Male organ used in urinating and mating.
Peritoneum. The membrane that encloses the internal organs (STOMACH, INTESTINES, LIVER, SPLEEN, PANCREAS).
Pesticide. A poison used to destroy pests of any sort.
Pica. Licking, chewing and eating of unusual objects (▷*Pica*).
Placenta. The sac inside which the FOETUS grows and is attached to the mother's UTERUS, through which it is nourished.
Plaster. A mixture of materials that hardens; used for immobilizing body parts.
Pleura. Membrane that lines the chest cavity.
Pleuropneumonia. Inflammation of the PLEURA and LUNGS (▷*Coughs, colds and pneumonia*).
Pneumonia. INFLAMMATION of the lungs (▷*Coughs, colds and pneumonia*).
Pododermatitis. INFLAMMATION of the skin of the foot.
Post mortem. After death; examination to discover the cause of death.
Post partum. After a birth.
Poultice. Soft, usually heated, preparation spread on a cloth and applied to a sore or INFLAMMATION (▷*Traditional medicines*).
Pox. A disease caused by a VIRUS (▷*Pox*).
Predator. Animal that eats other animals.
Pregnancy. The development of the young inside the mother.
Premolars. Cheek teeth in front of the MOLARS (▷*Estimating a camel's weight and age*).
Prognosis. A forecast on the probable outcome of a disease; the prospect for recovery. May be favourable, guarded, or unfavourable.
Prolapsed rectum. The lower portion of the intestinal tract (the RECTUM) comes out of the ANUS.
Prolapsed uterus. The UTERUS descends into the VAGINA and may be seen at the vaginal opening (▷*Prolapse of the vagina or womb*).
Prophylactic. Preventing disease.
Protozoon, protozoa. MICRO-ORGANISM consisting only of one cell. Some protozoa (e.g., trypanosomes) cause diseases.
Pulmonary. Pertaining to the LUNGS.
Purgative. Causing evacuation of dung from the INTESTINES.
Pus. A whitish fluid produced by inflamed tissue and infected wounds.

Quarantine. Keeping sick animals separated from healthy ones.

Rabid. Having RABIES (▷*Rabies*).
Rabies. A dangerous disease caused by a VIRUS (▷*Rabies*).
RBC. Red blood cell count: measure for the number of red blood cells in the blood (▷*Checking for diseases in the laboratory*).
Rectum. The last part of the gut before the ANUS.
Recumbency. Lying down.
Rehydration. The restoration of water to a body.
Repellent. Substance that repels or drives off other organisms, such as flies.
Reproductive tract. The organs involved in reproduction. In the female, the OVARIES, UTERUS, VAGINA and VULVA. In the male, the TESTICLES, vas deferens (the tube leading from the testicles to the penis), prostate and PENIS.
Resistance. The natural ability of an animal to remain unaffected by noxious agents in its environment; the acquired ability of disease-causing organisms to survive a chemical that normally kills them.
Respiratory tract. The organs involved in breathing. Includes the UPPER RESPIRATORY TRACT (nose, LARYNX, TRACHEA and BRONCHI) and LOWER RESPIRATORY TRACT (LUNGS and PLEURA) (▷*Coughs, colds and pneumonia*).
Retained placenta. A disease condition in which the PLACENTA is not expelled after calving, requiring treatment (▷*Retained afterbirth*).
Reticulum. Second STOMACH of a RUMINANT.
Retina. The back of the eye which is sensitive to the light.

Rhinitis. INFLAMMATION of the nose.

Rift Valley fever. A disease cause by a VIRUS (▷*Rift Valley fever*).

Ringworm. A skin disease caused by a FUNGUS (▷*Ringworm*).

Rumen. First STOMACH of a RUMINANT.

Ruminant. An animal (such as cattle, sheep, goats, buffaloes and camels) that has a STOMACH with four compartments (RUMEN, RETICULUM, OMASUM and ABOMASUM). Ruminants regurgitate undigested food from the RUMEN and chew it when at rest.

Ruminating. Chewing the CUD.

Rut. The periodic sexual excitement of male camels (▷*Rutting*).

***Saam*.** Rendille and Gabbra name for a disease in calves of unknown cause (▷*Saam*).

Saddle gall or sore. Skin and tissue damage and ABSCESS through badly fitted saddles (▷*Saddle sores*).

Saliva. Fluid produced in the mouth.

Salmonellosis. Disease caused by BACTERIA of the genus *Salmonella* (▷*Salmonellosis*).

Sarcoptic mange. MANGE.

s.c. SUBCUTANEOUS.

Scabies. MANGE.

Scalpel. Small surgical knife.

Sclera. The tough, usually white, outer coat of the eyeball.

Scrotum. The bag of skin around the TESTICLES.

Secretion. Liquid produced by a GLAND.

Sedative. Drugs that reduce anxiety and make the animal easier to handle.

Septicaemia. The existence of MICRO-ORGANISMS or poison in the blood.

Serum. The clear liquid that separates from the blood when it clots (▷*Checking for diseases in the laboratory*).

Sinus. Cavity; commonly refers to the cavities in the skull that are connected with the nasal cavity.

Specific agent. Remedy that has a special effect on a particular disease.

Spinal canal. Hole running through the backbone. It contains nerves and liquid.

Spinal cord. The bundle of nerves located in the SPINAL CANAL.

Spleen. Internal organ that stores and cleanses the blood.

Splint. Pieces of wood put around a body part to keep broken bones in place.

Sporadic. An outbreak of disease in a single or scattered location.

Spore. The inactive but infectious form of some BACTERIA (e.g., CLOSTRIDIUM); the reproductive form of some FUNGI and blood PARASITES.

Sprain. A violent and sudden twist of a joint or muscles.

***Staphylococcus*.** A type of disease-causing BACTERIA.

Sterile. Free from living germs; not fertile.

Sternal. Pertaining to the breast bone.

Sternal recumbency. Lying on the chest.

Stimulant. Increases or hastens body activity.

Stomach. The main organ where food is digested. In camels and other RUMINANTS, the stomach consists of four compartments: the RUMEN, RETICULUM, OMASUM and ABOMASUM.

Stomachic. Stimulates activity of the STOMACH.

Stomach tube. Long tube inserted into the mouth and used to put liquids directly into the STOMACH (▷*Administering medicines*).

Stomatitis. INFLAMMATION of the mouth.

***Streptococcus*.** A type of disease-causing BACTERIA.

Streptothricosis. DERMATOPHILOSIS (▷*Dermatophilosis*).

Stringhalt. Dislocated kneecap (▷*Dislocated kneecap*).

Styptic. Stops bleeding with an ASTRINGENT.

Subcutaneous, s.c. Under the skin (▷*Administering medicines*).

***Surra*.** TRYPANOSOMIASIS (▷*Trypanosomiasis*).

Suture. Stitch, stitching (in surgery).

Symptom. Functional evidence of disease or of a patient's condition.

Syndrome. The collection of symptoms associated with a particular disease.

Systemic. Pertaining to or affecting the body as a whole.

Tabanid. Type of biting fly.

Tar. A dark-brown or black, viscid liquid obtained from various pine-tree species or from bituminous coal.

Tendon. The end of a muscle which attaches it to the bone.

Testicles, testes. The male reproductive organs, in which the sperm grow.

Tetanus. A disease caused by *Clostridium tetani* BACTERIA (▷*Tetanus*).

Third eyelid. The NICTITATING MEMBRANE: a fold of the CONJUNCTIVA (▷*Eye problems*).

Tick. Type of external PARASITE (▷*Ticks*).

Tincture. Alcoholic extract of a plant drug.

Tonic. Produces healthy muscular condition and reaction.

Torticollis. Torsion of the neck, WRY NECK.

Tourniquet. A tight rope or bandage, used to restrict blood flow.

Trachea. Windpipe between mouth and lungs.

Tranquillizer. A medicine that calms or quietens an anxious patient.

Trocar. A pointed, needle-like instrument equipped with a CANNULA; used to puncture the wall of a body cavity to withdraw fluid or gas (▷*Bloat*).

Trypanosomiasis. Disease caused by trypanosome PARASITES (▷*Trypanosomiasis*).

Tsetse. Type of fly transmitting TRYPANOSOMIASIS.

Tumour. An unusual growth in the body.

Tympany. Excessive gas, BLOAT.

Ulcer. INFLAMMATION or sore on the skin or MUCOUS MEMBRANE, discharging pus.

Umbilical cord. Navel cord.

Umbilicus. NAVEL.

Upper respiratory tract. The nose, LARYNX (voice-box), TRACHEA (windpipe) and BRONCHI (air passages leading to the lungs).

Uterus. Womb, the organ inside a female where the young develops.

Vaccination. Applying a VACCINE.

Vaccine. A fluid that stimulates the production of antibodies in the body.

Vacutainer. Special tube used to collect blood (▷*How to collect samples for testing*).

Vagina. The portion of the female REPRODUCTIVE TRACT through which the baby animal must pass. It is separated from the UTERUS by the CERVIX.

Vermicide. Substance that kills worms or intestinal PARASITES.

Vermifuge. Substance that expels the worms or intestinal PARASITES; ANTHELMINTIC.

Verminous. Pertaining to, or due to, worms.

Vesicle. A small sac containing liquid.

Virus. A tiny MICRO-ORGANISM which causes disease.

Vitamin. Natural substance essential to the functions of the body.

Vulva. The opening below a female animal's tail to which the urinary and reproductive tracts are attached, which swells at time of OESTRUS and more so at calving time.

WBC. White blood cell count: measure for the number of white blood cells in the blood (▷*Checking for diseases in the laboratory*).

Wolf's tooth. First PREMOLAR on each side of the upper and lower jaw (▷*Estimating a camel's weight and age*).

Womb. UTERUS.

Wry neck. Camel disease causing the neck to be bent into an S-shape (▷*Wry neck*).

Zoonosis. Disease that can be transmitted from animals to people (▷*Diseases that people can catch from camels*).

Sources

Blood and Studdert (1988); FAO (1994); Forse (1999); IIRR (1994).

Bibliography and resources

This section lists books on camels, as well as important references on traditional veterinary medicine, simple veterinary practices and animal health in the tropics. It also lists resource organizations and websites devoted to camels.

References

Abbas, B. (1996) *Comparative Studies into the Ethnoveterinary Practices of Camel Pastoralists in Butana, Northeastern Sudan.* Pastoral and Environmental Network of the Horn of Africa (PENHA), London and Dryland Husbandry Project (OSSREA), Addis Ababa.

Acland, P.B.E. (1932) 'Notes on the camel in Eastern Sudan', *Sudan Notes and Records* 15, 119–49.

Agab, H. (1993) *The Epidemiology of Camel Diseases in Eastern Sudan, with Emphasis on Brucellosis.* MVSc thesis, University of Khartoum.

Agab, H. (1998) Traditional treatment methods of camels in eastern Sudan with emphasis on firing, *Journal of Camel Practice and Research* 5(1), 161–4.

Alhadrami, G. and Gawad, M.A. (1998) *Directory of Camel Researchers and Practitioners*, Animal Production Department, Faculty of Agricultural Sciences, United Arab Emirates University, Al-Ain, UAE.

Allen, W.R., Higgins, A.J., Maybew, I.G., Snow, D.H. and Wade, J.F. (1992) *Proceedings of the First International Camel Conference*, 2–6 February 1992, R&W Publications, Newmarket, Suffolk, UK.

Baerts, M., Lehmann, J., Ansay, M. and Kasonia, K. (1996) *A Few Medicinal Plants Used in Traditional Veterinary Medicine in Sub-Saharan Africa*, Louvain University Press, Belgium, and Technical Centre for Agricultural and Rural Cooperation (CTA), Wageningen, Netherlands. Published on the Internet at http://pc4.sisc.ucl.ac.be/prelude.html [accessed 4 March 2000].

Benjamin, M.M. (1978) *Outline of Veterinary Clinical Pathology*, 3rd edn, Iowa State University Press, Ames, Iowa.

Bernus, E. (1981) *Touaregs Nigériens*, Orstom, Paris.

Bizimana, N. (1994) *Traditional Veterinary Practice in Africa,* Gesellschaft für Technische Zusammenarbeit (GTZ), Eschborn, Germany.

Blood, D.C. and Studdert, V.P. (1988) *Baillière's Comprehensive Veterinary Dictionary*, Baillère Tindall, London.

Bollig, M. (1992) 'East Pokot camel husbandry', *Nomadic Peoples* 31, 34–50.

Bollig, M. (1995) 'The veterinary system of the pastoral Pokot', *Nomadic Peoples* 36/37, 17–34.

Carter, G.R. (1986) *Essentials of Veterinary Bacteriology and Mycology*, 3rd edn, Lea & Febiger, Philadelphia.

Catley, A. (1995) *Paravet Training Course – Phase 1. Notes for Trainers*, Save the Children (SCF UK)/ South East Rangelands Project, Jijiga, Ethiopia.

Catley, A. and Mohammed, A.A. (1995) 'Ethnoveterinary knowledge in Sanaag region, Somaliland (Part I): Notes on local descriptions of livestock diseases and parasites', *Nomadic Peoples* 36/37, 3–16.

Cauvet, C. (1925) *Le Chameau*, Librairie J-B, Baillière et Fils, Paris.

Cockrill, W.R. (1985) *The Camelid: An All Purpose Animal*, Parts I and II, Scandinavian Institute of African Studies, Uppsala.

Cross, H.E. (1917) *The Camel and its Diseases*, Ballière Tindall and Cox, London.

Curasson, G. (1947) *Le Chameau et ses Maladies*, Vigot Frères, Paris.

Dakkak, A. and Ouhelli, H. (1987) 'Helminth and helminthosis of the dromedary: A review of literature', *Revue Scientifique et Technique de l´Office International des Épizooties* 6(1), 447–61.

Domingo, I.V. (1998) 'Plants for animal heathcare'. *Footsteps* 34, 8–9.

Dorman, A.E. (1984) 'Aspects of the husbandry and management of the genus *Camelus*', *British Veterinary Journal* 140, 616–33.

El Amin, E.A. (1996) 'Parasites of the dromedary: A review'. *Parasitology Research in Africa*, Gray, G.D. and Uilenberg, G. (eds), Proceedings of an IFS workshop, Bobo-Dioulasso, Burkina Faso, 6–10 November 1995, IFS, Stockholm, pp. 319–40.

Evans, J., Simpkin, P. and Atkins, D. (1995) *Camel Keeping in Kenya, Range Management Handbook of Kenya* Vol. III, 8, Republic of Kenya, Ministry of Agriculture, Livestock Development and Marketing, Nairobi.

Fadl, M., Magzoub, M. and Burger, H.J. (1992) 'Prevalence of gastrointestinal nematode infection in the dromedary camel (*Camelus dromedarius*) in the Butana plains, Sudan', *Revue d'Élevage et de Médecine Vétérinaire des Pays Tropicaux* 45(3–4), 291–3.

FAO (1994) *A Manual for the Primary Animal Health Care Worker*, Food and Agriculture Organization of the United Nations, Rome.

Forse, B. (1999) *Where There is no Vet,* Macmillan, London.

Fowler, M.E. (1998) *Medicine and Surgery of South American Camelids*, 2nd edn, Iowa State University Press, Ames, Iowa.

Gahlot, T.K. (ed.) (2000) *Selected Topics on Camelids*, Camelid Publishers, Bikaner, India.

Gahlot, T.K. and Chouhan, D.S. (1992) *Camel Surgery*, Gyan Prakashan Mandir, Bikaner, India.

Grill, P.J. (1989) *Introducing the Camel: Basic Camel Keeping for the Beginner*, MCC/UNEP, Nairobi.

Higgins, A. (1983) 'Observations on the diseases of the Arabian camel (*Camelus dromedarius*) and their control: A review', *Veterinary Bulletin* 53(12), 1089–100.

Higgins, A. (1986) *The Camel in Health and Disease*, Baillière Tindall, London.

Hunter, A. (1996) *Animal Health*, Vols I and II, Macmillan Education, London.

IIRR (1994) *Ethnoveterinary Medicine in Asia: An Information Kit on Traditional Health Care Practices*, International Institute of Rural Reconstruction, Silang, Cavite, Philippines.

IIRR (1996) *Paraveterinary Medicine: An Information Kit on Low-Cost Health Care Practices*, International Institute of Rural Reconstruction, Silang, Cavite, Philippines.

ITDG and IIRR (1996) *Ethnoveterinary Medicine in Kenya: A Field Manual of Traditional Health Care Practices*, Intermediate Technology Development Group and International Institute of Rural Reconstruction, Nairobi.

Kaufmann, B. (1998) *Analysis of Pastoral Camel Husbandry in Northern Kenya*, Hohenheim Tropical Agriculture Series, Margraf Verlag, Weikersheim, Germany.

Klute, G. (1992) *Die schwerste Arbeit der Welt: Alltag von Tuareg-Nomaden*, Tickster Wissenschaft, München.

Köhler-Rollefson, I. (1991) 'Camelus dromedarius', *Mammalian Species* 375 (April 1991):1–8.

Köhler-Rollefson, I. (1996) *Kamelkultur und Kamelhaltung bei den indischen Raika: Ein Beitrag zum interkulturellen Vergleich von Mensch-Tier-Beziehungen,* Vet. med. Habilitation, University of Munich.

Köhler-Rollefson, I. (1996) 'Traditional management of health and disease in North Africa and India', *Ethnoveterinary Research and Development*, McCorkle, C., Mathias, E. and Schillhorn van Veen, T.W. (eds), Intermediate Technology Publications, London, pp. 129–36.

Köhler-Rollefson, I, Musa, B.E. and Achmed, M.F. (1991) 'The camel pastoral system of the Southern Rashaida in Eastern Sudan', *Nomadic Peoples* 24, 68–76.

Leese, A.S. (1927) *A Treatise on the One-Humped Camel in Health and Disease*, Haynes and Son, Stamford, Lincolnshire, UK.

Manefield, G.W. and Tinson, A.H. (1997) *Camels: A Compendium*, T.G. Hungerford Vade Mecum Series for Domestic Animals, Series C, no. 22, University of Sydney Post Graduate Foundation in Veterinary Science, Sydney.

Mathias, E., Rangnekar, D.V. and McCorkle, C.M. (eds) (1999) *Ethnoveterinary Medicine: Alternatives for Livestock Development*, Proceedings of an International Conference held in Pune, India, on 4–6 November 1997, Vol. 1: Selected Papers, BAIF Development Research Foundation, Pune, India.

McCorkle, C., Mathias, E. and Schillhorn van Veen, T.W. (eds) (1996) *Ethnoveterinary Research and Development*, Intermediate Technology Publications, London.

Monteil, V. (1952) *Essaie sur le Chameau en Sahara Occidental*, Centre IFAN-Mauritanie, Saint-Louis, Senegal.

Morgan, W.T.W. (1981) 'Ethnobotany of the Turkana: Use of plants by a pastoral people and their livestock in Kenya', *Economic Botany* 35, 96–130.

Nicolaisen, J. (1963) 'Ecology and culture of the pastoral Tuareg', *Nationalmuseets Skrifter Etnografisk Roeke* 9, National Museum of Copenhagen.

Pacholek, X. and Agab, H. (1993) *Therapeutic Guide of Camel Diseases*, Mission of the Sudanese–French Cooperation Project, Khartoum (in Arabic).

Projet Cameline (1999) *Traitement des Maladies du Dromadaire: Guide de l'Auxiliaire d'Élevage*, Projet de Renforcement Institutionnel et Technique de la Filière Cameline, Association Nigérienne pour la Dynamisation des Initiatives Locales (ONG KARKARA), Niamey, Niger.

Quesenberry, P. (1990) *The JTA Handbook of Animal Health for Nepal*, United Mission to Nepal, Kathmandu.

Rathore, G.S. (1986) *Camels and their Management*, Indian Council of Agricultural Research, New Delhi.

Richard, D. (1979) *Study of the Pathology of the Dromedary in Borana Awraja (Ethiopia)*, PhD thesis, IEMVT, Maisons-Alfort, France.

Royal Botanic Gardens, Kew (1999) *Survey of Economic Plants for Arid and Semi-Arid Lands (SEPASAL) Database*, published on the Internet at http://www.rbgkew.org.uk/ceb/sepasal/internet/ [accessed 4 March 2000].

Sato, S. (1980) 'Pastoral movement and the subsistence unit of the Rendille of northern Kenya: with special reference to camel ecology', *Senri Ethnological Studies* 6, 1–8.

Schwartz, H.J. and Dioli, M. (eds) (1992) *The One-Humped Camel (*Camelus dromedarius*) in Eastern Africa: A Pictorial Guide to Diseases, Health Care and Management*, Verlag Josef Margraf, Weikersheim, Germany.

Sewell, M.M.H. and Brocklesby, D.W. (eds) (1990) *Handbook on Animal Diseases in the Tropics*, 4th edn, Ballière Tindall, London.

Sloss, M.W. and Kemp, R.L. (1978) *Veterinary Clinical Parasitology*, 5th edn, Iowa State University Press, Ames, Iowa.

Smuts, M.M.S. and Bezuidenhout, A.J. (1987) *Anatomy of the Dromedary*, Clarendon Press, Oxford.

Soulsby, E.J.L. (1982) *Helminths, Arthropods and Protozoa of Domesticated Animals*, 7th edn, English Language Book Society and Baillière Tindall, London.

Stiles, D. and Kassam, A. (1991) 'An ethno-botanical study of Gabra plant use in Marsabit District, Kenya', *Journal of the East African Natural History Society and National Museum* 81.

Tibary, A. and Anouassi, A. (1997) *Theriogenology in Camelidae: Anatomy, Physiology, Pathology, and Artificial Breeding*, Actes Editions, Institut Agronomique et Vétérinaire Hassan II, Rabat-Instituts, Morocco.

Wanyama, J.B. (1997) *Confidently Used Ethnoveterinary Knowledge among Pastoralists of Samburu, Kenya*, Vols 1 and 2, Intermediate Technology Kenya, Nairobi.

Wernery, U. and Kaaden, O.-R. (1995) *Infectious Diseases of Camelids*, Blackwell Wissenschaftsverlag, Berlin.

White, R.J., Bark, H. and Bali, S. (1987) 'Xylazine and ketamine anaesthesia in the dromedary camel under field conditions', *Veterinary Record* 120, 110–3.

Wilson, R.T. (1984) *The Camel*, Longman, London.

Wilson, R.T. (1998) *Camels*, Tropical Agriculturalist Series, Macmillan/CTA, London.

Wolfgang, K.E. (1986) *Traditional Veterinary Concepts of Twareg Pastoralists in Central Niger*, Thesis, Tufts University School of Veterinary Medicine, Boston.

Journals and newsletters

The following journals and newsletters frequently contain information on camel health and management and ethnoveterinary medicine.

Appropriate Technology. Research Information Ltd, 222 Marylands Avenue, Hemel Hempstead HP2 7TD, UK. Tel +44-20-8328 2470; fax +44-1442-259395; email: info@resinf.co.uk

Australian Camel News. Published four times a year. PMB 118, William Creek, via Port August 5710, Australia. Email: acn@austcamel.com.au, internet http://www.austcamel.com.au/acn_home.htm.

Camel Newsletter. Published occasionally by CARD-N (Camel Applied Research and Development Network), c/o Arab Center for the Studies of Arid Zones and Dry Lands (ACSAD), PO Box 2440, Damascus, Syria. Tel +963-11-532 3039, 532 3087; fax +963-11-532 3063; email: ruacsad@rusys.eg.net. (Editor-in-chief, Muhammad F. Wardeh).

Compas Newsletter of Endogenous Development. Compas, PO Box 64, 3830 AB Leusden, Netherlands. Tel +31-33-494 3086; fax +31-33-494 0971; email: compas@etcnl.nl.

The Camel Caravan. Bimonthly publication on camel health care, reproduction, hand rearing, training, and management. The American Camel Company, Rt 1 Box 3648B, Sidney, MT 59270 USA. Tel/fax +1-406-798 3405; email: ygr@mcn.net.

The Exchange. Heifer Project International (HPI), PO Box 808, Little Rock, Arkansas, USA. Tel +1-501-376-6836; email: exchange@heifer.org.

Footsteps. Tearfund, 100 Church Rd, Teddington TW11 8QE, UK. Tel +44-1746-768750, fax +44-1746-764594; email: imc@tearfund.dircon.co.uk. (Editor, Isabel Carter).

Herders Magazine/Magazine des Eleveurs. Available from World Herders Council/Conseil Mondial des Eleveurs, BP 2453, 6002 Lucerne, Switzerland. Tel/fax +41-41-3610718; email: condial@bluewin.ch.

Honey Bee. Sristi, Indian Institute of Management, Vastrapur, Ahmedabad 380015, India. Tel +91-79-407241, fax +91-79-642 7896; email: honeybee@iimahd.ernet.in.

Indian Journal of Veterinary Surgery. Pantnagar, India.

Indian Veterinary Journal. 7 Chamiers Road, Nandanam, Chennai 600 035, India. Tel +91-44-435 1006, 433 2691; fax +91-44-433 8894; email: ivj@md3.vsnl.net.in.

Indigenous Knowledge and Development Monitor. Nuffic-CIRAN, PO Box 29777, 2502 LT The Hague, Netherlands. Tel +31-70-4260 324, fax +31-70-4260 329; email: ikdm@nuffic.nl.

Journal of Camel Practice and Research. Biannual journal published by Camel Publishing House, 67 Gandhi Nagar West, near Lalgarh Palace, Bikaner 334001, India. Tel +91-151-427 029, fax +91-151-527 673. (Editor, T.K. Gahlot).

LEISA: ILEIA Newsletter for Low External Input and Sustainable Agriculture. PO Box 64, 3830 AB Leusden, Netherlands. Tel +31-33-494 3086, fax +31-33-495 1779; email: ilea@ileia.nl.

Nomadic Peoples. Published twice a year by Berghahn Books, 3 Newtec Place, Magdalen Road, Oxford OX4 1RE, UK. Tel +44-1865-250 011, fax +44-1865-250 056; email: berghahnuk@aol.com.

Of Cattle and Camels: Pastoralist Newsletter. ACORD, Dean Bradley House, 52 Horseferry Road, London SW1P2AF. Tel +44-171-227-8600, fax +44-171-799-1868; email: info@acord.uk.

Le N'dama: Journal des Vétérinaires et Zootechniciens d'Afrique. Prelude, Sub-network Health, Animal Productions and Environment, c/o Michel Ansay, 15, rue N. Royer, 4367, Fize-le Marsal (CRISNEE), Belgium. Email: mansay@ulg.ac.be.

New Agriculturalist (online issue). http://www.new-agri.co.uk.

Revue Scientifique et Technique. Office International des Épizooties, 12, rue de Prony, 75017 Paris, France. Fax +33-1-42 67 09 87.

Tropical Animal Health and Production. Centre for Tropical Veterinary Medicine, University of Edinburgh, Easter Bush, Roslin, Midlothian, EH25 9RG, UK.

Organizations

Australia

Arid Zone Research Institute, South Stuart Highway, PO Box 8760, Alice Springs NT 0871, Australia.

Belgium

Instituut voor Biotechnology, Vrije Universiteit Brussel, Paardenstraat 65, B-1640 Sint Genesius Rode, Belgium.

Egypt

Faculty of Veterinary Medicine, Cairo University, Giza, Egypt.

France

Unité de Coordination pour l'Élevage Camelin, CIRAD-EMVT, Campus International de Baillarguet, BP 5035, 34032 Montpellier, Cedex, France. Tel +33-4-6759 3703; fax +33-4-6759 3825 (Director, Dr B. Faye).

Département d'Élevage et de Médecine Vétérinaire, CIRAD-EMVT, 10 rue Pierre-Curie, 94704 Maisons-Alfort, Cedex, France.

Germany

Kamelverein Fatamorgana eV, 72224 Rotfelden, Germany. Tel +49-7054-2899; fax +49-7054-7041.

Centre for Tropical Agriculture, Institute for Animal Production, Universität Hohenheim (480), D-70593 Stuttgart, Germany.

India

National Research Centre on Camel (NRCC), Jorbeer, PB No. 7, Bikaner 334001. Tel/fax +91-151-522183; email: nrccamel@x400.nicgw.nic.in (Director, Dr M.S. Sahani).

Department of Surgery and Radiology, College of Veterinary and Animal Science, Bikaner 334001, India.

Applied Camel Research Project, c/o Lokhit Pashu-Palak Sansthan, Ambedkar Nagar, Desuri Road, Sadri 306702, Pali District, Rajasthan, India. Tel +91-2934-85086; fax +91-2934-85563 (Director, Hanwant Singh Rathore).

Iraq

College of Veterinary Medicine, Baghdad University, Iraq.

Israel

Center for Comparative Medicine and Desert Research, Ben-Gurion University of the Negev, PO Box 653, Beersheva 84105 (Director, Professor R. Yagil, email: reuven@bgumail.bgn.ac.il).

Jordan

Faculty of Veterinary Medicine, Jordan University of Science and Technology, Irbid, Jordan.

Kenya

FARM Africa, Pastoralists Development Project, PO Box 795, Nanyuki, Kenya.

Intermediate Technology Development Group, PO Box 39493, Nairobi, Kenya. Tel +254-2-442 108.

Ol Maisor Ranch, PO Box 9, Rumuruti, Kenya.

Libya

Camel Research Unit, PO Box 80403, Tripoli, Libya. Fax +218-21-4831027.

Mauritania

Centre National d'Élevage et de Recherches Vétérinaires, BP 167, Nouakchott, Mauritania.

Laitière de Mauretanie, BP 2069, Nouakchott, Mauritania.

Morocco

Institut Agronomique et Vétérinarire Hassan II, BP 6202 Rabat Institut, Rabat, Morocco. Tel +212-7-779684; fax +212-7-779684; email: bengoumi@iam.net.ma.

Niger

Projet de Renforcement Institutionnel et Technique de la Filière Cameline, BP 510 Niamey, Niger. Tel/fax +227-733607; email: camelin@intnet.ne.

Nigeria

Department of Animal Science, Usmanu Danfodiyo University, PMB 2346, Sokoto, Nigeria.

Oman

Department of Camel Affairs, Diwan of Royal Court, Muscat 111, Sultanate of Oman.

Pakistan

Department of Clinical Medicine and Surgery, Faculty of Veterinary Science, University of Agriculture, Faisalabad, Pakistan. Tel +92-41-630131; fax +92-41-612425.

Saudi Arabia

Center for the Development of Rangelands and Animal Wealth, PO Box 322, Sakaka, Al Jouf, Saudi Arabia. Tel +966-46-330080, 46331348; fax +966-46-331088.

Faculty of Agriculture and Veterinary Medicine, King Saud University, PO Box 1482, Al-Gassim, Buraydah, Saudi Arabia.

College of Veterinary Medicine and Animal Resources, King Faisal University, PO Box 1757, Al Ahsa, Saudi Arabia.

Sudan

Faculty of Veterinary Science, University of Khartoum, PO Box 32, Khartoum North, Sudan.

Sweden

Department of Parasitology, National Veterinary Institute, PO Box 7073, S-75007, Uppsala, Sweden.

Scandinavian Institute of African Studies, Uppsala, Sweden.

Syria

Camel Applied Research and Development Network (CARDN), c/o Arab Center for the Studies of Arid Zones and Dry Lands (ACSAD), PO Box 2440, Damascus, Syria. Tel +963-11-532 3039, 532 3087; fax 532 3063; email: ruacsad@rusys.eg.net.

Tunisia

École Supérieure d'Agriculture, 7030 Mateur, Tunisia.

United Arab Emirates

Camel Research Centre, PO Box 110, Abu Dhabi, UAE.

Central Veterinary Research Laboratory, PO Box 597, Dubai, UAE. Tel +971-4-375 165; fax +971-4-368 638.

Websites

These websites contain links to other sites focusing on camels.

Australian Camel. http://www.austcamel.com.au/index.htm

CamelNet. http://www.camelnet.ethz.ch/

Liszt Camelid. http://www.liszt.com/cgi-bin/start.lcgi?list=CAMELID&info= u&server= listserv@home.ease.lsoft.com&type=u (Camelid discussion group)

Index

Page numbers in **bold** refer to the most important entry. See the *Glossary* (page 231) for additional technical terms not found in the index. See page 213 for the names of diseases in local languages, and page 217 for local names of plants.

www.ingramcontent.com/pod-product-compliance
Lightning Source LLC
Jackson TN
JSHW062158130125
77033JS00017B/576

* 9 7 8 1 8 5 3 3 9 5 0 3 1 *